Workbook for

Radiologic Science for Technologists

W9-BXY-596

Workbook for

Radiologic Science for Technologists

Tenth Edition

Stewart Carlyle Bushong, ScD, FACR, FACMP
Professor of Radiologic Science
Baylor College of Medicine
Houston, Texas

Frank Goerner, PhD
Assistant Professor of Medical Physics
Department of Radiology
University of Texas Medical Branch
Galveston, Texas

3251 Riverport Lane
St. Louis, Missouri 63043

WORKBOOK FOR RADIOLOGIC SCIENCE FOR TECHNOLOGISTS: ISBN: 978 -0-323-08137-5
PHYSICS, BIOLOGY, AND PROTECTION, TENTH EDITION

Notices

Knowledge and best practice in this field are constantly changing. As new research and experience broaden our understanding, changes in research methods, professional practices, or medical treatment may become necessary.

Practitioners and researchers must always rely on their own experience and knowledge in evaluating and using any information, methods, compounds, or experiments described herein. In using such information or methods they should be mindful of their own safety and the safety of others, including parties for whom they have a professional responsibility.

With respect to any drug or pharmaceutical products identified, readers are advised to check the most current information provided (i) on procedures featured or (ii) by the manufacturer of each product to be administered, to verify the recommended dose or formula, the method and duration of administration, and contraindications. It is the responsibility of practitioners, relying on their own experience and knowledge of their patients, to make diagnoses, to determine dosages and the best treatment for each individual patient, and to take all appropriate safety precautions.

To the fullest extent of the law, neither the Publisher nor the authors, contributors, or editors, assume any liability for any injury and/or damage to persons or property as a matter of products liability, negligence or otherwise, or from any use or operation of any methods, products, instructions, or ideas contained in the material herein.

International Standard Book Number: 978-0-323-08137-5

Marketing Manager: Jennifer Gianino
Senior Content Development Specialist: Luke Held
Executive Content Strategist: Jennifer Janson
Publishing Services Manager: Julie Eddy/Hemamalini Rajendrababu
Project Manager: Kelly Milford/Prasad Subramanian
Content Coordinator: Kate O'Toole
Cover Designer: Gopalakrishnan V

Printed in United States

Last digit is the print number: 9 8 7 6 5 4 3 2 1

Preface

Straightforward and fun, the workbook stimulates discussion while helping students review information and hone the skills necessary to become informed and competent radiologic technologists.

Similar to previous edition, the 10th edition starts with a section of Worksheets, followed by the Math Tutor section. The worksheets are organized by topic and numbered according to the textbook chapters. The worksheet numbers and descriptive titles make it easy to find worksheets to test specific topics or coordinate with the major concepts of a textbook chapter; they primarily contain multiple choice questions that can be quickly graded and returned. The Laboratory Experiments, formerly found in previous edition workbooks, have been moved to the Evolve site for ease of use; they can be found at http://evolve.elsevier.com. The answer keys have also been moved to the Evolve site.

Each worksheet features "Penguins" to aid in the successful completion of the exercises. The Penguin provides a concise summary of information that is relevant to the exercise questions. Lighthearted and to the point, Penguins make it easier than ever to review major text-book concepts.

The author wishes to thank the following reviewers for their valuable input: **Jeff Hamzeh, PhD,** Keiser University, **Deanna Butcher, MA, RT(R),** St. Cloud Hospital School of Diagnostic Imaging, **Lee Nakamura, MD,** University of Texas Medical Branch, **Nathan Priddy, MD,** University of Texas Medical Branch, and **Miguel Trelles, MD,** University of Texas Medical Branch.

As always, Elsevier welcomes your comments about this book or any of our other imaging sciences publications.

The author especially appreciates your comments regarding any of the material in this volume, including specific questions, Penguins, and Math Tutor. Please e-mail me at sbushong@bcm.tmc.edu so that together we can make this material even more instructive and "Physics even more Phun ."

Stewart Carlyle Bushong

Contents

Worksheet 1-1
Nature of Our Surroundings
Matter and Energy
Sources of Ionizing Radiation

 Some representative radiation levels are as follows:

In Our Daily Lives

Living next to a nuclear power station	5 μSv/yr (0.5 mrem/yr)
Cross-country jet flight	20 μSv (2 mrem)
Fallout at the height of atomic weapons testing	50 μSv (5 mrem)
Consumer products (e.g., smoke detectors, watch dials)	30 μSv/yr (3 mrem/yr)

Natural Background

Sea level	1 mSv/yr (100 mrem/yr)
Mountains	5 mSv/yr (500 mrem/yr)

The Healing Arts

99mTc thyroid image	100 μGy_t (10 mrad)
Genetically significant dose (GSD)	200 μGy_t (20 mrad)
Mean marrow dose	1 mGy_t (100 mrad)
Entrance skin exposure (ESE)	
Posterior-anterior (PA) chest examination	100 μGy_a (10 mR)
Panoramic dental x-ray	2 mGy_a (200 mR)
Lumbar spine examination	10 mGy_a/min (1000 mR)
Fluoroscopic examination	40 mGy_a/min (4000 mR/min)

Computed Tomography

Head examination	40 mGy_t (4000 mrad)
Body examination	20 mGy_t (2000 mrad)

Occupational Dose Limit	
Radiographer	50 mSv/yr (5000 mrem/yr)
Public	1 mSv/yr (100 mrem/yr)

MASS IS THE QUANTITY OF MATTER DESCRIBED BY ITS ENERGY EQUIVALENCE.

ENERGY IS THE ABILITY TO DO WORK.

RADIATION IS THE TRANSFER OF ENERGY.

EXERCISES

1. Which of the following items is considered to be matter?
   a. Airport surveillance x-rays
   b. Anode heat
   c. Cell phone signals
   d. Light from a movie projector
   e. Wet snow

2. Which of the following is the principal difference between mass and weight?
   a. Mass is measured in pounds (lb); weight is measured in kilograms (kg).
   b. Mass is the equivalence of energy; weight is the force exerted by gravity.
   c. There is no difference; mass and weight are equal.
   d. Weight does not change with position; mass does.
   e. Weight is energy; mass requires gravity.

3. Energy is defined as:
   a. A force exerted by a body
   b. Anything that occupies space and has shape
   c. The ability to do work
   d. The degree of gravity
   e. The quantity of matter

1

4. Which of the following examples best represents kinetic energy?
   a. A snowman
   b. A thrown snowball
   c. Anode mass
   d. The metal plates in a battery
   e. The terminals of a battery

5. Which of the following is an example of potential energy?
   a. A heated anode
   b. A mobile x-ray imaging system in motion
   c. An x-ray beam
   d. An x-ray imaging system
   e. Visible light

6. In Einstein's famous $E = mc^2$ equation, c stands for which of the following?
   a. Acceleration of mass
   b. Force
   c. Mass-energy equivalence
   d. The speed of light
   e. The theory of relativity

7. Radiation is:
   a. Energy transferred
   b. Isotropic emission
   c. Kinetic particles
   d. Mass with a charge
   e. Measured in joules

8. The milligray in air (mGy_t) relates to which of the following?
   a. A dose equivalent
   b. Ions produced in the air
   c. Isotropic emission
   d. Non-ionizing radiation
   e. Tissue-absorbed dose

9. Which of the following is an example of electromagnetic radiation?
   a. Alpha radiation
   b. Beta rays
   c. Sound
   d. Ultrasound
   e. Visible light

10. When ionization occurs, which of the following is true?
    a. The negative ion is electromagnetic radiation.
    b. The negative ion is the ion pair.
    c. The negative ion is the target atom.
    d. The positive ion is electromagnetic.
    e. The positive ion is the resulting atom.

11. X-rays are most like:
    a. Alpha rays
    b. Beta rays

c. Diagnostic ultrasound
d. Gamma rays
e. Radio waves

12. Which of the following is the largest source of human exposure to man-made radiation?
    a. Cosmic rays
    b. Medical diagnostic x-rays
    c. Nuclear power–generating stations
    d. Radioactive fallout
    e. Radioactive materials in consumer products

13. What is the approximate annual effective dose from natural environmental radiation at sea level?
    a. 50 μSv/yr (5 mrem/yr)
    b. 100 μSv/yr (10 mrem/yr)
    c. 500 μSv/yr (50 mrem/yr)
    d. 1 mSv/yr (100 mrem/yr)
    e. 5 mSv/yr (500 mrem/yr)

14. Which of the following results in the highest annual radiation dose?
    a. Cosmic rays
    b. Diagnostic x-rays
    c. Microwave radiation
    d. Nuclear power
    e. Radiation from inside the earth

15. Which of the following contributes more than 1 mGy_t per year to each of us?
    a. Consumer products
    b. Diagnostic x-rays
    c. Microwave oven radiation
    d. Radioactive fallout radiation
    e. Radioisotopes in nuclear medicine

16. The milligray in tissue (mGy_a) is related most closely to which of the following?
    a. Dose equivalent
    b. Radiation exposure
    c. The gray
    d. The joule
    e. The sievert

17. Which of the following is ionizing electromagnetic radiation?
    a. Beta rays
    b. Gamma rays
    c. Microwaves
    d. Radio waves
    e. Ultrasound

18. Which of the following is a unit of mass?
    a. Joule
    b. Kilogram
    c. mrad
    d. Pound
    e. Volt

Worksheet 1-2
Discovery of X-Rays
Development of Modern Radiology

- X-rays were discovered in 1895 by Roentgen.
- The cadmium tungstate (CdWO4) radiographic intensifying screen was developed by Edison and was first used in 1898.
- Clarence Dally, who was an assistant to Edison, died of radiation injuries in 1904.
- In 1913, Coolidge developed the modern heated filament x-ray tube.
- The National Council on Radiation Protection (NCRP) reduced the occupational dose limit to 50 mSv/yr in 1957.
- The image-intensifier tube became available in the early 1960s.
- Diagnostic ultrasound was introduced in the early 1960s.
- Computed tomography appeared in 1972.
- Magnetic resonance imaging was introduced for clinical use in 1980.
- The first federal imaging regulation—the Mammography Quality Standards Act (MQSA)—was passed in 1992.
- The first all-digital department of radiology (Baltimore Veterans Affairs Medical Center [VAMC]) opened in 1993.
- Solid-state digital image receptors were introduced in 1996.
- The Radiological Society of North America (RSNA) presented the first annual showing of Integrating the Healthcare Environment (IHE) in 1997.
- Multislice helical computed tomography appeared in 1998.
- Digital mammography was approved by the U.S. Food and Drug Administration (FDA) in 2000.
- Positron emission tomography (PET) assumed a role in clinical practice in 2002.
- Sixty-four-slice helical computed tomography was offered in 2004 by several vendors.
- Dual source computed tomography was introduced in 2005 (Siemens).
- Three hundred twenty-slice helical computed tomography available (Toshiba).

EXERCISES

1. Roentgen discovered x-rays with which device?
   a. Anode tube
   b. Coolidge tube
   c. Crookes tube
   d. Geissler tube
   e. Snook interrupterless transformer

2. The phosphor that Roentgen used in early experiments with x-rays was which of the following?
   a. Barium platinocyanide
   b. Cadmium tungstate
   c. Calcium tungstate
   d. Rare earth
   e. Zinc cadmium sulfide

3. How are x-ray tube voltages measured?
   a. Kilovolt
   b. Megavolt
   c. Microvolt
   d. Millivolt
   e. Volt

4. Which of the following early pioneers developed the fluoroscope?
   a. Alexander G. Bell
   b. J.J. Thomson
   c. Thomas Edison
   d. Wilhelm Roentgen
   e. William Crookes

5. Who first applied x-ray beam collimation and filtration in medical imaging?
   a. Wilhelm Roentgen
   b. William Coolidge
   c. William Crookes
   d. William Longfellow
   e. William Rollins

3

6. Which of the following is the type of x-ray tube that is used today?
   a. Coolidge tube
   b. Crookes tube
   c. Geissler tube
   d. Leonard tube
   e. Snook tube

7. The Bucky grid, which was introduced in 1921, does what?
   a. Improves contrast resolution
   b. Improves spatial resolution
   c. Provides x-ray collimation
   d. Reduces examination time
   e. Reduces patient exposure

8. Which of the following regarding radiation lethality is true?
   a. Clarence Dally was the first American to die because of x-ray exposure.
   b. No medical radiation deaths have occurred.
   c. Radiology has always been considered a completely safe occupation.
   d. The first x-ray–induced death did not occur until approximately 1920.
   e. The first x-ray–induced death occurred within a year of Roentgen's discovery.

9. Which of the following describes the Coolidge x-ray tube?
   a. It has a heated cathode.
   b. It has a rotating anode.
   c. It is not as good as the Crookes tube.
   d. It is not in use today.
   e. It was used by Roentgen when he discovered x-rays.

10. Roentgen originally identified x-rays as which of the following?
    a. Alpha rays
    b. Cathode rays
    c. Electrons
    d. X-heat
    e. X-light

11. What are the two simple, general types of x-ray imaging procedures?
    a. Digital and analog
    b. Electromagnetic and ultrasonic
    c. Radiographic and fluoroscopic
    d. Radiographic and tomographic
    e. Roentgenographic and ultrasonic

12. Which of the following provides dynamic x-ray images?
    a. Digital radiography
    b. Doppler ultrasonography
    c. Fluoroscopy
    d. Mammography
    e. Tomography

13. The film base for a radiograph made in 1920 would have been made of which of the following?
    a. Calcium tungstate
    b. Cellulose acetate
    c. Cellulose nitrate
    d. Glass
    e. Tungstate cadmium

14. X-ray beam collimation and filtration do which of the following?
    a. Compromise image quality
    b. Improve spatial resolution
    c. Reduce exposure time
    d. Reduce patient dose
    e. Result in patient discomfort

15. Which of the following imaging modalities was developed most recently?
    a. Computed tomography (CT)
    b. Diagnostic ultrasound
    c. Direct digital radiography
    d. Magnetic resonance imaging (MRI)
    e. Multislice helical CT

16. Which of the following radiation responses was not reported before 1910?
    a. Aplastic anemia
    b. Death
    c. Epilation
    d. Leukemia
    e. Skin erythema

Worksheet 1-3
Reports of Radiation Injury
Basic Radiation Protection
The Diagnostic Imaging Team

- Radiology is a safe occupation.
- The principal concerns about medical x-ray exposure are cancer and leukemia.
- The occupational dose limit for radiologic technologists is 50 mSv/yr (5000 mrem/yr).
- Remember the principle of ALARA: Maintain radiation exposure as low as reasonably achievable.
- The three cardinal principles of radiation protection are: (1) reduce time, (2) increase distance, and (3) use protective shielding where appropriate.
- Radiologic technologists must be certified by the American Registry of Radiologic Technologists (ARRT); medical physicists must be certified by the American Board of Medical Physics (ABMP) or American Board of Radiology (ABR); interpreting physicians should be ABR certified.

EXERCISES

1. One of the cardinal principles of radiation protection states that the radiographer should minimize which of the following?
   a. Distance
   b. kVp
   c. mAs
   d. Shielding
   e. Time

2. Which of the following is not included in the 10 basic radiation control principles of diagnostic radiology?
   a. Always wear a radiation monitor while at work.
   b. Collimate the x-ray beam to the appropriate field size.
   c. Use high-kVp technique.
   d. Use high-mA technique.
   e. Wear protective apparel during fluoroscopy.

3. If it is necessary to immobilize a patient during a radiographic examination, the most acceptable person to do this is a/an:
   a. 18-year-old brother of the patient
   b. 20-year-old female technologist
   c. 40-year-old male technologist
   d. 50-year-old female friend of the patient
   e. Hospital orderly

4. Which of the following is correctly stated for diagnostic radiology?
   a. Collimation is important only for chest examination.
   b. Copper is used most often as an x-ray filter.
   c. Gonad shields are as important for a 50-year-old woman as for a 20-year-old woman.
   d. The radiologic technologist may hold patients for some x-ray examinations.
   e. Radiographic intensifying screens reduce patient dose.

5. Which of the following will reduce personnel exposure the most?
   a. Collimation of the x-ray beam
   b. Filtration of the x-ray beam
   c. Recording of fluoroscopy time
   d. A high-kVp technique
   e. Use of protective barriers for radiographers

6. When abdominal radiography is conducted on a child, which of the following is true?
   a. Gonad shielding is not necessary.
   b. Increasing kVp will increase image contrast.
   c. The parent should hold the child if necessary, and protective apparel should be provided.
   d. The parent should hold the child if necessary, and protective apparel is not necessary.
   e. The technologist should hold the child if necessary.

7. All except which of the following help to reduce patient dose?
   a. Cones
   b. Filtration
   c. Gonadal shields
   d. Intensifying screens
   e. Radiographic grids

8. After termination of an x-ray exposure:
   a. No more x-rays are emitted.
   b. The patient continues to emit scatter radiation for a few seconds.
   c. The patient continues to emit scatter radiation for less than 1 second.
   d. The patient is momentarily radioactive.
   e. X-rays continue to be emitted for a few seconds.

5

9. During fluoroscopy, what should the radiographer always do?
   a. Leave the radiation monitor behind the fixed protective barrier.
   b. Position the radiation monitor under the protective apron.
   c. Remain as close to the patient as possible.
   d. Wear a radiation monitor when examined as a patient.
   e. Wear protective apparel.

10. The main reason for filtering the x-ray beam is to:
   a. Absorb heat.
   b. Absorb penetrating x-radiation.
   c. Focus the x-ray beam.
   d. Reduce patient dose.
   e. Sharpen the image.

11. Which of the following represents implementation of a radiation protection procedure?
   a. Avoid repeat examination.
   b. Collimate to the film size.
   c. Monitor processor performance.
   d. Remove filtration.
   e. Wear protective apparel at the control console.

12. Which of the following is an example of an x-ray beam collimator?
   a. Dead-man switch
   b. Elapsed timer
   c. Filter
   d. Positive-beam limitation (PBL)
   e. Radiographic grid

13. X-ray examination of the pelvis of a woman of reproductive capacity should be limited to which of the following times?
   a. The 10-day interval after onset of menses
   b. The 10-day interval before onset of menses
   c. The first 10 days of every month
   d. The last 10 days of every month
   e. There are no restrictions; any time is fine.

14. Which of the following is true regarding the discovery of ionizing radiation?
   a. It was predicted by Mendeleev's field theory.
   b. Radioactivity was discovered within a year of Roentgen's discovery.
   c. Roentgen's discovery occurred in 1906.
   d. The apparatus that Roentgen used was called a Coolidge tube.
   e. The first radiation fatality occurred in 1920.

15. Generally, x-ray examinations are reserved for which of the following?
   a. Asymptomatic patients
   b. Older patients
   c. Patients who are not pregnant
   d. Symptomatic patients
   e. X-ray personnel

16. Gonad shields should be used:
   a. For all examinations of all patients
   b. On all female patients
   c. On all male patients
   d. When the gonads are in or near the useful beam
   e. When the gonads are in the useful beam

17. Which of the following is the principal reason to avoid repeat examination?
   a. The cost of the procedure is doubled.
   b. The images may be confused.
   c. The patient is inconvenienced.
   d. The patient receives twice the radiation dose.
   e. The radiographer's workload is doubled.

Worksheet 1-4
Numeric Prefixes

 The numeric prefixes most often encountered in radiology are as follows:

Multiple	Prefix	Symbol
10^{-12}	pico-	p
10^{-9}	nano-	n
10^{-6}	micro-	μ
10^{-3}	milli-	m
10^{-2}	centi-	c
10^{3}	kilo-	k
10^{6}	mega-	M
10^{9}	giga-	G
10^{12}	tera-	T

EXERCISES

1. 10 kilometers (km) is equal to:
   a. 100 m
   b. 1000 m
   c. 10,000 m
   d. 100,000 m
   e. 1,000,000 m

2. A radiographic exposure that lasts $\frac{1}{10}$ s is equal to:
   a. 100 μs
   b. 1 ms
   c. 10 ms
   d. 100 ms
   e. 1000 ms

3. A posteroranterior (PA) chest examination is conducted at 120 kVp. The peak x-ray tube voltage is:
   a. 120 V
   b. 1200 V
   c. 12,000 V
   d. 120,000 V
   e. 1,200,000 V

4. A radiographic exposure made on the 200 mA station is equivalent to:
   a. 2000 μA
   b. 20,000 μA
   c. 200,000 μA
   d. 2,000,000 μA
   e. 20,000,000 μA

5. If you are 160 cm tall, your height is also:
   a. 0.16 m
   b. 16 mm
   c. 16,000 mm
   d. 1.6×10^{6} μm
   e. 1.6×10^{9} μm

6. Which of the following is *correct?*
   a. 1,000,000 eV = 1 keV
   b. 0.001 A = 1 pA
   c. 10^{-7} m = 1 nm
   d. 10 μA = 0.1 mA
   e. $\frac{1}{60}$ s = 17 ms

7. If your mass is 70 kg, it is also:
   a. 0.07 mg
   b. 7000 g
   c. 70,000 g
   d. 7,000,000 mg
   e. 70,000,000 μ\g

8. Which of the following scientific prefixes is *correct?*
   a. A $\frac{1}{120}$ s exposure is 8 ms.
   b. A 35 keV x-ray has 35×10^{6} eV of energy.
   c. 1 nm is 10^{-12} m.
   d. 1 μBq is 10^{-3} Bq.
   e. 10 kVp is 1000 Vp.

9. A KUB radiograph (radiography of the kidneys, ureters, and bladder) is made at 82 kVp/200 mA/0.25 s. This is equivalent to:
   a. 0.82×10^{3} kVp/2 $\times10^{-5} \times$ A/2.5 $\times 10^{4}$ ms
   b. 0.82×10^{4} kVp $\times$ 0.2 A $\times$ 25 ms
   c. 8.2×10^{6} mVp/2 $\times 10^{2}$ mA/2.5 $\times 10^{2}$ ms
   d. $8.2 \times 10^{7} \times$ Vp/2 $\times 10^{5} \times$ A/2.5 $\times 10^{6}$ μs
   e. 82×10^{3} Vp/2 $\times 10^{-1}$ A/250 ms

10. The normal source-to-image receptor distance (SID) for an upright chest radiograph is 180 cm. This is equivalent to:
    a. 1.8 m
    b. 18 mm
    c. 180 mm
    d. 1800 μm
    e. 18,000 μm

11. When the radiographic exposure time is ½ s, it is also:
    a. 50 ms
    b. 200 ms
    c. 500 ms
    d. 2000 ms
    e. 5000 ms

12. A fluoroscopic examination is conducted at 1.5 A. This is equivalent to:
    a. 15 mA
    b. 150 mA
    c. 1500 mA
    d. 15,000 mA
    e. 1500 μA

13. The normal x-ray tube potential for a mammogram is 26 kVp. This is equivalent to:
    a. 2.6×10^{-2} Vp
    b. 2.6×10^{-1} Vp
    c. 2.6×10^{2} Vp
    d. 2.6×10^{3} Vp
    e. 2.6×10^{4} Vp

14. The SID for a mobile radiograph is often 90 cm. This is equivalent to:
    a. 9×10^{-2} m
    b. 9×10^{-1} m
    c. 9×10^{0} m
    d. 9×10^{2} m
    e. 9×10^{3} m

15. A radiographic exposure requires 400 ms. This is also:
    a. 0.0004 s
    b. 0.004 s
    c. 0.04 s
    d. 0.4 s
    e. 4 s

16. A radiographic exposure is made at 600 mA, 200 ms. This is equivalent to:
    a. 1.2 mAs
    b. 1.2×10^{1} mAs
    c. 1.2×10^{2} mAs
    d. 1.2×10^{3} mAs
    e. 1.2×10^{4} mAs

17. A chest radiograph is conducted at 125 kVp. This is equivalent to:
    a. 1.25×10^{2} Vp
    b. 1.25×10^{3} Vp
    c. 1.25×10^{4} Vp
    d. 1.25×10^{5} Vp
    e. 1.25×10^{6} Vp

18. An average annual occupational radiation exposure for a radiographer is approximately 5 mSv. This is equivalent to:
    a. 5×10^{-3} Sv
    b. 5×10^{-2} Sv
    c. 5×10^{-1} Sv
    d. 5×10^{0} Sv
    e. 5×10^{2} Sv

19. A lateral chest radiograph will expose a patient to approximately O.2 mGy_a. This is equivalent to:
    a. 2×10^{1} $μGy_a$
    b. 2×10^{2} $μGy_a$
    c. 2×10^{3} $μGy_a$
    d. 2×10^{4} $μGy_a$
    e. 2×10^{5} $μGy_a$

20. The spectrum of visible light extends from approximately 400 nm to 700 nm. This is equal to:
    a. (4 to 7) $\times 10^{-4}$ m
    b. (4 to 7) $\times 10^{-5}$ m
    c. (4 to 7) $\times 10^{-6}$ m
    d. (4 to 7) $\times 10^{-7}$ m
    e. (4 to 7) $\times 10^{-8}$ m

Worksheet 1-5
Standard Units of Measurement

 The International System of Units (SI) has been adopted by nearly all countries. It incorporates seven **base units** as its foundation. The base units then are used to develop **derived units,** some of which are identified by **special names.** The radiologic units are examples of derived units with special names.

Seven SI Base Units

Quantity	Name	Symbol
Amount of substance	Mole	mol
Electric current	Ampere	A
Length	Meter	m
Luminous intensity	Candela	cd
Mass	Kilogram	kg
Temperature	Kelvin	K
Time	Second	s

SI-Derived Units with Special Names

Quantity	Name	Symbol	Expression in Terms of Base Units
Electric charge	Coulomb	C	A*s
Electric potential	Volt	V	m*kg/s*A
Energy, work	Joule	J	m*kg/s
Force	Newton	N	m*kg/s
Frequency	Hertz	Hz	1/s
Power	Watt	W	m*kg/s

EXERCISES

1. Which of the following is *not* a base quantity in the SI?
   a. Electric current
   b. Mass
   c. Radiation exposure
   d. Temperature
   e. Time

2. Which of the following is an SI base unit?
   a. Becquerel
   b. Coulomb
   c. Coulomb/kilogram
   d. Gray
   e. Kilogram

3. Which of the following standards of SI measure is *correct?*
   a. The foot was measured by King Henry VIII.
   b. The meter is related to the visible emission from the sun.
   c. The meter is the length of an engraved platinum-iridium bar.
   d. The second is based on the rotation of the earth around the sun.
   e. The second is based on the vibrations of cesium atoms.

4. Water has a mass density of 1 g/cm^3. Its density is also:
   a. $10^{-3} kg/m^3$
   b. $1 kg/m^3$
   c. $10 kg/m^3$
   d. $10^3 kg/m^3$
   e. $10^5 kg/m^3$

5. SI stands for which of the following?
   a. Inconsistent system
   b. Incorrect system
   c. Le Système Institutional
   d. Le Système International d'Unités
   e. System International

6. Which of the following is *not* a system of units?
   a. British
   b. CGS
   c. French
   d. MKS
   e. SI

7. Which of the following is an SI name for a base unit?
   a. Celsius
   b. Kilovolt
   c. Milliampere
   d. Newton
   e. Second

9

8. Which of the following is a unit of energy?
   a. Gray
   b. Joule
   c. Newton
   d. Rad
   e. Sievert

9. Which of the following is expressed in the proper units?
   a. Absorbed dose: Sv
   b. Activity: rem
   c. Dose equivalent: rad
   d. Exposure: Bq
   e. Exposure: C/kg

10. Which of the following is an SI-derived unit?
    a. Dyne
    b. Horsepower
    c. Joule
    d. Kelvin
    e. Roentgen

11. Which of the following has units of s^{-1}?
    a. Dose
    b. Exposure
    c. Frequency
    d. Time
    e. Velocity

12. The unit of measure that is the same for all systems of measure is the:
    a. Calorie
    b. Kilogram
    c. Meter
    d. Pound
    e. Second

13. A kilogram is the:
    a. Energy required to raise 1 lb of water 1° C
    b. Mass of a standard gold bar
    c. Mass of 1 lb of water
    d. Mass of 1000 cm^3 of water
    e. Temperature rise of 1 lb of water

14. What unit results when a coulomb is divided by a second?
    a. Ampere
    b. Hertz
    c. Ohm
    d. Rad
    e. Volt

15. What common radiologic unit results from the following? millicoulomb × second =
    a. ESE
    b. kVp
    c. mA
    d. PBL
    e. SID

16. The radiologic unit milliampere-second (mAs) is actually a measure of:
    a. Electric charge
    b. Electric potential
    c. Number of electrons
    d. Potential difference
    e. X-ray intensity

17. Which of the following is a unit of electric potential?
    a. Joule
    b. kVp
    c. mA
    d. mAs
    e. Newton

18. The fundamental unit of force is the:
    a. Coulomb
    b. Joule
    c. Newton
    d. Roentgen
    e. Volt

Worksheet 1-6
Radiologic Units

Radiation Exposure:
 Air kerma is the kinetic energy transferred from photons to electrons. Air kerma is measured in joules per kilogram (J/kg) where 1 J/kg = 1 Gy_a
 1 gray in air (Gy_a) = 1 J/kg (1 roentgen (R) = 2.58 = 10^{-4} coulombs per kilogram (C/kg) of air)

Radiation Absorbed Dose:
 Absorbed dose is the radiation energy absorbed per unit mass and has units of J/kg or Gy_t.
 1 Gy_t = 1 J/kg = 10^2 rad (1 radiation absorbed dose (rad) = 10^2 ergs per gram
 (erg/g) = 10^{-2} gray in tissue (Gy_t))

Equivalent Dose:
 The sievert is the unit of equivalent dose. It takes into account the effect of different types of radiation.
 1 Sv = 1 J/kg = 10^2 rem
 (1 roentgen equivalent man (rem = 10^2 ergs per gram (erg/g) = 10^{-2} sieverts (Sv))

Effective Dose:
 This measure of radiation intensity accounts for different tissue and organ radiosensitivity. It is used for radiation risk assessment and is expressed in sieverts (Sv); (rem).

Radioactivity:
 1 curie (Ci) = 3.7 × 10^{10} atoms disintegrating per second (s^{-1})
 3.7 × 10^{10} Becquerel (Bq)
 1 Bq = 1 s^{-1}

EXERCISES

1. A radiation monitoring report would express a radiographer's dose equivalent in which of the following?
   a. Becquerel
   b. Curie
   c. Gray
   d. Roentgen
   e. Sievert

2. A posterior-anterior (PA) chest radiograph delivers approximately what dose to the patient?
   a. 100 eV
   b. 100 J
   c. 100 mR
   d. 100 μGy_a
   e. 100 μGy_t

3. To produce death, mice must be irradiated with a total dose of approximately:
   a. 6 eV
   b. 6 Gy_a
   c. 6 Gy_t
   d. 6 J
   e. 6 Sv

4. The approximate output intensity of a radiographic x-ray tube is:
   a. 50 mCi/mAs
   b. 50 mJ/mAs
   c. 50 μGy_a/mAs
   d. 50 μGy_t/mAs
   e. 50 Sv/mAs

5. ^{99m}Tc is the *most* often used radionuclide in diagnostic nuclear medicine. It is used in quantities of:
   a. MBq
   b. Ci
   c. Gy_a
   d. J
   e. Sv

6. The mGy_a is a unit of measure that specifies which of the following?
   a. Absorption of x-rays
   b. Attenuation of x-rays
   c. Character of x-rays
   d. Intensity of x-rays
   e. Quality of x-rays

7. Which of the following adequately describes the use of the Gy_t?
   a. To measure energy absorbed by tissue
   b. To measure radiation exposure in air
   c. To measure the amount of radioactive material
   d. To measure the occupational exposure received by a radiographer
   e. To measure the output intensity of an x-ray machine

8. Which of the following is a classic radiologic unit?
   a. Ampere
   b. Coulomb/kilogram
   c. Joule
   d. Rem
   e. Sievert

9. If $20\ Gy_t$ is delivered to 2 g of soft tissue, 1 g of this tissue receives:
   a. $0.5\ Gy_t$
   b. $10\ g\text{-}Gy_t$
   c. $10\ Gy_t$
   d. $20\ g\text{-}Gy_t$
   e. $20\ Gy_t$

10. Absorbed dose can be measured in:
    a. ergs
    b. Gy
    c. J
    d. keV
    e. kg-Gy

11. Which of the following is *not* a unit of energy?
    a. Calorie
    b. Electron volt
    c. Erg
    d. Gray
    e. Joule

12. Which of the following statements is equivalent?
    a. $1\ Gy_t = 1\ J/kg$
    b. $1\ mCi = 37\ \mu C/kg$
    c. $1\ Sv = 100\ erg/g$
    d. $200\ mrad = 2\ cGy$
    e. $500\ mR = 5\ mGy_a$

13. Which of the following is a unit of radioactivity?
    a. Ci
    b. Gy
    c. J
    d. R
    e. Rad

14. Absorbed dose can be expressed in:
    a. Bq
    b. Ci
    c. Ergs
    d. eV
    e. J/kg

15. Which of the following demonstrates the proper use of air kerma?
    a. An angiographer receives an occupational exposure of $10\ mGy_a$.
    b. $100\ Gy_t$ of ^{131}I is administered to image the thyroid.
    c. Patient treatment dose with a linear accelerator unit is 6000 R.
    d. The dose limit (DL) for radiologic technologists is 50 mSv/yr.
    e. X-ray intensity from a linear accelerator unit is 2 Gy_a/min.

16. In diagnostic radiology, it is acceptable to assume that $1\ mGy_a$ is equal to:
    a. 1 Ci
    b. 1 erg
    c. 1 J
    d. 1 keV
    e. $1\ mGy_t$

17. In the SI system:
    a. Equivalent dose is expressed in Gy.
    b. kVp is equal to keV.
    c. 1 J is approximately equal to 1 MeV.
    d. 1000 rad is equivalent to 10 Gy.
    e. 1000 rad is equivalent to 100 Sv.

18. Dose rate could be expressed in units of:
    a. Ergs/g
    b. J/kg/min
    c. keV/min
    d. kVp/s
    e. Sv/min

19. When SI is used, radiation exposure is defined in units of coulombs/kilogram. With regard to this unit of measure, which of the following is *true?*
    a. *Coulomb* refers to electrons released in ionization.
    b. *Coulomb* refers to energy absorbed.
    c. *Kilogram* refers to mass of radiation.
    d. *Kilogram* refers to the radiation mass.
    e. Kilogram refers to the patient's mass.

Worksheet 1-7
Newton's Laws

 ■ **Newton's first law**—*Inertia:* When no force is acting on an object, it will continue in its present state of motion or rest.

■ **Newton's second law**—*Force:* The force required to change the state of motion of an object is directly proportional to the product of the mass of the object and the acceleration.

■ **Newton's third law**—*Reaction:* For every force, there is an equal but opposite force.

■ **Mass** is the property of matter that tends to keep a stationary object at rest or that resists a change in the motion of an object that is already moving (Newton's first law).

■ **Force** is a push or a pull. Newton's second law, which expresses the concept of force, is his greatest and is represented by the equation:

$$F = ma \text{ where}$$

Force (newtons [N]) = Mass (kg) × Acceleration (m/s²)

■ The weight of an object is actually the force of gravitational attraction on its mass. In mathematical terms:

$$W = mg$$

Weight (N) = Mass (kg) × Acceleration (m/s²)

EXERCISES

1. Which of the following is *not* a correct statement of Newton's laws?
   a. Acceleration is equal to initial velocity plus final velocity, divided by 2.
   b. Force is equal to mass times acceleration.
   c. Momentum is equal to mass times velocity.
   d. Velocity is equal to distance divided by time.
   e. Weight is equal to mass times acceleration.

2. Which of the following correctly states Newton's first law of motion?
   a. An object at rest will remain at rest unless acted on by an external force.
   b. An object with mass (*m*) and acceleration (*a*) is acted on by a force, given by the equation $F = ma$.
   c. For every action, there is an opposite and equal reaction.
   d. Matter and energy are related.
   e. The total momentum before any interaction is equal to the total momentum after the interaction.

3. Another name for velocity is:
   a. Energy
   b. Mass
   c. Speed
   d. Time
   e. Work

4. When you travel 50 mph, you are also going approximately:
   a. 80 km/hr
   b. 100 km/hr
   c. 1100 ft/min
   d. 2200 ft/min
   e. 3300 ft/min

5. Acceleration is also:
   a. The product of time and distance
   b. The rate of change of time with velocity
   c. The rate of change of velocity with distance
   d. The rate of change of velocity with time
   e. Time squared

6. An automobile travels 30 miles in 30 minutes. Its average velocity is approximately:
   a. 1 mile/min
   b. 33 miles/min
   c. 60 miles/min
   d. 88 miles/min
   e. 99 miles/min

7. The final speed of a dragster in a quarter mile race is 80 mph. The average velocity is:
   a. 4 miles/hr
   b. 8 miles/hr
   c. 16 miles/hr
   d. 32 miles/hr
   e. 40 miles/hr

8. A dragster requires 8 s to reach a speed of 80 mph. What is its acceleration?
   a. 1.1 m/s²
   b. 2.2 m/s²
   c. 3.3 m/s²
   d. 4.5 m/s²
   e. 5.5 m/s²

13

9. Inertia is:
   a. Mass times acceleration
   b. Newton's second law of motion
   c. Resistance to a change in motion
   d. Velocity divided by time
   e. Velocity times time

10. Which of the following statements refers to a vector quantity?
   a. The car was speeding north at 100 km/hr.
   b. The speed of light is 3×10^8 m/s.
   c. The standard man has a mass of 70 kg.
   d. The standard man weighs 70 kg.
   e. The units of the Planck constant are J-s.

11. A World Series fastball was clocked at 90 mph. How long did that ball take to travel the 90 feet to the plate?
   a. Less than 1 s
   b. 1 s
   c. Longer than 2 s
   d. 1.5 s
   e. 2 s

12. How many fundamental laws of motion did Newton formulate?
   a. 1
   b. 2
   c. 3
   d. 4
   e. 5

13. If someone were to fall off the edge of the south rim of the Grand Canyon, the force exerted would be measured in:
   a. kg
   b. J
   c. m/s
   d. mSv
   e. N

14. If the acceleration caused by gravity is 9.8 m/s^2, what is the gravitational force acting on a 50-kg sack pushed off the roof of a 50-story building?
   a. 0.2 N
   b. 5.1 N
   c. 40.2 N
   d. 80 N
   e. 490 N

15. How is momentum *best* described?
   a. For every action, there is an equal and opposite reaction
   b. It is the force of an object caused by the downward pull of gravity
   c. It is the product of the mass of an object and its velocity
   d. It is the relationship between matter and energy
   e. Objects falling to the earth accelerate at a constant rate

16. The total momentum before any interaction is:
   a. An equal and opposite reaction
   b. Decreased by the property of friction, so it is less after the interaction
   c. Equal to the total momentum after the interaction
   d. Greater than the total momentum during the interaction
   e. Less than the total momentum during the interaction

17. Which of the following is a unit of work?
   a. Gray
   b. Hertz
   c. Joule
   d. Newton
   e. Rad

Worksheet 1-8
Mechanics

 Mechanics is the physics of objects at rest (statics) and objects in motion (dynamics).

WORK

If one exerts a **force** (a push or pull) on a box and moves it across the floor, one does **work** on the box. The following is the formula for work:

$$W = Fd$$

The unit of work is the **joule** (J) if the force is measured in newtons and the distance in meters (1 J = 1 N × 1 m).

ENERGY

A system that is capable of doing work is said to have energy. Energy is the ability to do work, and it can take many forms, including heat energy, electric energy, nuclear energy, and mechanical energy. Mechanical energy may be potential or kinetic:

1. **Potential energy (PE):** The energy of an object is a result of its position. For example, a brick raised over your head or a coiled spring has potential energy.
2. **Kinetic energy (KE):** The energy of an object is a result of its motion.

$$KE\ \tfrac{1}{2}\ mv^2$$

The basic unit of energy is the **joule.** Other units are also used:

1 electron volt (eV) = 1.6×10^{-19} J
1 erg = 10^{-7} J
1 British thermal unit (BTU) = 1.06 J
1 foot-pound (ft-lb) = 1.36 J
1 kilowatt-hour (kW-hr) = 3.6×10^6 J

POWER

Power is the rate at which work is done. The following is the formula for power:

$$P = W/t$$

The unit of power is the **watt** (1 watt = 1 J/s). A commonly used unit of power is the **kilowatt,** which is equal to 1000 watts. Another frequently used unit of power is **horsepower** (hp):

$$1\ hp = 746\ watts$$

EXERCISES

A radiographer lifts a box onto a platform. Choose one or more of the following choices (a through f) to use as you complete Exercises 1 to 5.
a. The distance the box is lifted
b. The force used by the man to lift the box
c. The mass of the box
d. The size of the box
e. The time required to lift the box
f. The velocity of the box

1. The **KE** of the box depends on _____.
2. The man's **power** output depends on _____.
3. The **PE** of the box depends on _____.
4. The total **energy** used depends on _____.
5. The **work** done depends on _____.

6. Which of the following statements about work is *true?*
   a. It can be measured in watts.
   b. It depends on time.
   c. It has units the same as energy.
   d. It is measured in newtons.
   e. It is performed when a large weight is held motionless.

7. A one-bedroom apartment might use 1000 kW-hr of electricity. The kilowatt-hour is a unit of:
   a. Energy
   b. Force
   c. Heat
   d. Potential energy
   e. Power

8. KE is directly proportional to:
   a. A vector quantity
   b. Acceleration
   c. Force
   d. Mass
   e. Velocity

9. Which of the following units of energy is *most* fundamental?
   a. Calorie
   b. Electron volt
   c. Erg
   d. Joule
   e. Kilowatt hour

10. Which of the following is the primary method of heat dissipation from the rotating anode of an x-ray tube?
    a. Conduction
    b. Convection
    c. Convention
    d. Radiation
    e. Reduction

11. Which of the following statements about energy is *true?*
    a. Energy is a force.
    b. Energy is a form of power.
    c. Energy is the ability to do work.
    d. Energy is the rate of doing work.
    e. X-rays can be described by their potential energy.

12. How much work is done in lifting a 1 kg box of film from the floor to a shelf that is 2 m high? (*Hint:* 1 kg = 2.2 lb = 9.8 N)
    a. 1 J
    b. 2.2 J
    c. 4.5 J
    d. 19.6 J
    e. 9 N

13. A car with a 300 hp engine is very fast. The power of the engine is equivalent to how many kilowatts?
    a. 0.4 kW
    b. 2.5 kW
    c. 25 kW
    d. 224 kW
    e. 300 kW

14. Heat is transferred from a glass-enclosed fireplace primarily by:
    a. Conduction
    b. Convection
    c. Convention
    d. Radiation
    e. Temperature

15. A 1 degree change is equal in thermal energy for which two scales?
    a. Absolute and kelvin
    b. Celsius and absolute
    c. Celsius and Fahrenheit
    d. Celsius and kelvin
    e. Fahrenheit and kelvin

16. Which British unit is equivalent to the newton?
    a. Foot-pound
    b. Gram
    c. Joule
    d. Kilogram
    e. Pound

Worksheet 2-1
Centuries of Discovery

 ■ The concept of an atom has existed through time and developed into the elements of the periodic table.

THE PERIODIC TABLE

■ The periodic table is a systematic grouping of the elements that is based on similarity of chemical properties.
■ The vertical columns are called **groups**. The horizontal rows are **periods**.
■ As you proceed from left to right in a period, the number of easily removable electrons, called **valence electrons**, increases by one from one group to the next.

EXERCISES

1. Which of the following statements is *true* regarding our understanding of atomic structure?
   a. Rutherford described the nuclear atom.
   b. Rutherford identified cathode rays as particles, and constituents of all are correct atoms.
   c. Rutherford is known as the "Father of Radioactivity."
   d. Rutherford is responsible for the periodic table.
   e. Rutherford was an epicurean and envisioned the atom as something familiar to him—plum pudding.

2. In the rendering of the atom by J. J. Thomson:
   a. Electrons were in orbits.
   b. Electrons were distributed throughout the nucleus as plums in a pudding.
   c. Eyes and hooks represented electrons.
   d. He called it the "cathode ray atom."
   e. Uniform positive electrification was theorized.

3. The periodic table presents the elements in the order of:
   a. Atomic charge
   b. Atomic mass
   c. Atomic number
   d. Natural occurrences
   e. Number of isotopes

4. Approximately how many known elements are there?
   a. 50
   b. 100
   c. 150
   d. 200
   e. 300

5. The only element that is *not* placed in any group on the periodic table is:
   a. Helium
   b. Hydrogen
   c. Plutonium
   d. Tungsten
   e. Uranium

6. The horizontal rows in the periodic table are called:
   a. Articles
   b. Compounds
   c. Groups
   d. Molecules
   e. Periods

7. As you move from left to right across the periodic table, what happens to the number of outer-shell electrons from one element to the next?
   a. It decreases by 1.
   b. It decreases by 2.
   c. It increases by 1.
   d. It increases by 2.
   e. It remains constant.

8. Which group in the periodic table contains elements that have only one electron in the outer shell?
   a. Actinide metals
   b. Alkali metals
   c. Halogens
   d. Rare earths
   e. Vapors

9. Which of the following is a transitional element?
   a. Barium
   b. Carbon dioxide
   c. Iodine
   d. Tungsten
   e. Xenon

10. Atoms with all electron shells filled are:
    a. Chemically stable
    b. Chemically very reactive
    c. Found in group 1 of the periodic table
    d. Gases
    e. Radioactive

11. Atoms with three electrons in the outer shell:
    a. Are compounds
    b. Are molecules
    c. Are probably inert gases
    d. Are probably radioactive
    e. Have three valence electrons

12. In the periodic table of the elements, the group number identifies the:
    a. Electron spin state
    b. Number of electrons in the outer shell
    c. Principal quantum number of the outermost shell
    d. Total number of electrons in the atom
    e. Valence state of the atom

13. All of the following are elements, *except:*
    a. Carbon
    b. Molybdenum
    c. Oxygen
    d. Steel
    e. Tungsten

14. How many atoms are there in one molecule of sodium bicarbonate ($NaHCO_3$)?
    a. 1
    b. 3
    c. 4
    d. 6
    e. 8

15. Which of the following physicists had a major part in describing the atom as we know it today?
    a. Becquerel
    b. Bohr
    c. Curie
    d. Einstein
    e. Roentgen

16. Which of the following statements is *true?*
    a. A 6000-yard golf course is approximately 10^4 m long.
    b. A football field is approximately 10^3 m long.
    c. An atomic nucleus has a diameter of approximately 10^{-10} m.
    d. In 1 year, light can travel approximately 10^{16} m.
    e. The wavelength of a 100 keV x-ray is approximately 10^{-8} m.

17. The periodic chart of elements is attributed to:
    a. Dimitri Mendeleev
    b. Ernest Rutherford
    c. J. J. Thomson
    d. John Dalton
    e. Niels Bohr

18. Rutherford made what significant contribution to science?
    a. Description of the electron shells
    b. Description of the nuclear atom
    c. Discovery of artificial radioactivity
    d. Discovery of negatively charged electrons
    e. Periodic table of the elements

Worksheet 2-2
Fundamental Particles
Atomic Structure

 Matter is composed of atoms. Atoms are composed of fundamental particles called **protons, neutrons,** and **electrons.** The positively charged protons and uncharged neutrons make up the **nucleus** of the atom. The negatively charged electrons revolve around the nucleus in definite orbits, just as the planets orbit the sun.

The electron is the lightest of the fundamental particles. The mass of the proton is 1836 times larger than the mass of the electron. The neutron mass is 1839 times larger than that of the electron.

The closer electrons are to the nucleus, the more tightly bound they are. The number of electrons in any shell increases to a maximum of $2n^2$, where n is the shell number. No matter how large the atom becomes, however, it normally has the same number of electrons as protons. If this is not the case, the atom is an **ion.**

EXERCISES

1. If $^{129}_{53}I$ is a stable, electrically neutral atom, then how many neutrons are there in such an atom?
   a. 53
   b. 76
   c. 129
   d. 182
   e. The question does not give enough information.

2. When oxygen ($^{16}_{8}O$) combines with two atoms of hydrogen ($^{1}_{1}H$) to form water, the resultant molecule has a total of:
   a. 8 electrons
   b. 10 protons
   c. 16 electrons
   d. 18 protons
   e. 20 nucleons

3. The atomic mass number of an atom is given by the number of:
   a. Electrons
   b. Neutrons
   c. Protons
   d. Protons plus neutrons
   e. Protons plus neutrons plus electrons

4. The atomic number:
   a. Has the symbol "A"
   b. Has the symbol "N"
   c. Is the number of neutrons
   d. Is the number of protons
   e. Is the number of protons plus neutrons

5. Isotopes are atoms:
   a. In the same molecule
   b. Of the same element
   c. That are ions
   d. That contain the same number of neutrons plus protons
   e. With the same number of nucleons

6. Electrons in the M-shell:
   a. Have lower binding energy than those in the N-shell
   b. Never exceed 8 in number
   c. Do not exceed 18 in number
   d. Do not exist in an atom of tungsten (W)
   e. Probably are closer to the nucleus than those in the L-shell

7. $^{12}_{6}C$ and $^{14}_{6}C$ have the same:
   a. A number
   b. N number
   c. Number of neutrons
   d. Number of nucleons
   e. Number of protons

8. The binding energy of an electron to a nucleus:
   a. Increases with increasing distance from the nucleus
   b. Is higher for an L-shell electron than for an M-shell electron
   c. Is higher for a low-Z atom than for a high-Z atom
   d. Is higher for an N-shell than for an M-shell
   e. Depends on the size of an electron

9. How many nucleons does $^{131}_{53}$I have?
   a. 53
   b. 78
   c. 131
   d. 184
   e. 237

10. The number of protons in the nucleus is called the:
    a. Atomic number
    b. Elemental charge
    c. Ionization state
    d. Mass
    e. Valence

11. A neutron has approximately:
    a. $\frac{1}{2000}$ atomic mass unit (amu) and no charge
    b. 1 amu and no charge
    c. 1 amu and a charge of 1
    d. 4 amu and a charge of 2
    e. 4 amu and no charge

12. How many different types of nucleons are there?
    a. 1
    b. 2
    c. 3
    d. 4
    e. 6

13. Which of the following is a fundamental particle?
    a. Alpha
    b. Beta
    c. Electron
    d. Gamma
    e. Hydrogen

14. What is the maximum number of electrons allowed in the outermost shell of an atom in the third period, n = 3?
    a. 2
    b. 8
    c. 18
    d. 32
    e. 50

15. Tungsten $^{184}_{74}$W has how many neutrons?
    a. 74
    b. 110
    c. 184
    d. 258
    e. 332

16. What is the maximum number of electrons permitted in the N-shell?
    a. 8
    b. 18
    c. 24
    d. 32
    e. 50

17. Regarding atomic nomenclature:
    a. Atomic mass is the number of neutrons.
    b. Atomic mass is the number of protons.
    c. Atomic mass is the number of protons minus neutrons.
    d. Atomic mass number determines chemical properties.
    e. Atomic mass number is a whole number.

18. The following atoms are all stable; which has the highest K-shell electron binding energy?
    a. Al (aluminum)
    b. Hg (mercury)
    c. S (sulfur)
    d. Sr (strontium)
    e. Tc (technetium)

Worksheet 2-3
Atomic Nomenclature
Combinations of Atoms

The atomic mass number and the precise mass of an atom are not the same. Atoms of various elements may combine to form structures called molecules. Quantities of a given molecule are called a chemical compound.

Certain naturally occurring and artificially produced atoms can emit radiation spontaneously. Such atoms are said to be **radioactive.** Radioactivity is the result of instability in the nucleus. Three types of radiation come from the nucleus of a radioactive atom: **alpha (α) particles, beta (β) particles, and gamma (γ) rays.**

- Alpha particles consist of two protons and two neutrons.
- Beta particles are actually electrons that are emitted from the nucleus.
- Gamma rays are the product of electromagnetic radiation of high energy and high penetrability (much like x-rays).

EXERCISES

Match the following.

_____ 1. Alpha particle	a. A particle accelerator used to produce radioisotopes
_____ 2. Beta particle	b. A particle with a charge of -1.602×10^{-19} C
_____ 3. Cyclotron	c. A stable atom that can be made radioactive
_____ 4. Gamma ray	d. A substance composed of atoms with unstable nuclei
_____ 5. Gold	e. An atom that is naturally radioactive
_____ 6. Isotope	f. Atoms with the same number of protons but different numbers of neutrons
_____ 7. Radioactive	g. Radiation that cannot penetrate a sheet of paper material
_____ 8. Radioactivity	h. Spontaneous emission of energy or particles from unstable nuclei
_____ 9. Radioisotope	i. Uncharged radiation; highly penetrating
_____ 10. Uranium	j. Usually produced by particle accelerators from common elements

11. When a radioisotope emits a beta particle:
    a. A gamma ray is always emitted.
    b. A neutron is converted to a proton.
    c. A proton is converted to a neutron.
    d. An electron is converted to a beta particle.
    e. An x-ray is always emitted.

12. Which of the following pairs of atoms are isobars?
    a. ^{129}I and ^{131}I
    b. ^{131}I and ^{198}Hg
    c. ^{2}H and ^{3}H
    d. ^{3}He and ^{3}H
    e. ^{131}I and ^{137}Cs

13. Potassium ($^{40}_{19}$K) is a naturally occurring radioisotope that decays by beta emission. Therefore, the daughter atom:
    a. Has a mass of approximately 19 amu
    b. Will also be radioactive
    c. Will have 19 neutrons
    d. Will have 40 nucleons
    e. Will have 90 protons

14. Isotopes are:
    a. Atoms that have an identical mass and atomic number
    b. Atoms that have the same atomic mass number but different atomic numbers
    c. Atoms that have the same atomic number but different atomic mass numbers
    d. Molecules that consist of identical atoms
    e. Molecules that have the same number of atoms

15. The number of disintegrations per second in 2 mCi of ^{99m}Tc is:
    a. 3.7×10^{7}
    b. 3.7×10^{10}
    c. 3.7×10^{12}
    d. 7.4×10^{7}
    e. 7.4×10^{10}

16. With regard to $^{90}_{38}Sr + ^{2}_{3}$:
    a. The atomic number is 90.
    b. The symbolism indicates that this is a radioactive nuclide.
    c. The valence is 3.
    d. There are 90 neutrons in the nucleus of this atom.
    e. There are a total of 36 electrons in one such atom.

17. Beta emission:
    a. Occurs only with heavy elements
    b. Occurs only with light elements
    c. Occurs only with radioisotopes with long half-lives
    d. Results in the gain of a proton
    e. Results in the loss of 1 amu

18. Alpha emission:
    a. Occurs only with light elements
    b. Occurs only with radioisotopes with long half-lives
    c. Results in the gain of a proton
    d. Results in the loss of 2 amu
    e. Results in the loss of 4 amu

19. After beta emission, the nucleus has:
    a. Decreased in A number by 1
    b. Decreased in Z and A numbers by 1
    c. Decreased in Z number by 1
    d. Increased in A number by 1
    e. Increased in Z number by 1

20. 1 Ci is equivalent to disintegration of how many atoms every second?
    a. 3×10^8
    b. 3×10^{10}
    c. 3.7×10^8
    d. 3.7×10^{10}
    e. 2.2×10^{12}

21. 10 mCi is equivalent to:
    a. $3.7\ 10^8$ Bq
    b. 10^{-6} Ci
    c. 3.7×10^{10} d/s
    d. 10^{-2} nCi
    e. 2.2×10^{12} d/min

22. Which of the following statements about atoms is *true?*
    a. $A = Z + N$
    b. $A = Z - N$.
    c. An alpha emission contains four units of mass and four units of charge.
    d. In a radioactive atom, the number of protons does not equal the number of electrons.
    e. Nucleons are electrons, protons, and neutrons.

23. Which of the following pairs of atoms are isotones?
    a. $^{1}_{1}H$ and $^{2}_{1}H$
    b. $^{130}_{56}Ba$ and $^{132}_{56}Ba$
    c. $^{130}_{53}I$ and $^{131}_{54}Xe$
    d. ^{99}Tc and ^{99m}Tc
    e. $^{133}_{54}Xe$ and $^{133}_{55}Cs$

24. Isomers are atoms that have different:
    a. Energy states
    b. Filled electron shells
    c. Numbers of neutrons
    d. Numbers of protons
    e. States of ionization

25. Radioisotopes:
    a. Are ionized
    b. Are made with x-rays
    c. Are stable atoms
    d. Have closed electron shells
    e. Have unstable nuclei

Worksheet 2-4
Radioactivity

Radioactivity is due to natural or artificially induced instability in the nucleus of an atom. To become stable, the nucleus decays by emitting alpha, beta, or gamma radiation. Radioactivity is measured in curies or Becquerels: preferably Becquerels.

$$1 \text{ curie (Ci)} = 3.70 \times 10^{10} \text{ disintegrations/s}$$
$$1 \text{ becquerel (Bq)} = 1 \text{ disintegration/s}$$

The quantities of radioactive material used for medical imaging are megabecquerels (MBq) and millicuries (mCi).

$$100 \text{ MBq} = 2.7 \text{ mCi.}$$
$$10 \text{ mCi} = 370 \text{ MBq}$$

Radioactivity decreases with time. The time required for the activity of a sample to decay to half of its original value is called the radioactive half-life ($t_{1/2}$).

EXERCISES

1. Radioactive half-life is the time:
   a. It takes for half of the dose to be delivered
   b. It takes for half of the mass to disappear
   c. It takes for one atom to disintegrate
   d. Required for radioactivity to reach one half of its original value
   e. When half of the quantity now present remains

2. How many half-lives must elapse before the remaining activity is less than 0.1% of the original activity?
   a. 4 half-lives
   b. 6 half-lives
   c. 8 half-lives
   d. 10 half-lives
   e. 12 half-lives

3. Given a 50 μCi (0.19 MBq) sample of ^{131}I ($t_{1/2}$ = 8 days), the radioactivity will be 3 μCi after approximately how many days?
   a. 24 days
   b. 32 days
   c. 36 days
   d. 40 days
   e. 44 days

4. A 10 mCi quantity of technetium ^{99m}Tc ($t_{1/2}$ = 6 hr) is available at 8:00 AM. At noon on that same day, the radioactivity will be closer to:
   a. 1 mCi than to 3 mCi
   b. 3 mCi than to 5 mCi
   c. 5 mCi than to 8 mCi
   d. 10 mCi than to 8 mCi
   e. 15 mCi than to 10 mCi

5. ^{14}C ($t_{1/2}$ = 5730 yr) is used for radiocarbon dating. Approximately how old is a tree specimen that contains 3 nCi/g (110 Bq/g) if the original concentration of radioactivity is known to be 12 nCi/g (444 Bq/g)?
   a. 5730 years
   b. Approximately 11,000 years
   c. Approximately 17,000 years
   d. Younger than 5730 years
   e. Older than 17,000 years

6. 100 mCi (3.7 GBq) of an unknown radionuclide has a half-life of 15 days. Therefore:
   a. 400 mCi should have been available 15 days earlier.
   b. In 15 days, only 25 mCi will remain.
   c. In 1 month, 25 mCi will have decayed.
   d. In 1 month, only 75 mCi will remain.
   e. In 3½ months, the activity will be less than 1 mCi.

7. How much ^{99m}Tc ($t_{1/2}$ = 6 hr) decays in 24 hours?
   a. 3%
   b. 6%
   c. 14%
   d. 86%
   e. 94%

8. In approximately how many half-lives will the activity of 10 mCi (0.37 GBq) of I ($t_{1/2}$ = 8 days) be reduced to 0.1 mCi (3.7 MBq)?
   a. 3.3 half-lives
   b. 10 half-lives
   c. 12.5 half-lives
   d. 50 half-lives
   e. 100 half-lives

9. Which of the following statements about a given radioisotope is *true?*
   a. As the number of atoms decreases, the half-life decreases.
   b. The half-life increases as the decay constant increases.
   c. The number of radioactive atoms decreases linearly with time.
   d. The percentage of atoms decaying per unit of time decreases.
   e. The percentage of atoms decaying per unit of time is constant.

10. If the half-life of $^{131}_{53}$I is 8 days, approximately how much $^{131}_{53}$I remains of an original shipment of 50 μCi (1.9 MBq) after 24 days?
    a. 25 nCi
    b. 25 nCi
    c. 3 μCi
    d. 6 μCi
    e. 12 μCi

11. 10 mCi of ^{99m}Tc is a normal patient dose for imaging. How many Becquerels is this?
    a. 2.2×10^8 Bq
    b. 3.7×10^8 Bq
    c. 2.2×10^{11} Bq
    d. 3.7×10^{11} Bq
    e. 3.7×10^{12} Bq

12. $^{131}_{53}$I has a half-life of 13 hours. If 150 μCi (5.7 MBq) is available at noon on Wednesday, approximately how much will remain at 5:00 PM on Friday?
    a. 10 μCi
    b. 20 μCi
    c. 30 μCi
    d. 40 μCi
    e. 50 μCi

13. The radioactivity of an unknown radioisotope is measured to be 40 μCi (15 MBq) at 9:00 am on Monday. Another measurement at 9:00 pm on Tuesday yields a result of 2.5 μCi (0.1 MBq). What is the half-life of the radioisotope?
    a. 3 hours
    b. 6 hours
    c. 9 hours
    d. 12 hours
    e. 18 hours

14. Use the following graph to estimate the percentage

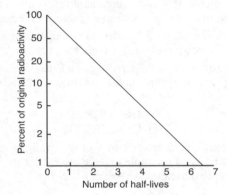

of radioactivity that remains after 2½ half-lives.
    a. 2.5%
    b. 5%
    c. 16%
    d. 50%
    e. 75%

15. The shape of the radioactive decay curve is:
    a. A concave-down curve on linear paper
    b. A concave-up curve on semilog paper
    c. A straight line on linear paper
    d. A straight line on semilog paper
    e. Linear and nonthreshold

Worksheet 2-5
Types of Ionizing Radiation

- Radiation is the transfer of energy from one position or medium to another.
  - There are two types of radiation: ionizing and non-ionizing.
- There are two sources of radiation: naturally occurring radiation and man-made radiation.
- Ionizing radiation is any radiation that is capable of removing an orbital electron from an atom.
- There are two types of ionizing radiation: particulate and electromagnetic.

I. Particulate
  a. Alpha (α) particles
  b. Beta (β) particles
  c. Other nuclear particles

II. Electromagnetic
  a. Gamma (γ) rays
  b. X-rays

EXERCISES

1. The difference between electrons and beta particles is:
   a. Beta particles are ionizing.
   b. Beta particles have higher energy.
   c. Electrons have higher mass.
   d. Electrons have higher velocity.
   e. Their origin

2. In the air:
   a. A gamma ray does not normally travel farther than 10 m.
   b. Alpha particles have a range of 1 to 10 cm.
   c. Alpha particles travel farthest.
   d. An x-ray does not normally travel farther than 1 m.
   e. Beta particles have a range of 1 to 10 mm.

3. The amount of energy acquired when an electron is accelerated by a potential difference of 1 V is:
   a. 1 Ci
   b. 1 eV
   c. 1 J
   d. 1 μGy_a
   e. 1 μGy_t

4. Alpha particles:
   a. Are similar to hydrogen nuclei
   b. Are useful in nuclear medicine
   c. Contain two electrons
   d. Have an A number of 4
   e. Have a Z number of 4

5. Of the following radiations, the *most* penetrating is a:
   a. 10 keV x-ray
   b. 100 keV gamma ray
   c. 0.01 MeV x-ray
   d. 2.1 MeV beta particle
   e. 4.8 MeV alpha particle

6. The difference between x-rays and gamma rays is:
   a. Gamma rays always have higher energy than x-rays.
   b. Gamma rays have a higher mass.
   c. Gamma rays travel faster.
   d. Their origin
   e. X-rays produce bremsstrahlung radiation and gamma rays do not.

7. X-rays have:
   a. 1 amu and are neutral
   b. A negative charge and no rest mass
   c. No mass and a charge of −1
   d. No mass and a charge of +2
   e. No mass and no charge

8. Given the general characteristics of ionizing radiation:
   a. All photons travel in straight lines, even in the presence of a magnetic field.
   b. As x-ray energy increases, so does linear energy transfer (LET).
   c. The neutron is a chargeless particle and is therefore non-ionizing radiation.
   d. The range of a beta particle in tissue can extend to a depth of 10 cm.
   e. The range of gamma rays in air normally does not exceed 1 m.

9. Which of the following types of radiation are emitted from outside of the nucleus?
   a. Alpha particles
   b. Beta particles
   c. Gamma rays
   d. Neutrinos
   e. X-rays

10. As compared with particulate radiation, electromagnetic radiation:
    a. Has a higher electrostatic charge
    b. Has higher linear energy transfer (LET)
    c. Is heavier
    d. Is more densely ionizing
    e. Is more penetrating

11. When electromagnetic radiation is compared with particulate radiation, it is *true* that:
    a. They both interact by ionization and excitation.
    b. Particulate radiation exists only at the speed of light.
    c. They are equally penetrating.
    d. They have equal mass.
    e. They have nearly equal LET.

12. Particulate ionizing radiation:
    a. Can include any type of subatomic particle
    b. Has greater range than electromagnetic radiation
    c. Includes ultrasound
    d. Travels at the speed of light
    e. Usually has low LET

13. Electromagnetic ionizing radiation:
    a. Comes from both inside and outside of the nucleus
    b. Has a lower velocity than light
    c. Has a lower velocity than particulate radiation
    d. Includes alpha and beta particles
    e. Includes therapeutic ultrasound

14. X-rays and gamma rays are examples of electromagnetic radiation. In addition, they both have:
    a. No electrostatic charge
    b. Small mass
    c. The same origin
    d. The velocity of ultrasound
    e. Variable velocity

15. Which of the following is an example of ionizing radiation?
    a. Energetic protons
    b. Microwaves
    c. MRI
    d. Therapeutic ultrasound
    e. Ultraviolet radiation

16. How does the energy of a gamma ray compare with the energy of an x-ray?
    a. The question does not give enough information.
    b. They are equal.
    c. The energy of gamma rays is greater than the energy of x-rays.
    d. The energy of gamma rays is less than the energy of x-rays.
    e. The energy of gamma rays is much greater than the energy of x-rays.

17. What are the two principal classes of ionizing radiation?
    a. Diagnostic and particulate
    b. MRI and electromagnetic
    c. MRI and ultrasound
    d. Particulate and electromagnetic
    e. Particulate and ultrasound

18. Which of the following is *not* ionizing radiation?
    a. Auger electrons
    b. Beta particles
    c. Neutrons
    d. Therapeutic ultrasound
    e. X-rays

Worksheet 3-1
Photons

 An x-ray photon is a quantum of electromagnetic energy.

The wave equation is as follows:

$$v = \lambda \times f \ or \ \text{Velocity} = \text{Wavelength} \times \text{Frequency}$$

Electromagnetic radiation always travels at the speed of light (3×10^8 m/s), so $v = c$ and, for electromagnetic radiation, $c = \lambda \times f$. The unit of frequency is the hertz (1 Hz = 1 cycle per second).

At a given velocity, wavelength and frequency are inversely proportional.

EXERCISES

1. X-ray wavelength is:
   a. Directly proportional to frequency
   b. Directly proportional to velocity
   c. Inversely proportional to frequency
   d. Inversely proportional to velocity
   e. Usually designated by "c"

2. Which of the following is *true* for both a 100 keV x-ray and a 10 keV gamma ray?
   a. They have equal frequencies.
   b. They have equal negative charges.
   c. They have equal wavelengths.
   d. They have the same origin.
   e. They have zero mass.

3. A frequency of 1 MHz is:
   a. 1 cycle per second
   b. 10^2 cycles per second
   c. 10^3 cycles per second
   d. 10^6 cycles per second
   e. 10^9 cycles per second

4. When the frequency of electromagnetic radiation is increased tenfold:
   a. The velocity decreases to $\frac{1}{10}$.
   b. The velocity increases times 10.
   c. The wavelength remains constant.
   d. The wavelength decreases to $\frac{1}{10}$.
   e. The wavelength increases times 10.

5. A single unit of electromagnetic radiation is also called a/an:
   a. Ion
   b. Photon
   c. Proton
   d. Quark
   e. Strange

6. Light has a constant velocity of $c = 3 \times 10^8$ m/s. Therefore:
   a. Its energy increases with increasing wavelength.
   b. Its frequency decreases with increasing wavelength.
   c. Its mass increases with increasing frequency.
   d. Its velocity is also 3×10^{12} cm/s.
   e. Its velocity is also 3×10^{12} mm/s.

7. The frequency of electromagnetic radiation is:
   a. Measured in disintegrations per second
   b. Measured in hertz
   c. Measured in meters per second
   d. Proportional to the wavelength
   e. Proportional to velocity

8. When one uses the sine wave as a model:
   a. Amplitude and frequency are directly proportional.
   b. Amplitude and wavelength are directly proportional.
   c. The distance from one peak to the next is the wavelength.
   d. The distance from one valley to the next is the frequency.
   e. The energy is proportional to amplitude.

9. Given the sine wave model of electromagnetic radiation:
   a. Amplitude and velocity are inversely related.
   b. Frequency and velocity are inversely related.
   c. Frequency times amplitude is a constant.
   d. Frequency times velocity is a constant.
   e. Frequency times wavelength is a constant.

10. Which of the following has a constant value for all electromagnetic radiation?
    a. Frequency
    b. Mass
    c. Origin
    d. Velocity
    e. Wavelength

11. The velocity of light is:
    a. 3×10^8 cm/s
    b. 3×10^{10} cm/s
    c. 3×10^{12} cm/s
    d. 3.7×10^{10} m/s
    e. 3.7×10^8 m/s

12. The amplitude of a sine wave is its:
    a. Frequency
    b. Minimum to maximum
    c. Velocity
    d. Wavelength
    e. Zero to maximum

13. The frequency of a sine wave is:
    a. The distance from crest to crest
    b. The distance from crest to valley
    c. The minimum to maximum
    d. The number of seconds that pass per crest
    e. The number of valleys that pass per second

14. The wave equation is described as follows:
    a. The product of frequency and velocity is constant.
    b. Velocity is frequency divided by wavelength.
    c. Velocity is wavelength divided by frequency.
    d. Wavelength is the product of velocity and frequency.
    e. Wavelength is velocity divided by frequency.

15. The velocity of ultrasound in tissue is 1540 m/s. If a 1 MHz transducer is used, what will be the wavelength of the ultrasound?
    a. 15.4 µm
    b. 1.54 mm
    c. 1540 mm
    d. 15.4 cm
    e. 1540 m

16. A 1 tesla MRI device operates at a radiofrequency of 42 MHz. What is the wavelength of this radiation?
    a. 4.2 mm
    b. 7.1 mm
    c. 42 cm
    d. 7.1 m
    e. 42 m

If the figure below represents a wave traveling at 25 cm/s, compute the following:

17. How many cycles occur in 1 s (frequency)?
    a. 1
    b. 2
    c. 3
    d. 4
    e. 5

18. How much time is necessary for two cycles?
    a. 0.1 s
    b. 0.2 s
    c. 0.3 s
    d. 0.4 s
    e. 0.8 s

19. What is the wavelength?
    a. 5 cm
    b. 10 cm
    c. 15 cm
    d. 20 cm
    e. 25 cm

Worksheet 3-2
Electromagnetic Spectrum

The electromagnetic (EM) spectrum includes many types of EM radiation that extend over 35 orders of magnitude from low-energy radio waves to high-energy x-rays and y-rays. Each region of the EM spectrum can be identified by energy, wavelength, or frequency through the following equations:

$$E = hf = hc/l \text{ and } c = lf$$

Traditionally, x-rays are identified by their energy, visible light by its wavelength, and radio waves by their frequency.

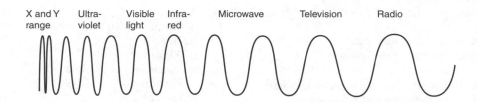

EXERCISES

1. A photon that has energy of approximately 1 eV is *most* likely:
   a. A gamma ray
   b. A radio emission
   c. An x-ray
   d. Therapeutic ultrasound
   e. Visible light

2. When the EM spectrum is considered, photons of a radio broadcast have relatively:
   a. High energy and long wavelengths
   b. High energy and short wavelengths
   c. High frequency and low energy
   d. Low energy and long wavelengths
   e. Low energy and short wavelengths

3. When white light is refracted through a prism, the following colors are emitted. Which has the longest wavelength?
   a. Blue
   b. Orange
   c. Red
   d. Ultraviolet
   e. Yellow

4. Invisible photons on the long-wavelength side of the visible-light spectrum can create a problem in the darkroom. Which of the following types of light are these photons likely to be?
   a. Green light
   b. Infrared light

   c. Laser light
   d. Maser light
   e. Ultraviolet light

5. The principal difference between x-rays and gamma rays is their:
   a. Energy
   b. Frequency
   c. Origin
   d. Velocity
   e. Wavelength

6. Radiation emitted from a standard radio broadcast antenna:
   a. Has a higher frequency than gamma rays
   b. Has a higher frequency than microwaves
   c. Has relatively high energy
   d. Is EM radiation
   e. Is sound

7. For any EM radiation:
   a. An increase in frequency results in an increase in energy.
   b. An increase in velocity results in an increase in energy.
   c. An increase in velocity results in an increase in frequency.
   d. An increase in wavelength results in an increase in energy.
   e. An increase in wavelength results in higher frequency.

29

8. EM radiation:
   a. Exists at zero velocity
   b. Exists only if its velocity is 3 × 108 m/s
   c. Has energy represented by amplitude
   d. Has mass that increases with increasing velocity
   e. Is usually shown as a square wave

9. If an x-ray imaging system is operated at 40 kVp, then:
   a. 20 keV x-rays are emitted
   b. All x-rays are emitted at 40 keV
   c. Non-ionizing x-rays are emitted
   d. X-rays up to 80 keV are emitted
   e. Zero-energy x-rays are emitted

10. A photon of red light:
    a. Comes from a nucleus
    b. Has a higher frequency than an x-ray
    c. Has a longer wavelength than a photon of green light
    d. Has more energy than blue light
    e. Has the same energy as microwaves

11. Which of the following characteristics is the same for both ultraviolet radiation and microwaves?
    a. Amplitude
    b. Energy
    c. Frequency
    d. Velocity
    e. Wavelength

12. Visible light cannot be:
    a. Absorbed
    b. Diffracted
    c. Reflected
    d. Refracted
    e. Weighed

13. X-rays can be:
    a. Attenuated
    b. Compacted
    c. Ionized
    d. Subdivided
    e. Weighed

14. The EM spectrum includes:
    a. Particulate radiation at the speed of light
    b. Radiation described by the following formula:
       Wavelength = Frequency × Velocity
    c. Radiation with physical properties determined by mass
    d. X-rays and radar with the speed of light in a vacuum
    e. X-rays, gamma rays, electrons, and neutrons that are used in medicine

15. Which of the following types of radiation would be classified as EM?
    a. 5 MHz therapeutic ultrasound
    b. 30 m radio broadcast
    c. 1000 Hz sound
    d. Beta radiation
    e. Heat convected from a radiator

16. Which of the following is an example of EM radiation?
    a. Alpha rays
    b. Diagnostic ultrasound
    c. Positrons
    d. Protons
    e. Ultraviolet light

17. Examples of EM radiation would *not* include:
    a. 1.5 T, 63 MHz MRI
    b. Cell phone signals
    c. Forced-air heat
    d. Light from an exit sign
    e. Phosphorescence from a watch dial

18. Which of the following is *not* an example of EM radiation?
    a. Gamma rays
    b. Grenz rays
    c. Laser radiation
    d. Star light
    e. Ultrasonic diathermy

Worksheet 3-3
Wave-Particle Duality

 E = hf (Quantum mechanics)

$$E = hf$$

where E = energy in joules and $h = 6.63 \times 10^{-34}$ J-s, f represents frequency, and h is the Planck constant. $E = mc^2$ (relativity).

$$E = mc^2$$

where E = energy in joules and $c = 3 \times 10^8$ m/s, the velocity of an x-ray.

To understand the true nature of photon radiation, both wave and particle concepts must be retained, because wavelike properties are exhibited in some experiments and particle-like properties are exhibited in others.

Photons interact with matter most easily when the matter is approximately the same size as the photon wavelength. X-rays behave as though they are particles. Visible light and radio-television emissions behave as waves.

EXERCISES

1. Which of the following is *not* a characteristic of the wave model of radiation?
   a. Collision
   b. Deflection
   c. Reflection
   d. Refraction
   e. Transmission

2. Which of the following *most* closely represents the term *attenuation?*
   a. Absorption of x-rays
   b. Deflection of x-rays
   c. Light absorbed in black glass
   d. Light reflected from a mirror
   e. Light transmitted through frosted glass

3. When a radiograph is viewed, one might properly state that:
   a. Bony structures are radiolucent.
   b. Fat is radiopaque.
   c. Fat is radioreflective.
   d. Lung tissue is radiolucent.
   e. Soft tissue is radiopaque.

4. The development of modern quantum mechanics is attributed to:
   a. Albert Nobel
   b. Ernest Rutherford
   c. Max Planck
   d. Niels Bohr
   e. William Coolidge

5. According to quantum mechanics, the energy of an x-ray is:
   a. Dependent on its origin
   b. Dependent on its velocity
   c. Directly proportional to its wavelength
   d. Inversely proportional to its wavelength
   e. Proportional to its amplitude

6. The expression that relates x-ray energy and wavelength through the Planck constant is:
   a. $E = hf$
   b. $E = hc$
   c. $E = hc/\lambda$
   d. $E = h/c\lambda$
   e. $E = \lambda c/h$

7. Which of the following statements about visible light is *true?*
   a. It can travel with any velocity up to 3×10^8 m/s.
   b. It is deflected by a magnetic field.
   c. It sometimes behaves like a wave.
   d. Its energy is directly proportional to its wavelength.
   e. The photoelectric effect demonstrates the wave model.

8. Visible light:
   a. Consists of short-wavelength red radiation and long-wavelength blue radiation
   b. Has a higher frequency than ultraviolet light
   c. Has a shorter wavelength than microwaves
   d. Has a wavelength range of 1 to 100 mm
   e. Interacts with matter in the same way that x-rays do

9. Which of the following terms is *not* associated with visible-light interaction?
   a. Absorption
   b. Reflection
   c. Refraction
   d. Transmission
   e. Vaporization

10. Which statement about visible light is *correct?*
    a. Black glass is lucent.
    b. If matter completely absorbs visible light, it is transparent.
    c. If matter attenuates visible light, it is opaque.
    d. If visible light is transmitted but attenuated, the matter is transparent.
    e. If visible light is transmitted unattenuated, the matter is lucent.

11. In radiographs of bony structures embedded in soft tissue, the bone is:
    a. Radiolucent
    b. Radiopaque
    c. Radiorefracted
    d. Translucent
    e. Transopaque

12. Which of the following statements about photon interaction is *true?*
    a. Air is transparent and radiopaque.
    b. Frosted glass is transparent.
    c. Lead is radiopaque.
    d. Soft tissue is radiopaque.
    e. Window glass is opaque.

13. Which type of electromagnetic radiation is *not* used for medical imaging?
    a. Gamma rays
    b. Microwaves
    c. Radiofrequency
    d. Visible light
    e. X-rays

14. When compared with visible light, x-rays have a greater:
    a. Charge
    b. Frequency
    c. Mass
    d. Velocity
    e. Wavelength

15. Which of the following types of electromagnetic radiation interact with matter such as a particle?
    a. Gamma rays
    b. Infrared radiation
    c. Microwaves
    d. Radiofrequencies

16. At what level should visible light interact *most* readily?
    a. Atomic
    b. Molecular
    c. Nucleon
    d. Organ
    e. Tissue

17. Compared with red light, green light has a greater:
    a. Charge
    b. Energy
    c. Mass
    d. Velocity
    e. Wavelength

18. The equivalent mass of an x-ray may be computed using:
    a. $m = hc/\lambda$
    b. $m = hc/f$
    c. $m = h\lambda/c^2$
    d. $m = hf/c^2$
    e. $m = hf\lambda/c^2$

19. A surface of which color reflects the *most* light?
    a. Black
    b. Blue
    c. Green
    d. Red
    e. White

Worksheet 3-3 **Wave-Particle Duality**

Worksheet 3-4
Inverse Square Law

 Radiation intensity decreases rapidly as the distance from the source increases. The intensity of radiation is inversely proportional to the square of the distance from the source to the object.

Inverse square law:

$$I_1/I_2 = d_2{}^2/d_1{}^2 = (d_2/d_1)^2$$

where I_1 is the intensity at distance d_1 from the source, and I_2 is the intensity at distance d_2 from the source.

EXERCISES

1. A source of ^{99m}Tc produces a radiation intensity of 1.5 μGy_a/hr (150 mR/hr) at 10 m. At what distance does the exposure rate equal 10 μGy_a/hr?
   a. 3.3 m
   b. 3.9 m
   c. 5.0 m
   d. 6.7 m
   e. 8.2 m

2. If the exposure rate 1 m from a source is 9 mR/hr (90 μGy_a/h), what is the exposure rate 3 m from the source?
   a. 90 μGy_a/hr
   b. 30 μGy_a/hr
   c. 10 μGy_a/hr
   d. 9 μGy_a/hr
   e. 1 μGy_a/hr

3. The inverse square law states that:
   a. Intensity and distance are proportional.
   b. Intensity is directly proportional to the square of the distance.
   c. Intensity is inversely proportional to the square of the distance.
   d. The square of the intensity is directly proportional to the distance.
   e. The square of the intensity is inversely proportional to the distance.

4. The inverse square law is a result of:
   a. Absorption
   b. Attenuation
   c. Divergence
   d. Scatter
   e. Transmission

5. The inverse square relationship applies to which of the following sources?
   a. Gamma ray
   b. Plane
   c. Point
   d. Ultrasound
   e. X-ray

6. Which of the following emissions is likely to obey the inverse square law?
   a. Heat from an iron skillet
   b. Infrared radiation from a patient
   c. Skylight
   d. Visible light from a 2 m fluorescent bulb
   e. X-rays from a mobile imaging system

7. To apply the inverse square law, one must know:
   a. Energy, distance, and intensity
   b. One distance and one intensity
   c. The frequency or the wavelength of radiation
   d. Two distances and one intensity
   e. Two intensities and two distances

8. If the distance from a point source is tripled, the intensity will be:
   a. Nine times
   b. One half
   c. One ninth
   d. One third
   e. Three times

9. If an instrument positioned 1 m from a point source is moved 50 cm closer to the source, the radiation intensity will:
   a. Decrease by a factor of 2
   b. Decrease by a factor of 4
   c. Increase by a factor of 2
   d. Increase by a factor of 4
   e. Remain constant

10. The distance from the earth to the sun is approximately 150 million km. If the earth were orbiting the sun at 50 million km, the solar intensity on the surface of the earth would be:
    a. 3 times more intense
    b. 9 times more intense
    c. 12 times more intense
    d. 27 times more intense
    e. The same

11. A linear source of radium is 15 mm long. Such a source of radiation obeys the inverse square law at approximately what minimum distance from the source?
    a. At contact
    b. 15 mm
    c. 25 mm
    d. 75 mm
    e. 105 mm

12. How far from a 1 m fluorescent bulb must one be before its light approximately obeys the inverse square law?
    a. 1 m
    b. 2 m
    c. 3 m
    d. 5 m
    e. 7 m

13. A ^{137}Cs source used for instrument calibration has an intensity of 1 mGy$_a$/hr (100 mR/hr) at 20 cm. What would the intensity be 40 cm from the source?
    a. 0.08 mGy$_a$/hr
    b. 0.12 mGy$_a$/hr
    c. 0.25 mGy$_a$/hr
    d. 0.5 mGy$_a$/hr
    e. 0.75 mGy$_a$/hr

14. The exposure rate from a ^{60}Co source used in radiation therapy is 1 Gy$_a$/min (100 R/min) at 80 cm. What would the exposure rate be 40 cm from the source?
    a. 0.25 Gy$_a$/min
    b. 0.50 Gy$_a$/min
    c. 1.0 Gy$_a$/min
    d. 2.0 Gy$_a$/min
    e. 4.0 Gy$_a$/min

15. A radiographic technique produces a patient dose of 2 mGy$_a$ (200 mrad) at a source-to-skin distance (SSD) of 80 cm. What would be the patient dose at an SSD of 160 cm if the technique remains the same?
    a. 0.5 mGy$_a$
    b. 0.8 mGy$_a$
    c. 1.0 mGy$_a$
    d. 2.0 mGy$_a$
    e. 4.0 mGy$_a$

16. A radiographic technique produces an exposure of 2 mGy$_a$ (200 mR) at a source-to-image receptor distance (SID) of 100 cm. What would the exposure be at an SID of 180 cm?
    a. 0.31 mGy$_a$
    b. 0.55 mGy$_a$
    c. 0.62 mGy$_a$
    d. 1.11 mGy$_a$
    e. 1.25 mGy$_a$

17. A radiograph produced at an SID of 100 cm results in an exposure of 1 mGy$_a$ (100 mR). What would be the exposure if the SID were reduced to 90 cm?
    a. 0.72 mGy$_a$
    b. 0.81 mGy$_a$
    c. 0.90 mGy$_a$
    d. 1.11 mGy$_a$
    e. 1.23 mGy$_a$

Worksheet 3-5
X-Ray Photons

X-rays also may be thought of as bundles of energy called **quanta** or **photons**. These x-ray photons travel at the speed of light, have direction, possess no mass or charge, and have electric and magnetic components that vary in a sinusoidal fashion. X-rays adhere to the following mathematical relationships:

$$c = \lambda \qquad E = mc^2$$
$$E = hf \qquad \lambda(nm) = \frac{1.24}{keV}$$
$$E = \frac{hc}{\lambda}$$

EXERCISES

1. Which of the following terms is associated with diagnostic imaging?
   a. Diffraction x-rays
   b. Grenz x-rays
   c. Megavoltage x-rays
   d. Superficial x-rays
   e. Supervoltage x-rays

2. Which of the following terms does *not* apply to an x-ray?
   a. Absorption
   b. Attenuation
   c. Diffraction
   d. Penetration
   e. Reflection

3. Given two x-rays, one of 50 keV and the other of 70 keV, the 70 keV x-ray:
   a. Is most likely radioactive
   b. Most likely came from a nucleus
   c. Has a higher velocity
   d. Has a longer wavelength
   e. Has a higher frequency

4. In the normal representation of an x-ray:
   a. Energy is amplitude.
   b. Mass is indicated by c.
   c. Velocity is the speed of light.
   d. Velocity varies from zero to the speed of light.
   e. Wavelength changes from short to long and back to short again.

5. The energy of an x-ray photon is directly proportional to its:
   a. Frequency
   b. Mass
   c. Velocity
   d. Velocity squared
   e. Wavelength

6. In a vacuum, x-rays travel with a velocity of:
   a. 186,000 km/hr
   b. 186,000 mph
   c. 3×10^{10} m/s
   d. 3×10^{10} cm/s
   e. 3.7×10^{10} cm/s

7. Which of the following is greater for a 30 keV x-ray than for a 60 keV x-ray?
   a. Charge
   b. Frequency
   c. Mass
   d. Velocity
   e. Wavelength

8. Which of the following electromagnetic radiations is in the diagnostic x-ray region?
   a. 78 eV
   b. 12,000 eV
   c. 65 keV
   d. 36 MeV
   e. 14 meV

9. The photon energy of an x-ray whose wavelength is 10 nm may be obtained *most* easily from which of the following?
   a. $E = mc^2$
   b. $E = hf$
   c. $E = hc/\lambda$
   d. $E = \lambda n$
   e. $E = \lambda/hc$

10. When x-rays are described, it can be said that:
    a. They are deflected by a very strong magnet.
    b. They can combine with other x-rays to form an atom.
    c. They can create molecules.
    d. They have a longer wavelength than radio waves.
    e. They travel in straight lines.

11. X-ray photons:
    a. Are part of the ultrasonic spectrum
    b. Are relatively long wavelength electromagnetic radiation
    c. Have a higher frequency than visible light
    d. Have a longer wavelength than radiofrequencies
    e. Have the same velocity as ultrasound

12. The energy of an x-ray:
    a. Can be computed from its mass
    b. Depends on its charge
    c. Increases with increasing wavelength
    d. Is a function of the Einstein constant
    e. Is inversely proportional to its wavelength

13. The model used to describe an x-ray photon:
    a. Consists of an S wave
    b. Has a radiofrequency field and a visual field
    c. Has an electrical field and an ultrasonic field
    d. Has an ultrasonic field and a magnetic field
    e. Is a sine wave

14. The Planck constant has units of:
    a. J
    b. J-eV
    c. J-kg
    d. J-s
    e. N-s

15. Which of the following characteristics is the same for both x-ray photons and light photons?
    a. Amplitude is the same.
    b. Energy is the same.
    c. Frequency is the same.
    d. Velocity is the same.
    e. Wavelength is the same.

16. X-rays:
    a. Have a mass of 1 amu and are neutral
    b. Have a negative charge and zero rest mass
    c. Have a positive charge and zero rest mass
    d. Have zero rest mass and a charge of plus two
    e. Have zero rest mass and are neutral

17. In the model of an x-ray:
    a. The amplitude of the sine wave is related to its energy.
    b. The frequency of the sine wave is related to its velocity.
    c. The wavelength of the sine wave is related to its velocity.
    d. Two sine waves are positioned perpendicular to each other.
    e. Two sine waves are superimposed.

18. Diagnostic x-rays are:
    a. High-energy electromagnetic radiation
    b. Long wavelength electromagnetic radiation
    c. Observed with varying velocity
    d. Photons with intermediate mass
    e. Photons with low frequency

19. An x-ray also can be correctly called a:
    a. Mass
    b. Photon
    c. Pronon
    d. Proton
    e. Quantity

Worksheet 3-6
Matter and Energy

 Matter (mass) is defined by its energy equivalence.

Einstein expressed the equivalence of mass and energy with the following equation:

$$E = mc^2$$

In the equation, if E is energy in joules, then c (the speed of light) must be 3×10^8 m/s, and m (the mass) must be measured in kilograms.

EXERCISES

1. Which of the following equations can be used to compute the mass equivalence of an x-ray photon?
   a. $m = Ec^2$
   b. $m = zv^2$
   c. $m = E/c^2$
   d. $m = \frac{1}{2} E^2$
   e. $m = Ev$

2. Which of the following equations can be used to compute the mass equivalence of an x-ray if its frequency is known?
   a. $m = E/c^2$
   b. $m = Ec^2$
   c. $m = hf/c^2$
   d. $m = h/\lambda f$
   e. $m = \frac{1}{2} c^2$

3. In the case of mass-energy conversions:
   a. Nuclear fission is an example.
   b. The inverse square law applies.
   c. The law of conservation of energy is violated.
   d. The law of conservation of matter is violated.
   e. The wave equation is an example.

4. In Einstein's relativistic equation, $E = mc^2$:
   a. c represents the velocity of ultrasound.
   b. If the mass is measured in kilograms and the velocity in meters per second, energy will be measured in joules.
   c. If the mass is measured in grams, the velocity must be measured in meters per second.
   d. If the velocity is 3×10^8 m/s, mass should be in grams.
   e. If the velocity is given as 186,000 miles/s, the energy will be in newtons.

5. When Einstein's relativistic equation is used to compute the energy equivalence of matter, it is usual to express such energy in:
   a. Calories
   b. Coulombs
   c. Ergs
   d. Joules
   e. Newtons

6. Energy can be:
   a. Created but not destroyed
   b. Destroyed but not created
   c. Expressed in newtons
   d. Measured in grays
   e. Transformed into matter

7. The energy equivalence of an electron at rest is 511 keV. It is also:
   a. 511 eV
   b. 511 MeV
   c. 0.51 eV
   d. 0.51 MeV
   e. 5.1 MeV

8. When various types of radiation are compared:
   a. The mass equivalence of a television broadcast is greater than that of red light.
   b. The mass equivalence of an FM broadcast is greater than that of ultraviolet light.
   c. The mass equivalence of blue light is greater than that of red light.
   d. The mass equivalence of microwaves is greater than that of x-rays.
   e. The mass equivalence of red light is greater than that of ultraviolet light.

9. If the entire mass of an electron ($m = 9.1 \times 10^{-31}$ kg) could be converted into an x-ray, its energy would be approximately:
   a. 4.15×10^{-15} eV-s
   b. 4.15×10^{-15} keV-s
   c. 511,000 eV
   d. 511 eV
   e. 5.1 MeV

10. 1 amu equals 1.66×10^{-27} kg. Its energy equivalence is:
    a. 1.5×10^{-10} J
    b. 1.5×10^{-7} J
    c. 1.5 kJ
    d. 1.5 mJ
    e. 1.5 nJ

11. What is the mass equivalence of a 35 keV x-ray?
    a. 6.3×10^{-31} kg
    b. 6.3×10^{-32} kg
    c. 6.3×10^{-33} kg
    d. 6.3×10^{-34} kg
    e. 6.3×10^{-35} kg

12. The SI unit for energy is the:
    a. Dyne
    b. Electron volt
    c. Erg
    d. Joule
    e. Newton

13. The energy of a 70 keV x-ray can be expressed as:
    a. 1.1×10^{-16} J
    b. 1.1×10^{-14} J
    c. 1.1×10^{-12} J
    d. 1.1×10^{-10} J
    e. 1.1×10^{-9} J

14. The equivalence of mass and energy is described by:
    a. The Bohr constant
    b. Einstein's theory
    c. Joule's laws
    d. Newton's laws
    e. Planck's theory

15. The energy of diagnostic x-rays is similar to that of which of the following radiations?
    a. Diffraction x-rays
    b. Grenz x-rays
    c. Megavoltage radiation
    d. Orthovoltage x-rays
    e. Superficial x-rays

16. In the equation E = hf, the *h:*
    a. Has units of energy
    b. Is a variable
    c. Stands for the Einstein constant
    d. Stands for the Bohr constant
    e. Relates photon energy to frequency

17. The Planck constant (h) has units of:
    a. eVs
    b. eVm/s
    c. JeV
    d. Jm
    e. Jm/s

18. Longer wavelength x-rays have:
    a. Higher energy
    b. Higher mass
    c. Higher velocity
    d. Lower energy
    e. Lower velocity

Worksheet 4-1
Electrostatics

 Matter has mass and energy equivalence. Matter may also have electric charge.

Electrostatics is the study of stationary electric charges:

- Electrified objects have excess charges.
- Objects can be electrified by contact, friction, or induction.
- Opposite charges attract; like charges repel.
- The magnitude of the attraction or repulsion is given by Coulomb's law:

$$F = k\,\frac{Q_a Q_b}{d^2}$$

where F is the force in newtons (attractive or repulsive), Q_a and Q_b are electrostatic charges in coulombs, d is separation distance in meters, and k is the proportionality constant ($k = 9.0 \times 10^9\,N - m^2/C^2$).

EXERCISES

1. What is the principal reservoir for excess electric charge?
   a. Clouds
   b. Lightning rod
   c. The atmosphere
   d. The earth
   e. Water pipes

2. Regarding the movement of an electric charge from one atom to another:
   a. Both positive and negative charges can move.
   b. It must occur in a large atom.
   c. Only positive charges move.
   d. Usually inner-shell electrons move.
   e. Usually outer-shell electrons move.

3. Electric energy can be converted into:
   a. Chemical energy by an x-ray imaging system
   b. Electromagnetic energy by a battery
   c. Mechanical energy by a battery
   d. Nuclear energy in a nuclear reactor
   e. Thermal energy by a lamp

4. Electrostatics:
   a. Concerns resting electric charges
   b. Concerns the mass energy conversion of electrons
   c. Governs the movement of electric charges in a conductor
   d. Is the conversion of kinetic energy
   e. Is the study of photon radiation

5. Coulomb's law states that electrostatic force is:
   a. Dependent on milliampere-seconds
   b. Directly proportional to the square of the distance between charges
   c. Directly proportional to the square of the product of charges
   d. Inversely proportional to the product of charges
   e. Inversely proportional to the square of the distance between charges

6. Which of the following is a method of electrification?
   a. Diffraction
   b. Excitation
   c. Induction
   d. Resonance
   e. Transmission

7. Static electricity:
   a. Can make one's hair stand on end
   b. Can produce x-rays
   c. Can result in magnetism
   d. Is the basis for transformer operation
   e. Is the study of electric currents

8. The unit of electrostatic charge is the:
   a. Ampere
   b. Coulomb
   c. Electron volt
   d. Newton
   e. Volt

9. The principal electrostatic law states that:
   a. A neutron will repel a neutron.
   b. A proton will repel a neutron.
   c. An electron will repel a neutron.
   d. An electron will repel a proton.
   e. An electron will repel an electron.

10. Objects become electrified because of:
    a. An excess of neutrons
    b. An excess of protons
    c. The transfer of electrons
    d. The transfer of neutrons
    e. The transfer of protons

39

11. The phenomenon of lightning occurs when:
    a. Adjacent clouds are electrically neutral.
    b. Adjacent clouds have negative electrification.
    c. Adjacent clouds have positive electrification.
    d. One cloud is positively electrified and an adjacent one is negatively electrified.
    e. Thunder is heard.

12. Which of the following would be included as one of the four basic electrostatic laws?
    a. Archimedes principle
    b. Conversion to magnetism
    c. Einstein's law
    d. Electric charge concentration
    e. Planck's law

13. An electrostatic force is created when a/an:
    a. Electrostatic charge exists
    b. Neutron approaches a neutron
    c. Neutron approaches an electron
    d. Proton approaches a neutron
    e. Proton approaches a proton

14. A radiographic tube is operated at 500 mA. How many electrons per second is this?
    a. 3.2×10^9
    b. 3.2×10^{18}
    c. 6.3×10^9
    d. 6.3×10^{17}
    e. 6.3×10^{18}

15. The unit of electrostatic force is the:
    a. Coulomb
    b. Electron volt
    c. Joule
    d. Newton
    e. Rad

16. Which of the following are *not* affected by electrostatically charged matter?
    a. Alpha particles
    b. Beta particles
    c. Electrons
    d. Protons
    e. X-rays

17. How many electrons are contained in 0.5 μC?
    a. 3.2×10^6
    b. 3.2×10^{12}
    c. 6.3×10^6
    d. 6.3×10^{12}
    e. 6.3×10^{18}

18. When a copper conductor becomes electrified (choose all that apply):
    a. A kink in the wire will have higher surface electrification.
    b. Excess electrons are uniformly distributed throughout the wire.
    c. It becomes heated.
    d. Negative charges concentrate on the surface, and positive charges are distributed throughout.
    e. The distribution of protons on its surface is uniform.

19. The unit of electric potential is the:
    a. Ampere
    b. Coulomb
    c. Newton
    d. Ohm
    e. Volt

20. Two positive 0.5 C charges are positioned 1.0 m apart. The force acting between them is:
    a. Attractive
    b. Exponential
    c. Neutral
    d. Repulsive
    e. Variable

40

Worksheet 4-2
Electrodynamics

 Electrodynamics is the study of electric charge in motion. A conductor is any material through which electrons flow easily. An insulator is any material that does not allow electron flow. A semiconductor is a material that under some conditions behaves as an insulator and under other conditions behaves as a conductor. A superconductor conducts electrons with no electrical resistance.

OHM'S LAW

Ohm's law: $V = IR$ where V is the electric potential in volts, I is the electric current in amperes, and R is the electric resistance in ohms (Ω).

Series Circuits

Total resistance: $R_T = R_1 + R_2 + R_3 \ldots$

Total current: $I_T = I_1 + I_2 + I_3 \ldots$

Total voltage: $V_T = V_1 + V_2 + V_3 \ldots$

Parallel Circuits

Total resistance: $\dfrac{1}{RT} = \dfrac{1}{R1} + \dfrac{1}{R2} + \dfrac{1}{R} + \ldots$

Total current: $I_T = I_1 + I_2 + I_3 + \ldots$

Total voltage: $V_T = V_1 = V_2 = V_3 \ldots$

EXERCISES

1. Which of the following is the best electric insulator?
   a. Aluminum
   b. Copper
   c. Nickel
   d. Water
   e. Wood

2. The ratio of the electric potential across a circuit element to the current flowing through that element is called:
   a. Current
   b. Energy
   c. Power
   d. Resistance
   e. Voltage

3. The electrical resistance of wire increases as the diameter of the:
   a. Insulator decreases
   b. Insulator increases
   c. Power supply increases
   d. Wire decreases
   e. Wire increases

4. When an electric current flows through a wire with resistance (R), energy is:
   a. Absorbed as heat
   b. Absorbed as light
   c. Generated as heat
   d. Generated as x-rays
   e. Transformed to mass

5. When electrons move in a copper wire:
   a. Resistance to the electron flow exists.
   b. Ionization occurs.
   c. The condition is called electromagnetic force.
   d. The condition is called electrostatics.
   e. They move down the middle of the wire.

6. The number of volts required to cause a current of 40 A in a circuit having a resistance of 5 Ω is:
   a. 5 V
   b. 8 V
   c. 40 V
   d. 45 V
   e. 200 V

7. The unit of electric potential is the:
   a. Ampere
   b. Coulomb
   c. Joule
   d. Ohm
   e. Volt

8. Ohm's law states that:
   a. Electric current is the product of voltage and resistance.
   b. Electric power is equal to current squared times voltage.
   c. Electric power is equal to voltage times current.
   d. The electric potential is equal to current squared times resistance.
   e. The electric potential is the product of current and resistance.

9. The flow of 1 C/s in a conductor is equal to:
   a. 1 Ω
   b. 1 A
   c. 1 eV
   d. 1 kVp
   e. 1 V

10. In a series circuit:
   a. Ohm's law fails.
   b. Only three circuit elements are allowed.
   c. The total current is the sum of the individual currents.
   d. The total resistance is the sum of the individual resistances.
   e. The voltage drop across each circuit element is the same.

11. In electrodynamics, which of the following is a *correct* expression?
   a. I = Qt
   b. R = I²V
   c. R = IV
   d. V = IR
   e. V = I/R

12. Which of the following is normally measured in volts?
   a. Electric potential
   b. Electromagnetic force
   c. Electromagnetic potential
   d. Electromagnetic radiation
   e. Electrostatic force

13. Milliampere-seconds (mAs) is a unit of:
   a. Electric current
   b. Electric potential
   c. Electromagnetic force
   d. Electromotive force
   e. Electrostatic charge

14. Electric insulators:
   a. Consist of materials such as silicon and germanium
   b. Convert electric energy to electromagnetic energy
   c. Convert electric energy to heat
   d. Inhibit movement of electric charge
   e. Permit movement of electric charge

15. 1 A is equal to:
   a. 1 Ω/s
   b. 1 C/s
   c. 1 eV/s
   d. 1 J/s
   e. 1 V/s

Worksheet 4-3
Alternating and Direct Currents

 ■ Direct current (DC), which is usually provided by a battery, flows in one direction.
■ Alternating current (AC) supplies power at 60 Hz.
■ Electric power is measured in watts (W).

$$P = VI$$

Power (W) = Voltage (V) × Current (I)

and

$$P = I^2R$$

Power (W) = (Current [I]² × Resistance [R])

and

$$E = Pt$$

Electric energy (J) = Power (W) × Time (s)

EXERCISES

Exercises 1 to 6 refer to the following figure:

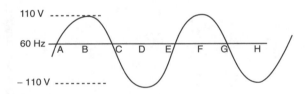

1. The length of time that elapses between A and E is:
   a. ½ s
   b. ⅟₃₀ s
   c. ⅟₆₀ s
   d. ⅟₁₂₀ s
   e. ⅟₂₄₀ s

2. One full cycle extends from:
   a. A to C
   b. B to F
   c. C to E
   d. D to E
   e. D to F

3. Considering the positive voltage pulse E to G, how many such pulses occur each second?
   a. 15
   b. 30
   c. 60
   d. 120
   e. 240

4. Given this waveform:
   a. The voltage at C is 60 Hz.
   b. The voltage at D is 60 Hz.
   c. The voltage at E is 110 V.
   d. The voltage at E is zero.
   e. The voltage at H is zero.

5. When one compares the figure segment from A to B with that from to B to C:
   a. Electron flow is fastest at B.
   b. Electrons are flowing faster from A to B than from B to C.
   c. Electrons are flowing in opposite directions at A and C.
   d. Electrons are speeding up from A to B and slowing down from B to C.
   e. The electric potential is higher at A than it is at C.

6. When one compares the segment from A to C with that from C to E:
   a. Electron flow is in opposite directions at B and D.
   b. Electrons are flowing more slowly between C and E.
   c. Electrons have more potential between A and C.
   d. Maximum electron velocity is at A, C, and E.
   e. The electromotive force is higher at B than it is at D.

7. The distinct difference between alternating current (AC) and direct current (DC) is that:
   a. DC can attain higher current.
   b. DC can attain higher voltage.
   c. DC electron flow is in one direction.
   d. DC electron flow varies in amplitude.
   e. DC has higher electrical resistance.

8. If a 60 W lightbulb is operated at 120 V, the current flowing through the bulb is approximately:
   a. 0.5 A
   b. 1 A
   c. 50 A
   d. 100 A
   e. 500 A

9. An x-ray imaging system has a 30 kW generator. If the maximum tube voltage is 150 kV, what is the available tube current?
   a. 200 mA
   b. 400 mA
   c. 600 mA
   d. 2 A
   e. 5 A

10. If a sine curve is used to represent 60 Hz AC, then:
    a. During the negative half-cycle, there is no electron flow.
    b. The amplitude of the curve is directly related to wavelength.
    c. The time from a positive peak to the next negative valley is 8 ms.
    d. The time from zero crossing to maximum amplitude is one cycle.
    e. The time from zero crossing to maximum amplitude is one-half cycle.

11. When electricity exists as 60 Hz AC:
    a. Electrons flow in one direction in alternating bursts.
    b. Electrons flow randomly in both directions.
    c. The number of electrons is proportional to the voltage.
    d. The velocity of electron flow is proportional to the current.
    e. The velocity of electron flow is proportional to the voltage.

12. In the United States, normal household electric power is:
    a. 50 V, 120 Hz, three phase
    b. 60 V, 120 Hz, single phase
    c. 120 V, 50 Hz, three phase
    d. 120 V, 60 Hz, single phase
    e. 120 V, 60 Hz, three phase

13. The unit of electric power is the:
    a. Hertz
    b. Joule
    c. Newton
    d. Volt
    e. Watt

14. Electricity is purchased on the basis of the kilowatt hours one consumes. The kilowatt hour also can be expressed in the unit:
    a. Amperes per second
    b. Joule
    c. Newton
    d. Volt
    e. Watts per ampere

15. Which of the following equations can be used to calculate electric power (P) consumption?
    a. $P = I^2V$
    b. $P = IR$
    c. $P = IV$
    d. $P = VR$
    e. $P = V/R$

16. A hair dryer is rated at 1000 W. Approximately what current will it produce on a normal 120 V, 60 Hz AC household supply?
    a. 8 A
    b. 10 A
    c. 80 A
    d. 110 A
    e. 800 A

Worksheet 4-4
Magnetism

- There are three states of magnetism: ferromagnetic, paramagnetic, and diamagnetic. Strongly magnetized material is ferromagnetic. Weakly magnetized material is paramagnetic. Nonmagnetic material is diamagnetic.
- The degree of magnetism increases as the number of unpaired electrons in an atom increases.
- Magnetic permeability is the property of a material to attract magnetic field lines.
- Magnetic susceptibility is the ease with which a material can be rendered magnetic.

EXERCISES

1. Which of the following is a physical property that we cannot sense?
   a. Acceleration
   b. Electric current
   c. Heat
   d. Magnetism
   e. Mass

2. An example of a magnetic domain is:
   a. A bar magnet
   b. A nucleus
   c. A permanent magnet
   d. An electromagnet
   e. The earth

3. If a bar magnet were suspended in space and another bar of nonmagnetic material were brought close to it, what would happen?
   a. Nothing
   b. The bar magnet would be attracted.
   c. The bar magnet would become demagnetized.
   d. The bar magnet would rotate.
   e. The imaginary magnetic field lines would be deviated.

4. If two bar magnets suspended in space were brought together, what would happen?
   a. Nothing
   b. One would rotate.
   c. The north pole of one would point to the north pole of the other.
   d. They would rotate and attract.
   e. They would rotate and repel.

5. A lodestone is an example of:
   a. A magnetic domain
   b. A natural magnet
   c. An electromagnet
   d. Demagnetized matter
   e. Paramagnetism

6. Which of the following would likely be classified as ferromagnetic material?
   a. Air
   b. Glass
   c. Iron
   d. Lead
   e. Water

7. If two magnets are bought together, north-to-north poles will _____, whereas north-to-south poles will _____.
   a. Attract; attract
   b. Attract; repel
   c. Not interact; interact
   d. Repel; attract
   e. Repel; repel

8. Most magnets:
   a. Are affected by another magnetic field
   b. Are diamagnetic
   c. Are naturally occurring if used in science and technology
   d. Have north, south, and neutral poles
   e. Have positive, negative, and neutral poles

9. Most magnetic materials are:
   a. Also radioactive
   b. Attracted to copper
   c. Bar shaped
   d. Shaped like a horseshoe
   e. Still magnetic when broken

10. A navigational compass:
    a. Has a north pole that is attracted to the equator
    b. Has a north pole that is attracted to the magnetic north pole of the earth
    c. Has both a north and a south pole
    d. Is usually made of glass
    e. Will not work at the equator

11. Which of the following is a classification of magnetism?
    a. Coulombic
    b. Diploic
    c. Electromagnetism
    d. Paramagnetism
    e. Polar magnetism

12. The earth's magnetic field is strongest:
    a. At the equator
    b. At the poles
    c. In deep space
    d. In near space
    e. In the atmosphere above the equator

13. The physical laws of magnetism:
    a. Include the conversion to electricity
    b. Include the conservation of magnetism
    c. Require that there be a south pole for every north pole
    d. Require that there be a south pole for every north pole but only for magnets of certain shapes
    e. Specify a force that increases with increasing distance from the magnet

14. Which of the following can create a magnetic field?
    a. A neutron at rest
    b. A quantum of visible light
    c. A spinning proton
    d. A stable atom
    e. An x-ray

15. The force between the poles of two bar magnets:
    a. Depends on the permeability of matter separating the magnets
    b. Is inversely proportional to the strength of each magnet
    c. Obeys a law similar in form to the Planck law
    d. Obeys the inverse square law
    e. Varies directly with the distance between them

16. When iron is fabricated into a magnet, magnetic domains:
    a. Align
    b. Cancel
    c. Disappear
    d. Induce
    e. Magnify

17. Magnetism has some properties similar to those of electrostatics, such as:
    a. Both can be converted to mass.
    b. Both can be sensed by touch.
    c. Both involve proton-type radiation.
    d. Both obey the inverse square law.
    e. Both refer to iron substances.

18. Magnetism:
    a. Can be converted to electricity
    b. Depends on monopolar atoms
    c. Is defined as a property that can attract glass, wood, or metal
    d. Is present in some naturally occurring ores
    e. Requires electricity

19. When a charged particle moves in a straight line, a magnetic field is:
    a. Created along the direction of particle motion
    b. Created and has the same sign as the particle
    c. Created perpendicular to the particle motion
    d. Erased
    e. Reversed

Worksheet 4-5
Electromagnetic Effect
Electromagnetic Induction

A current-carrying coil of wire creates a magnetic field. If an iron core is inserted, the magnetic field becomes many times more intense because the magnetic permeability of iron is greater than that of air. Such a device is called an **electromagnet**. Electromagnets are used in some x-ray imaging systems as switches.

EXERCISES

1. An electron moving in a conductor:
   a. Causes the conductor to behave as a bar magnet
   b. Causes the conductor to bend
   c. Produces a magnetic field in the conductor
   d. Produces a magnetic field perpendicular to the conductor
   e. Produces light in the conductor

2. The voltaic pile:
   a. Consists of a magnet and a conductor
   b. Consists of a pile of charges
   c. Consists of zinc and copper plates sandwiched together
   d. Is a modern dry-cell battery
   e. Was invented by Faraday

3. Electromotive force (EMF):
   a. Is an electrical mechanical force
   b. Is expressed in joules
   c. Is expressed in volts
   d. Stands for electromagnetic field
   e. Was discovered by Hans Oersted

4. The experimental link connecting electric and magnetic forces was discovered by:
   a. Edison
   b. Faraday
   c. Lenz
   d. Oersted
   e. Volta

5. The device designed to measure electron flow in a conductor is known as a/an:
   a. Ammeter
   b. Choke coil
   c. Electromagnet
   d. Solenoid
   e. Voltmeter

6. The fact that an electric current is induced if the conductor is in a changing magnetic field:
   a. Is known as Faraday's law
   b. Is known as Ohm's law
   c. Is the statement of the second law of electromagnetics
   d. Was discovered by Lenz
   e. Was discovered by Volta

7. The term *electromagnetic induction* refers to the production of:
   a. A magnetic field
   b. A static charge
   c. An electric current
   d. An electromagnet
   e. Electromagnetic radiation

8. A difference between self-induction and mutual induction is that:
   a. Mutual induction is the basis for an electric motor and self-induction is the basis for a transformer.
   b. Mutual induction requires two coils and self-induction requires only one.
   c. Only self-induction can create EMF.
   d. Self-induction requires two coils and mutual induction requires only one.
   e. There is no difference.

9. The magnetic field produced by an electromagnet has:
   a. Alternating poles
   b. Neither a north nor a south pole
   c. Only a north pole
   d. Only a south pole
   e. Properties similar to a bar magnet

10. One law of electromagnetics states that:
    a. An electric current is induced in a circuit if some part of that circuit is in a magnetic field.
    b. Electrostatics can be converted to magnetism.
    c. The induced current flows in the opposite direction of the inducing action.
    d. The right-hand rule is used to determine the direction of the induced current.
    e. There are two basic types of induction: primary and secondary.

11. The magnetic field produced:
    a. By a solenoid is more intense than that produced by an electromagnet
    b. By AC is stronger than that produced by DC.
    c. By an AC source is constant
    d. In a transformer is based on mutual induction
    e. In an electromagnet is most intense in the plane perpendicular to its axis

12. An electromagnet:
    a. Cannot be turned off
    b. Has an air core
    c. Is a coil of wire wound around an iron core
    d. Produces a magnetic field with or without an electric current
    e. Produces a monopolar magnetic field

13. Given a closed loop of wire with no electron flow, an electric current can be induced if:
    a. A changing magnetic field is present.
    b. A constant magnetic field is present.
    c. No magnetic field is present.
    d. The loop is cycled open/close.
    e. The loop is opened.

14. When an AC source is connected to a coil of wire:
    a. A constant magnetic field is generated.
    b. A front EMF is produced.
    c. An opposite EMF is induced.
    d. Electromagnetic radiation is produced.
    e. Mutual induction occurs.

15. When an electric current is induced by mutual induction, such current flows:
    a. According to Faraday's law
    b. According to Lenz's law
    c. According to Oersted's law
    d. In the primary coil
    e. In the secondary coil

16. Which of the following scientists is associated with the early development of electromagnetism?
    a. Edison
    b. Faraday
    c. Marconi
    d. Planck
    e. Roentgen

17. A modern dry-cell battery is a source of:
    a. Coulomb per joule
    b. Joule per coulomb
    c. Newton per coulomb
    d. Ohm per volt
    e. Volt per ohm

18. When the right-hand rule is applied to a straight wire, the thumb indicates the direction of the:
    a. Circuit resistance
    b. Electric current
    c. Electric field
    d. Electric potential
    e. Magnetic field

Worksheet 4-6
Electric Generators and Motors

 A coil of wire is called a solenoid. When the coil of wire is wrapped around an iron core, the generated magnetic field is intensified. Such a device is an electromagnet.

Electric generators and motors are electromechanical devices. The former converts mechanical energy to electric energy; the latter converts electric energy to mechanical energy.

Electric motors operate by passing an electric current through a loop of wire while in the presence of a magnetic field. The interaction between the electric current and the fixed magnetic field causes the loop to rotate, thereby producing mechanical energy. The induction motor, which is a type of electric motor, is used in all rotating anode x-ray tubes.

EXERCISES

1. Which of the following is *most* related to electromechanical devices?
   a. Edison's law of electromechanics
   b. Faraday's experiment
   c. Lenz's first law of electromagnetics
   d. Oersted's experiment on mutual induction
   e. The voltaic pile

2. In an electric generator:
   a. A coil of wire is rotated in a magnetic field.
   b. A transformer is charged.
   c. Alternating current (AC) is changed to direct current (DC).
   d. Chemical energy is converted to electrical energy.
   e. Electrical energy is converted to mechanical energy.

3. The electric generator is *most* closely associated with experiments conducted by:
   a. Edison
   b. Faraday
   c. Lenz
   d. Oersted
   e. Volta

4. Which of the following statements about generators and motors is *always true?*
   a. They are electromagnets.
   b. They both require commutators.
   c. They convert energy from one form into another.
   d. They have both primary and secondary windings.
   e. They require direct electric contact between primary and secondary coils.

5. In an electric motor:
   a. A coil of wire is mechanically rotated.
   b. A commutator ring is not necessary.
   c. AC is changed to DC.
   d. A transformer is discharged.
   e. Electric current is supplied to a coil of wire.

6. Which of the following would be classified as electromechanical devices?
   a. Generators and motors
   b. Generators and rectifiers
   c. Motors and rectifiers
   d. Transformers and electromagnets
   e. Transformers and rectifiers

7. The main difference between an AC and a DC electric generator is:
   a. The type of commutator ring
   b. A magnet
   c. A source of electromotive force
   d. A transformer
   e. A voltmeter

8. The electric current produced by an AC generator has:
   a. Alternating positive and negative intensity
   b. Constant negative intensity
   c. Constant positive intensity
   d. Pulsating negative intensity
   e. Pulsating positive intensity

9. An induction motor is used in an x-ray imaging system to:
   a. Control current
   b. Measure mAs
   c. Provide rectification
   d. Rotate the anode
   e. Vary voltage

10. In an induction motor, the only part to be rotated is the:
    a. Cathode
    b. Electromagnet
    c. Rotor
    d. Stator
    e. Wire loop

49

11. A fluoroscope is operated at 95 kVp, 2 mA. What is its power consumption?
    a. 47.5 W
    b. 190 W
    c. 47.5 kW
    d. 97 kW
    e. 190 kW

12. What power is required for a radiographic exposure at 76 kVp, 500 mA?
    a. 19 W
    b. 38 W
    c. 576 W
    d. 19 kW
    e. 38 kW

13. A 110 V heater requires 15 A. What is the power consumption?
    a. 15 W
    b. 110 W
    c. 125 W
    d. 1650 W
    e. 1800 W

14. How much current will a 60 W lightbulb draw from a 120 V receptacle?
    a. 60 mA
    b. 500 mA
    c. 1 A
    d. 15 A
    e. 120 A

15. Electric current waveforms are graphs of:
    a. Electric current versus resistance
    b. Electric current versus time
    c. Electric current versus voltage
    d. Electric voltage versus current
    e. Electric voltage versus resistance

16. Theoretically, conduction electrons come to rest momentarily:
    a. At the peak of the waveform
    b. At the valley of the waveform
    c. At zero crossing
    d. Just before either a peak or a valley
    e. They never come to rest

17. Electric ranges, air conditioners, and furnaces require 220 V, 60 Hz AC. Therefore, compared with most household appliances, they require which of the following?
    a. A higher electric potential
    b. A higher operating frequency
    c. A lower electric potential
    d. Greater conductivity
    e. Greater semiconductivity

18. Which of the following has an associated magnetic field?
    a. Helium atom
    b. Hydrogen atom
    c. Hydrogen nucleus
    d. Neutron
    e. Stationary electron

19. When iron is brought near a permanent magnet, the lines of the magnetic field are:
    a. Attracted to the iron
    b. Attracted to the magnet
    c. Repelled by the iron
    d. Repelled by the magnet
    e. Unaffected

Worksheet 4-7
The Transformer

A transformer consists of two electromagnets with a common iron core. A voltage impressed on the primary coil will generate a voltage in the secondary coil, provided that the power is AC. The transformer law is as follows:

$$\frac{V_s}{V_p} = \frac{N_s}{N_p}$$

where the subscript s refers to the secondary coil, the subscript p refers to the primary coil, N is the number of turns of the coil, and V is the voltage. The ratio Ns/Np is known as the **turns ratio**.

In an x-ray imaging system, there are usually three transformers: the variable-voltage autotransformer, the high-voltage step-up transformer, and the step-down filament transformer.

EXERCISES

1. The transformer changes:
   a. Electric current to voltage
   b. Electric energy to electromagnetic energy
   c. Electric energy to mechanical energy
   d. Mechanical energy to electric energy
   e. The amplitude of the voltage

2. A transformer operates:
   a. On AC but not on DC
   b. On both DC and AC
   c. On DC but not on AC
   d. Only above its critical current
   e. Only on a constant voltage

3. If a transformer produces a large secondary current from a small primary current:
   a. Power will be increased.
   b. The turns ratio will be greater than 1.
   c. The turns ratio will be less than 1.
   d. The voltage will be larger on the secondary side than on the primary side.
   e. There will be more windings on the secondary side than on the primary side.

4. The symbol for a transformer is:

5. The principal application of a transformer in an x-ray imaging system is to:
   a. Change AC to DC
   b. Change DC to AC
   c. Change frequency
   d. Change voltage
   e. Produce x-rays

6. The output current in a step-up transformer is:
   a. Higher than the input current
   b. Independent of the input current
   c. Independent of the turns ratio
   d. Lower than the input current
   e. The same as the input current

7. A transformer with a turns ratio of 1000:1 is:
   a. A step-down transformer
   b. A step-up transformer
   c. An autotransformer
   d. Used to increase current
   e. Used to reduce voltage

8. When a step-up transformer is in use:
   a. The primary winding has more turns than the secondary winding.
   b. The secondary current is greater than the primary current.
   c. The secondary voltage is greater than the primary voltage.
   d. X-ray tube current is selected.
   e. The turns ratio is equal to 1.

9. When a transformer is designed, the change in current is:
   a. Dependent on the supply voltage
   b. Directly proportional to the voltage change
   c. In the same direction as the voltage change
   d. Inversely proportional to the turns ratio
   e. Proportional to the turns ratio

10. Which of the following is a transformer design used in x-ray imaging systems?
   a. Capacitor type
   b. Filament type
   c. Rectifier type
   d. Rotating type
   e. Shell type

11. An autotransformer:
    a. Contains a single coil that serves as both primary and secondary coils
    b. Controls x-ray tube current
    c. Is a shell type of transformer
    d. Is an electromechanical device
    e. Is used to control frequency

12. Which of the following statements about transformers is *correct*?
    a. If there were equal numbers of primary and secondary coil turns, the turns ratio would be zero.
    b. In the shell-type transformer, the primary and secondary coils are wound on different cores.
    c. Laminated transformer cores are more efficient than unlaminated ones.
    d. The autotransformer controls current.
    e. The high-voltage transformer in an x-ray imaging system is the autotransformer.

13. A transformer "transforms" or changes electric:
    a. Frequency
    b. Impedance
    c. Power
    d. Resistance
    e. Voltage

14. Transformers have iron cores to intensify the:
    a. Electric current
    b. Electric potential
    c. Electric power
    d. Electric voltage
    e. Magnetic field

15. Primary to secondary coupling in a transformer is enhanced by:
    a. 60 Hz
    b. AC
    c. An iron core
    d. DC
    e. EMF

16. If DC is applied to the primary coil of a step-up transformer, what is the result in the secondary coil?
    a. AC
    b. Increased current
    c. Increased magnetic field
    d. Increased voltage
    e. Nothing

17. The *turns ratio* is defined as:
    a. Number of secondary windings ÷ primary windings
    b. Primary iron core ÷ secondary iron core
    c. Primary voltage ÷ secondary voltage
    d. Primary windings ÷ number of secondary windings
    e. Secondary current ÷ primary current

18. Which of the following accurately represents the transformer law?
    a. $Is/I_p = N_p/N_s$
    b. $Is/Ip = Ns/Np$
    c. $Is/Ip = Vs/Vp$
    d. $Ip/Is = Vp/Vs$
    e. $Ip/Is = Np/Ns$

19. What is the transformer that looks like a square donut called?
    a. Auto
    b. Closed-core
    c. High-frequency
    d. Induction
    e. Shell-type

Worksheet 5-1
Operating Console
Control of Kilovolt Peak (kVp)

- Peak kilovoltage (kVp) is controlled by a series of electric taps on the autotransformer.
- The autotransformer has only one winding.
- The autotransformer can function in the step-up or the step-down mode.
- The transformer law can be used to calculate the secondary voltage:

$$\frac{V_s}{V_p} = \frac{N_s}{N_p}$$

where V_p refers to primary voltage, V_s is secondary voltage, N_p refers to the number of windings enclosed by primary taps, and N_s is the number of windings enclosed by secondary taps.

EXERCISES

1. Power to the primary side of the high-voltage transformer comes from the:
   a. Filament transformer
   b. Line-voltage compensator
   c. Primary side of the autotransformer
   d. Rectifier
   e. Secondary side of the autotransformer

2. The output voltage from the autotransformer is:
   a. Always less than the input voltage
   b. Always more than the input voltage
   c. Fed directly to the rectifiers
   d. Inversely proportional to the turns ratio
   e. Proportional to the turns ratio

3. The autotransformer converts:
   a. Chemical energy to electric energy
   b. Electric energy to chemical energy
   c. Electric energy to electric energy
   d. Magnetic energy to electric energy
   e. Mechanical energy to electric energy

4. The autotransformer operates on the principle of:
   a. Coulomb's law
   b. Edison's law
   c. Faraday's law
   d. Newton's law
   e. Oersted's law

5. The principal purpose of the high-voltage transformer is to do which of the following?
   a. Adjust voltage
   b. Increase voltage
   c. Rectify voltage
   d. Reduce voltage
   e. Stabilize voltage

6. The voltage supplied to an x-ray imaging system is 220 V. The voltage used by the x-ray tube is produced by which of the following?
   a. Autotransformer
   b. Exposure timer
   c. Filament transformer
   d. High-voltage transformer
   e. Rheostat

7. 220 V is supplied to 800 primary turns of an autotransformer. What will be the output voltage across 200 secondary turns?
   a. 27.5 V
   b. 55 V
   c. 880 V
   d. 1760 V
   e. 3520 V

8. The autotransformer has only one:
   a. Coil
   b. Meter
   c. Rectifier
   d. Switch
   e. Turns ratio

9. The principal purpose of the autotransformer is to:
   a. Adjust voltage
   b. Increase voltage
   c. Rectify voltage
   d. Reduce voltage
   e. Stabilize voltage

10. Which of the following is directly connected to the autotransformer?
    a. Filament
    b. kVp meter
    c. mA meter
    d. Rectifier
    e. X-ray tube

53

11. Taps on the windings of an autotransformer may be used to select which of the following?
    a. Exposure time
    b. Focal spot
    c. Line compensation
    d. mA
    e. Rectification

12. 440 V is supplied to 1000 primary turns of an autotransformer. If the desired output voltage is 100 V, how many secondary turns must be tapped?
    a. 100
    b. 227
    c. 454
    d. 4400
    e. 10,000

13. The autotransformer can be used to do which of the following?
    a. Control exposure time
    b. Convert AC to DC
    c. Convert DC to AC
    d. Increase kVp
    e. Increase mA

14. If V stands for voltage and T for the number of turns enclosed between the taps of an autotransformer, then the autotransformer law is which of the following?
    a. $V_p/V_s = T_p/T_s$
    b. $V_pT_p = T_sV_s$
    c. $V_pV_s = T_pT_s$
    d. $V_s/V_p = T_p/T_s$
    e. $V_s = V_p$

15. In the design of an autotransformer:
    a. A single coil serves as both the primary and the secondary coils.
    b. The exposure timer is on the primary side.
    c. The major kVp adjustment and the line-voltage compensator are on the secondary side.
    d. The major kVp adjustment is on the primary side and the minor kVp adjustment is on the secondary side.
    e. There are separate primary and secondary coils.

16. Selection of kVp:
    a. Involves two series of autotransformers
    b. Requires rectified voltage
    c. Requires that constant voltage be supplied to the autotransformer
    d. Uses meters and switches that are at high kVp
    e. Uses the step-up transformer

17. Line compensation:
    a. Adjusts the line frequency to 60 Hz
    b. Compensates for rectification
    c. Is necessary for proper exposure timing
    d. Is necessary to convert AC to DC
    e. Is required to stabilize voltage

18. Which of the following is used to determine the voltage before exposure?
    a. A filament transformer
    b. A postreading voltmeter
    c. A voltmeter
    d. A step-up transformer
    e. An autotransformer

Worksheet 5-2
Operating Console
Control of Milliamperage (mA)

The x-ray tube current is controlled by an electric filament circuit that is separate from that of the high-voltage circuit. The circuit elements of importance for supplying and controlling the tube mA are the autotransformer, the precision resistors, the filament transformer, and the filament.

The mA meter, although physically located on the operating console, is electrically connected to the secondary side of the high-voltage transformer through a center tap to electrical ground. This allows for direct measurement of the tube current without the possibility of electric shock.

Thermionic emission is the release of electrons from a heated filament. A correction circuit is incorporated to control the **space charge effect**.

EXERCISES

1. One coulomb per second (C/s) is equivalent to 1 A, and 1 C is equal to 6.3×10^{18} electrons. Therefore, operation at 100 mA would result in a current of:
   a. 6.3×10^{16} electrons
   b. 6.3×10^{16} electrons/s
   c. 6.3×10^{17} electrons
   d. 6.3×10^{17} electrons/s
   e. 6.3×10^{18} electrons

2. The filament transformer:
   a. Has four windings
   b. Increases current
   c. Increases voltage
   d. Is an autotransformer
   e. Must have precision resistors

3. The filament transformer is usually:
   a. A part of the autotransformer
   b. Located with the high-voltage generator
   c. An autotransformer
   d. Located in the operating console
   e. A step-down transformer

4. A posterior-anterior (PA) chest requires a technique of 125 kVp at 4 mAs. The total number of electrons used to make the exposure is:
   a. 2.5×10^{15}
   b. 2.5×10^{16}
   c. 2.5×10^{17}
   d. 6.3×10^{16}
   e. 6.3×10^{17}

5. The filament circuit:
   a. Begins at the filament and ends at the filament transformer
   b. Begins at the autotransformer and ends at the filament
   c. Controls kVp
   d. Is located entirely in the operating console
   e. Is located in all three of the major components of an x-ray imaging system: the console, the high-voltage generator, and the x-ray tube

6. A filament transformer has a turn ratio of 1:20. What current must be supplied to the primary windings if 5 A is required by the filament?
   a. 125 mA
   b. 200 mA
   c. 250 mA
   d. 50 A
   e. 100 A

7. The filament transformer in the previous question is supplied with 150 V to the primary side. What is the secondary voltage?
   a. 750 mV
   b. 3000 mV
   c. 1.5 V
   d. 7.5 V
   e. 30 V

8. The unit mAs:
   a. Could be expressed in coulombs
   b. Could be expressed in coulombs/second
   c. Is a unit of electric current
   d. Is a unit of electromotive force (EMF)
   e. Is electron/s

9. An exposure technique of 100 mA at 100 ms compared with 50 mA at 50 ms results in:
   a. Eight times the total number of electrons
   b. Fewer projectile electrons
   c. Four times the total number of electrons
   d. Three times the total number of electrons
   e. Twice the total number of electrons

10. The control of focal spot size depends on:
    a. The filament that is energized
    b. The mA station selected
    c. The secondary taps of the autotransformer
    d. The target angle selected
    e. The turns ratio of the filament transformer

11. The meter that monitors x-ray tube current is:
    a. Connected to the autotransformer
    b. Connected to the secondary side of the step-down transformer
    c. Grounded to the primary center tap of the step-up transformer
    d. Physically located on the control console
    e. The same as the filament current monitor

12. X-ray tube current is usually measured in which of the following?
    a. Amperes (A)
    b. Ampere-seconds (As)
    c. Microamperes (μA)
    d. Milliamperes (mA)
    e. Milliampere-seconds (mAs)

13. A filament current of 5 A is necessary for thermionic emission. What electron flow is this?
    a. 3.2×10^{15} electrons/s
    b. 3.2×10^{16} electrons/s
    c. 3.2×10^{17} electrons/s
    d. 3.2×10^{18} electrons/s
    e. 3.2×10^{19} electrons/s

14. The filament transformer is designed:
    a. As a step-up transformer
    b. To operate on DC power
    c. With a turns ratio less than 1
    d. With a turns ratio greater than 1
    e. With an mA meter grounded to the center tap

15. Which of the following would be *correct* to use for expressing x-ray tube current?
    a. Coulombs
    b. Coulombs/second
    c. Electron volts
    d. Kilovolt peak
    e. Kilovolts/second

16. The design of fixed mA stations requires the use of which of the following?
    a. A center-tapped meter
    b. DC power
    c. Major and minor taps
    d. Precision resistors
    e. Primary and secondary windings

17. Operation at 100 mA for 1 s results in which of the following?
    a. 6.3×10^{16} electrons
    b. 6.3×10^{17} electrons/s
    c. 6.3×10^{17} electrons
    d. 6.3×10^{18} electrons/s
    e. 6.3×10^{18} electrons

18. A filament transformer has 800 primary windings and is supplied with 200 mA. If the secondary coil has 100 windings, what will be the secondary current?
    a. 25 mA
    b. 100 mA
    c. 400 mA
    d. 1600 mA
    e. 3200 mA

Worksheet 5-3
Operating Console
Exposure Timers

 Exposure timers are precision devices that start and stop x-ray production. There are four basic types of exposure timers:

1. **Mechanical timers:** These operate by spring action, similarly to a hand-wound alarm clock. These timers are not very accurate, and they are not used on modern equipment.
2. **Synchronous timers:** These timers use a synchronous motor that operates at 60 rps. Their shortest possible exposure time is $\frac{1}{60}$ s.
3. **Electronic timers:** This type of timer operates on an electronic resistive-capacitive circuit based on the time required to charge a capacitor. These timers are accurate, allow exposures as short as 1 millisecond (ms), and can be used for serial radiography.
4. **mAs timers:** These timers are electronic timers that monitor the product of mA and time, and terminate the exposure when the proper mAs is reached.

Automatic exposure control (AEC) incorporates a radiation-measuring device that terminates the x-ray exposure when enough x-radiation has reached the image receptor.

EXERCISES

1. A radiographic technique calls for a 50 ms exposure, but the exposure control has only fractional notation. Which of the following should be selected?
   a. $\frac{1}{60}$ s
   b. $\frac{1}{40}$ s
   c. $\frac{1}{20}$ s
   d. $\frac{1}{10}$ s
   e. $\frac{1}{4}$ s

2. A radiographic technique calls for a 400 mA, $\frac{1}{20}$ s exposure. What is the mAs?
   a. 5 mAs
   b. 10 mAs
   c. 20 mAs
   d. 40 mAs
   e. 80 mAs

3. If an x-ray imaging system is operated at 600 mA, 50 ms, the total mAs will be which of the following?
   a. 6 mAs
   b. 30 mAs
   c. 60 mAs
   d. 300 mAs
   e. 600 mAs

4. A radiographic technique of 100 mA at $\frac{1}{4}$ s has been used. If one changes to the 500 mA station, the appropriate exposure time for the same mAs is which of the following?
   a. $\frac{1}{4}$ s
   b. $\frac{3}{20}$ s
   c. $\frac{1}{20}$ s
   d. $\frac{1}{5}$ s
   e. $\frac{1}{10}$ s

5. Operation at 300 mA for $\frac{1}{20}$ s is equivalent to operation at 900 mA for:
   a. 8 ms
   b. 17 ms
   c. 60 ms
   d. 200 ms
   e. 500 ms

6. The control of exposure time is always:
   a. Automatically set
   b. Determined by kVp
   c. On the primary side of the autotransformer
   d. On the primary side of the high-voltage transformer
   e. On the secondary side of the filament circuit

7. The exposure timer on a three-phase radiographic imaging system will:
   a. Be automatic
   b. Be electronic
   c. Be synchronous
   d. Limit exposure to $\frac{1}{60}$ s or longer
   e. Limit exposure to 8 ms and no shorter

8. An automatic exposure control (AEC) device:
   a. Can use a photomultiplier tube on the entrance side of the patient
   b. Can use an ionization chamber between the patient and the image receptor
   c. Cannot control exposures shorter than $\frac{1}{120}$ s
   d. Does not require a manual timer
   e. Works only with three-phase and high-frequency power

9. With an automatic exposure control (AEC) device:
   a. Exposures less than 100 ms are not possible.
   b. It is not necessary to depress the exposure control.
   c. The exposure starts and stops automatically.
   d. Technique selection is not necessary.
   e. A backup timer is required.

10. The shortest exposure possible with single-phase equipment is $\frac{1}{120}$ s. How many milliseconds is that?
    a. 8 ms
    b. 17 ms
    c. 35 ms
    d. 50 ms
    e. 120 ms

11. Mammography sometimes requires exposures as long as 1.5 s. This is equivalent to which of the following?
    a. 15 ms
    b. 100 ms
    c. 150 ms
    d. 1000 ms
    e. 1500 ms

12. The shortest exposure possible with three-phase equipment is 1 ms. What fraction of a second is that?
    a. $\frac{1}{50}$
    b. $\frac{1}{100}$
    c. $\frac{1}{120}$
    d. $\frac{1}{500}$
    e. $\frac{1}{1000}$

13. There are 30 video frames each second for a fluoroscopic CRT dynamic image. What is the length for each frame?
    a. 1 ms
    b. 10 ms
    c. 16 ms
    d. 33 ms
    e. 60 ms

14. The human eye cannot visualize faster than approximately five views each second. What is the integration time of the human eye?
    a. 1 ms
    b. 10 ms
    c. 20 ms
    d. 100 ms
    e. 200 ms

15. A radiographic technique calls for 86 kVp/200 mAs using the 800 mA station. What is the exposure time?
    a. 10 ms
    b. 25 ms
    c. 100 ms
    d. 250 ms
    e. 500 ms

16. mA is a unit of electric current, and mAs is a unit of:
    a. Electric charge
    b. Electric potential
    c. Reciprocal kVp
    d. X-ray beam quality
    e. X-ray beam quantity

Worksheet 5-4
High-Voltage Generator
High-Voltage Generation

 The high-voltage section of the x-ray imaging system contains the following:

- The **high-voltage transformer** ($N_s/N_p > 1$), which converts low voltage from the autotransformer to the required kVp.
- The **filament transformer** ($N_s/N_p > 1$), which reduces the voltage from the autotransformer to about 10 V for heating the filament. At the same time, the filament current is regulated to the range of 4 to 10 A.
- A **rectifier circuit** that converts the alternating voltage into a direct voltage before use by the x-ray tube.

The accompanying figure shows the change in voltage waveform at each stage of generation.

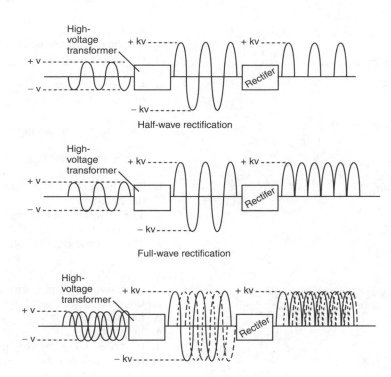

Half-wave rectification

Full-wave rectification

Three-phase rectification

Voltage Waveform	Pulses per Second	Percentage Ripple
Half-wave	60	100
Full-wave	120	100
Three-phase, six-pulse	360	13
Three-phase, 12-pulse	720	4
High frequency	Up to 1000	1

EXERCISES

1. Which of the following is contained in a typical high-voltage generator?
   a. Diode rectifiers
   b. Autotransformer
   c. Exposure switch
   d. kVp meter
   e. mA meter

2. A change in the voltage waveform from the primary side to the secondary side of the high-voltage transformer produces a change in:
   a. Amplitude
   b. Frequency
   c. Phase
   d. Velocity
   e. Wavelength

3. In half-wave rectification, each inverse half cycle in the primary circuit corresponds to how many voltage pulses across the x-ray tube?
   a. None
   b. One
   c. Two
   d. Four
   e. Twelve

4. Which of the following is higher for a single-phase high-voltage generator than for a three-phase high-voltage generator?
   a. kVp
   b. Purchase price
   c. Rotor speed
   d. Voltage ripple
   e. X-ray quality

5. Which of the following is a disadvantage of three-phase power compared with single-phase power?
   a. Higher capital cost
   b. Higher electrical operating costs
   c. Limited kVp
   d. Longer minimum exposure time
   e. Softer radiation

6. The disadvantage of a self-rectified circuit is:
   a. Its complexity
   b. Its cost
   c. Its limitation of use to dental imaging systems
   d. Its limited exposure time
   e. Its requirement of DC power

7. An exposure of $\frac{1}{10}$ s:
   a. At 50 mA is 50 mAs
   b. At 100 mA is 1000 mAs
   c. Is 120 ms
   d. Produces six pulses in full-wave rectification
   e. Produces twice as much radiation if full-wave rectified than if half-wave–rectified

8. Full-wave rectification:
   a. Has less ripple compared with half-wave rectification
   b. Is one example of self-rectification
   c. Produces higher kVp than half-wave rectification
   d. Requires at least four rectifiers
   e. Requires at least twelve rectifiers

9. A rectifier:
   a. Can be a semiconductor
   b. Converts DC to AC
   c. Increases current
   d. Increases voltage
   e. Increases x-ray intensity

10. Concerning the transformers used in the x-ray circuit:
    a. The filament transformer is also an autotransformer.
    b. The filament transformer usually is located in the console.
    c. The high-voltage transformer is a step-up device.
    d. They convert AC to DC.
    e. They operate only on DC.

11. Which of the following is an advantage of three-phase power over single-phase power?
    a. Improved spatial resolution
    b. Increased kVp
    c. Increased mAs
    d. Increased x-ray intensity per mAs
    e. Lower capital cost

12. Oil is used in the high-voltage section of an x-ray imaging system for which of the following functions?
    a. Electrical insulation
    b. Reduction of rotor friction
    c. Reduction of voltage ripple
    d. Thermal conduction
    e. Voltage rectification

Worksheet 5-5
High-Voltage Generator
Rectification

 Nearly everything electric in a hospital operates on alternating current (AC) power. However, in radiology, the most important component of an x-ray imaging system, the x-ray tube, requires direct current (DC).

Circuit elements in the high-voltage generator of the x-ray imaging system, called **rectifiers,** transform the AC to DC. The process of conversion from AC to DC is called **rectification.**

Some types of x-ray imaging systems, primarily dental and portable systems, are capable of transforming AC into DC themselves, while simultaneously producing x-rays. Such a circuit is said to be **self-rectified.** Self-rectification results in half-wave rectification. **Full-wave rectification** is most often used in conventional x-ray imaging systems, and such a circuit requires a minimum of four rectifiers. To full-wave rectify **three-phase power,** a minimum of 6 rectifiers is required for a six-pulse unit, and 12 are required for a 12-pulse unit. Today most x-ray generators are high frequency and thus create a relatively constant potential voltage waveform.

EXERCISES

1. Which of the following principles of rectification produces the maximum efficiency of x-ray production?
   a. Four-diode rectification
   b. Half-wave rectification
   c. High frequency rectification
   d. Self-rectification
   e. Two-diode rectification

2. To generate three-phase, six-pulse power, at least how many rectifiers are necessary?
   a. 4
   b. 6
   c. 8
   d. 12
   e. 16

3. A semiconductor rectifier:
   a. Has a heated anode
   b. Has a heated cathode
   c. Is a solid-state device
   d. Is an electromechanical device
   e. Is used only for mammography

4. If a single rectifier is inserted into a circuit that conducts 60 Hz AC so that it suppresses the positive portion of the waveform, then the output waveform will contain:
   a. 60 negative pulses per second
   b. 60 positive pulses per second
   c. 120 negative pulses per second
   d. 120 positive pulses per second
   e. Variable pulses, depending on frequency

5. The voltage ripple associated with various x-ray generators is:
   a. 70.7% for single-phase, full-wave rectification
   b. 100% for self-rectification
   c. Higher for self-rectification than for half-wave rectification
   d. Highest with high frequency
   e. Less for single-phase than for three-phase power

6. A rectifier:
   a. Converts AC to DC
   b. Converts DC to AC
   c. Increases voltage
   d. Refers to a type of electromagnetic device
   e. Refers to a type of electromechanical device

7. Inspect the following circuit, and identify which diodes pass current at the same time:

   a. 1 and 2
   b. 3 and 4
   c. 1 and 3
   d. 1 and 4

8. Near the p-n junction of a semiconductor diode, one will find:
   a. A filtered anode
   b. A heated anode
   c. A heated cathode
   d. A p type of material containing excess electrons
   e. An n type of material containing excess electrons

9. A semiconductor diode:
   a. Allows current to flow only from n type of material to p type
   b. Allows current to flow only from p type of material to n type
   c. Contains carriers that are also called proton traps
   d. Contains holes that are also called proton traps
   e. Is also called an electromechanical rectifier

10. In a circuit that contains a single rectifier:
    a. Electron flow is pulsed but uninterrupted.
    b. Electrons flow in one direction but not the other.
    c. The result is constant potential DC.
    d. Twice as many electrons flow in the output coil as in the input coil.
    e. Voltage is increased.

11. If 60 Hz AC power is full-wave rectified, output voltage consists of:
    a. 60 pulses per second
    b. 90 pulses per second
    c. 120 pulses per second
    d. 70% ripple
    e. Zero ripple

12. The current from a common household wall receptacle in the United States is:
    a. 50 Hz AC
    b. 50 Hz DC
    c. 60 Hz AC
    d. 60 Hz DC
    e. Constant potential.

13. Thermionic emission refers to:
    a. Electron emission from a heated source
    b. Heat conduction
    c. Heat emission from an electric conductor
    d. Heat radiation
    e. Ionization with heat

14. Which of the following is the symbol for a diode?

15. The main advantage of full-wave rectification over half-wave rectification is:
    a. Higher-energy x-rays
    b. Higher kVp
    c. Higher mA
    d. Less voltage ripple
    e. A greater number of x-rays per cycle

16. How many overlapping pulses are generated in 1 s for three-phase, six-pulse power?
    a. 60
    b. 120
    c. 360
    d. 720
    e. 2160

Match the approximate voltage ripple with each of the following. Some answers may be used more than once.

_____ 17. Full-wave rectified   a. 1%

_____ 18. High frequency   b. 4%

_____ 19. Three-phase, six-pulse   c. 13%

_____ 20. Three-phase, 12-pulse   d. 71%

_____ 21. Self-rectified   e. 100%

Worksheet 5-5   **High-Voltage Generator**

Worksheet 6-1
Internal Components
The X-Ray Tube Cathode

The cathode is the negative side of the x-ray tube. Its major components are the **filament** and the **focusing cup.** The filament is a small coil of wire, usually of thoriated tungsten, that provides electrons for the production of x-rays. The focusing cup directs the beam of electrons to the target on the anode.

Tungsten vaporization with deposition on the inside of a glass enclosure x-ray tube is the most common cause of x-ray tube failure.

EXERCISES

1. The three principal parts of an x-ray imaging system are:
   a. Anode, cathode, and focusing cup
   b. Anode, cathode, and high-voltage generator
   c. X-ray tube, control console, and high-voltage generator
   d. X-ray tube, high-voltage generator, and image receptor
   e. X-ray tube, protective housing, and high-voltage generator

2. The primary purpose of the glass envelope of an x-ray tube is to:
   a. Control leakage radiation
   b. Control off-focus radiation
   c. Cool the tube
   d. Ensure against electric shock
   e. Provide a vacuum

3. The protective housing of an x-ray tube is designed to:
   a. Control isotropic x-ray emission
   b. Control scatter radiation
   c. Limit operation to 100 kVp or less
   d. Reduce the hazard of leakage radiation
   e. Reduce the hazard of scatter radiation

4. A diagnostic x-ray tube is an example of which of the following?
   a. Cathode
   b. Diode
   c. Tetrode
   d. Anode
   e. Electrode

5. The large filament is used during radiography when the heat load is:
   a. High, and visibility of detail is important
   b. High, and visibility of detail is less important
   c. Low, and high kVp is required
   d. Low, and visibility of detail is important
   e. Low, and visibility of detail is less important

6. In most x-ray tubes, there are two filaments to:
   a. Ensure saturation current
   b. Produce higher energy x-rays
   c. Provide two electrodes
   d. Provide two focal spots
   e. Reduce space charge effects

7. The focusing cup:
   a. Is on the positive side of the x-ray tube
   b. Is slightly positive with respect to the filament
   c. Is the grid in a grid-controlled x-ray tube
   d. Is usually made of thoriated tungsten
   e. Selects the filament

8. Once filament temperature becomes adequate, a further small rise in filament temperature will cause tube current to:
   a. Decrease just a bit
   b. Decrease very much
   c. Increase just a bit
   d. Increase very much
   e. Not change

9. The cathode beam of an x-ray tube is the:
   a. Current that heats the filament
   b. Focused electron beam within the tube
   c. Off-focus radiation
   d. Primary x-ray beam
   e. Secondary radiation

10. The x-ray tube current:
    a. Controls x-ray energy
    b. Flows through both filaments at the same time
    c. Is controlled by the filament current
    d. Is the current that flows through the filament
    e. Usually varies from 50 to 1000 A

11. Most x-ray tubes used for radiography:
    a. Are dual-focus tubes
    b. Do not emit leakage radiation
    c. Have a fixed anode
    d. Operate in the space charge–limited mode
    e. Use tungsten filaments that do not vaporize

12. The cathode is:
    a. A diode
    b. Designed to supply heat
    c. One of the two parts of a diode
    d. Part of the target
    e. Positively charged

13. When a filament burns out:
    a. It should be replaced within 30 days.
    b. The filament current goes to maximum.
    c. The filament current goes to zero.
    d. The tube current is maximum.
    e. The x-ray intensity is maximum.

14. The space charge effect:
    a. Is more pronounced at high kVp
    b. Is more pronounced at low mA
    c. Limits kVp
    d. Occurs in the vicinity of the anode
    e. Occurs in the vicinity of the cathode

15. The x-ray tube filament:
    a. Conducts approximately 5 A
    b. Conducts current only when an exposure is made
    c. Is a diode
    d. Is the space charge
    e. Is usually copper

16. If saturation is achieved and the filament current is fixed, tube current:
    a. Decreases with use
    b. Falls with increasing kVp
    c. Remains fixed
    d. Rises with increasing exposure time
    e. Rises with increasing kVp

17. X-ray tube current:
    a. Depends on exposure time
    b. Depends on voltage
    c. Increases when the kVp is decreased
    d. Is measured in milliamperes rather than amperes
    e. Is zero when filament current is above thermionic emission

Examine the filament emission chart above and answer Exercises 18 and 19.

18. What is the full-wave tube current when the filament current is 4.6 A and the tube voltage is 70 kVp?

19. To obtain 125 mA half-wave–rectified x-ray tube current at 100 kVp, what must the filament current be?

Worksheet 6-2
Internal Components
The X-Ray Tube Anode

The x-ray tube anode serves four principal functions: (1) **electrical conduction** of the x-ray tube current, (2) **mechanical support** for the target, (3) **thermal conduction** of heat, and (4) **x-ray production.** The active portion of the anode, in which x-rays are produced, is the target. Almost all targets are made of tungsten (usually alloyed with rhenium). However, some that are used exclusively for mammography have molybdenum or rhodium targets.

The area of the target on which the projectile electrons interact is the **focal spot.** All diagnostic x-ray tubes have an inclined anode to take advantage of the **line-focus principle.**

Tungsten is the element of choice for the target for general radiography for three main reasons: atomic number (Z = 74), thermal conductivity, and high melting point.

EXERCISES

1. A stationary-anode x-ray tube:
   a. Incorporates the line-focus principle
   b. Is used to produce very short exposures
   c. Limits leakage radiation
   d. Provides for greater heat dissipation
   e. Usually has a very small focal spot

2. The heel effect occurs because of:
   a. A focusing cup
   b. Reduced tube current
   c. The shape charge effect
   d. The shape of the filament
   e. X-ray absorption in the anode

3. The main reason for using the line-focus principle is to:
   a. Increase heat capacity
   b. Increase x-ray intensity
   c. Reduce exposure time
   d. Reduce focal-spot size
   e. Reduce heel effect

4. Rotating anode x-ray tubes:
   a. Have a copper target embedded in a tungsten anode
   b. Have a tungsten target embedded in a copper anode
   c. Have target angles that are less than 10 degrees
   d. Incorporate the line-focus principle
   e. Produce higher energy x-rays

5. X-ray intensity is higher on the cathode side than on the anode side because of which of the following?
   a. The focusing cup
   b. The line-focus principle
   c. The space charge effect
   d. X-ray absorption in the anode
   e. X-ray deflection from the anode

6. Which of the following target angles is characteristic of a rotating anode x-ray tube?
   a. 1 degree
   b. 10 degrees
   c. 20 degrees
   d. 50 degrees
   e. 100 degrees

7. Small target angles result in which of the following?
   a. Better collimation
   b. Increased heat capacity
   c. Less heel effect
   d. Small focal-spot size
   e. Small space charge

8. Molybdenum is used for anode stem material because of which of the following?
   a. It has a high atomic number.
   b. It has a shiny surface and reflects electrons well.
   c. It has longer life.
   d. It is a good heat conductor.
   e. It is a poor thermal conductor.

9. Tungsten is the choice material for x-ray anodes because of its:
   a. High atomic number
   b. High rpm
   c. High x-ray intensity
   d. Low atomic number
   e. Low rpm

10. The effective focal spot is:
    a. Larger than the actual focal spot
    b. Largest on the anode side of the central axis
    c. Smaller than the actual focal spot
    d. Smallest on the cathode side of the central axis
    e. The same size as the actual focal spot

65

11. The heel effect:
    a. Is more pronounced when large target angles are used
    b. Is reduced with a focusing cup
    c. Occurs only with rotating anode x-ray tubes
    d. Requires that the cathode be positioned to the thicker anatomy
    e. Suggests that the cathode be up during posteroanterior (PA) chest radiography

12. What is a prominent engineering difficulty in the manufacture of high-speed rotating anodes?
    a. Balance of the rotor
    b. Control of space charge effects
    c. Marriage to the focusing cup
    d. Proper target angle
    e. Target-face polish

13. Which of the following is a component of an electromagnetic induction motor?
    a. Cathode
    b. Filament
    c. Stator
    d. Target angle
    e. Target disk

14. Necessary properties of x-ray target material include which of the following?
    a. High melting point
    b. High rotation speed
    c. Low atomic number
    d. Low coefficient of friction
    e. High electrical resistance

15. Which of the following is an advantage of the rotating anode tube over the stationary anode tube?
    a. Higher heat capacity
    b. Higher kVp capacity
    c. Longer exposure time
    d. Reduced heel effect
    e. The line-focus principle

16. The anode angle of an x-ray tube is increased to give which of the following?
    a. Smaller focal spot
    b. Higher heat capacity
    c. Proper focusing of the electron beam
    d. Proper reflection
    e. Uniform x-ray intensity

17. Which of the following components of a diagnostic x-ray tube is on the positive side of the tube?
    a. The cathode
    b. The filament
    c. The focusing cup
    d. The grid
    e. The stator

18. As the anode target angle increases:
    a. Effective focal-spot size increases
    b. Heel effect becomes more pronounced
    c. kVp increases
    d. Radiation intensity on the central ray increases
    e. Target rotating speed increases

19. A stationary anode will *most* likely be used in which of the following?
    a. Chest radiography
    b. Dentistry
    c. General radiography
    d. Interventional radiology
    e. Mammography

Worksheet 6-3
X-Ray Tube Failure
X-Ray Tube Rating Charts

 The three types of tube rating charts are the radiographic rating chart, the anode cooling chart, and the housing cooling chart.

The **radiographic rating chart** shows which single radiographic techniques are within the safe limits of operation for a particular x-ray tube. The **anode cooling chart** displays the thermal capacity of the anode and the time required for the heated anode to cool. The **housing cooling chart** gives the maximum heat capacity of the x-ray tube housing, as well as the time required for that housing to cool. Thermal energy absorbed by the anode is measured in **heat units (HU)**.

$$1 \text{ J} = 1 \text{ kV} \times 1 \text{ mA} \times 1 \text{ s}$$

$$1 \text{ HU} = \text{kVp} \times \text{mA} \times \text{Seconds for single-phase power} = 0.7 \text{ J}$$

$$1 \text{ HU} = 1.4 \text{ kVp} \times \text{mA} \times \text{Seconds for three-phase and high-frequency power}$$

$$1 \text{ HU} = 1.4 \text{ J for three-phase and high-frequency power}$$

EXERCISES

Use the charts on page 68 to answer questions 1 through 21.

1. The high-speed rotor (10,000 rpm) permits longer exposure times than the low-speed rotor at single-phase operation (3400 rpm).
   a. True
   b. False

2. If the intersection of time and kVp falls on an mA curve, that mA is safe.
   a. True
   b. False

3. Most of the troublesome heat generated in an x-ray tube occurs at the filament.
   a. True
   b. False

4. Generally, a small focal spot allows longer exposure times than a large focal spot.
   a. True
   b. False

5. The radiographic rating chart reports the time that should elapse between exposures.
   a. True
   b. False

6. It is *not* possible to exceed the heat capacity of the housing without first exceeding that of the anode.
   a. True
   b. False

7. A tube can become "gassy" because of anode overheating and the release of gas.
   a. True
   b. False

8. The radiographic rating chart is designed primarily to protect the filament.
   a. True
   b. False

9. Rotor speed does *not* influence heat capacity.
   a. True
   b. False

10. Heat units (HU) can be expressed as exposure rate in R/min (Gy_a/min).
    a. True
    b. False

Which of the following conditions of exposure are safe, and which are unsafe?

11. 100 kVp, 150 mA, 500 ms; 3400 rpm, 0.6 mm focal spot
    a. Safe
    b. Unsafe

12. 100 kVp, 150 mA, 500 ms; 3400 rpm, 1.2 mm focal spot
    a. Safe
    b. Unsafe

13. 100 kVp, 150 mA, 500 ms; 10,000 rpm, 0.6 mm focal spot
    a. Safe
    b. Unsafe

0.6 mm focal spot—3400 rpm

1.2 mm focal spot—3400 rpm

0.6 mm focal spot—10,000 rpm

1.2 mm focal spot—10,000 rpm

14. 100 kVp, 150 mA, 500 ms; 10,000 rpm, 1.2 mm focal spot
    a. Safe
    b. Unsafe

15. 100 kVp, 700 mA, 1000 ms; 10,000 rpm, 1.2 mm focal spot
    a. Safe
    b. Unsafe

16. 60 kVp, 200 mA, 100 ms; 3400 rpm, 0.6 mm focal spot
    a. Safe
    b. Unsafe

17. 120 kVp, 200 mA, 700 ms; 10,000 rpm, 0.6 mm focal spot
    a. Safe
    b. Unsafe

18. 80 kVp, 300 mA, 2000 ms; 3400 rpm, 0.6 mm focal spot
    a. Safe
    b. Unsafe

19. 120 kVp, 150 mA, 10 ms; 3400 rpm, 0.6 mm focal spot
    a. Safe
    b. Unsafe

20. 105 kVp, 700 mA, 100 ms; 10,000 rpm, 1.2 mm focal spot
    a. Safe
    b. Unsafe

21. How many heat units are produced by the following radiographic technique: 100 kVp, 150 mA, 500 ms, single phase, 3400 rpm, 0.6 mm focal spot?

68

Use the following charts to answer questions 22 through 25.

Anode thermal characteristics

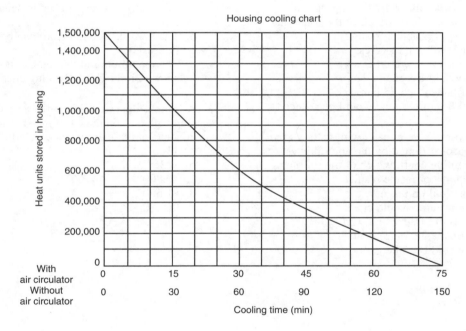

Housing cooling chart

22. What is the maximum number of heat units that the anode can absorb?
23. How long would it take the tube to cool down completely from maximum heat as determined in the previous question?
24. If an anode absorbs 200,000 HU, how long will it take to cool completely?
25. If an anode absorbs 180,000 HU, how long will it be before another 180,000 HU can be absorbed?

Select the *one* correct answer from the following:

26. To determine whether any set of tube rating charts is applicable for a given x-ray tube, one should:
    a. Check to see that the operating console will allow operation at 150 kVp because this is the maximum indicated on all radiographic rating charts.

b. Determine whether the operating console allows all of the mA settings indicated for the radiographic rating chart.

c. Identify the type of tube, the anode rotation, the focal-spot size, and the type of generator to make certain that all of these match the specifications on the chart.

d. Make an exposure at a radiographic technique that exceeds the maximum permitted by the charts, and check to see whether the interlock circuit prevents the exposure.

e. Warm the tube with five rapid exposures.

27. Which of the following would be allowed according to the 1.2 mm/10,000 rpm radiographic rating chart on page 68?
a. 68 kVp/800 mA/500 ms
b. 82 kV/1000 mA/200 ms
c. 88 kV/1000 mA/50 ms
d. 90 kVp/800 mA/500 ms
e. 108 kVp/600 mA/1000 ms

28. If a single exposure were made with factors *slightly* exceeding those permitted by the appropriate radiographic rating chart, which of the following would be the *most* probable result?
a. The anode would pit or crack.
b. The glass envelope would crack.
c. The rotor would freeze and stop.
d. The tube filament would burn out.
e. The useful life of the tube would be reduced.

29. If a single exposure were made with factors *greatly* exceeding those permitted by the appropriate radiographic rating chart, which of the following would be the *most* probable result?
a. The anode would pit or crack.
b. The glass envelope would crack.
c. The rotor would freeze and stop.
d. The tube filament would break.
e. The tube would become gassy.

30. Which of the following conditions will *not* damage an x-ray tube?
a. Exceeding the anode heat storage capacity
b. Exceeding the heat storage capacity of the tube housing
c. Exceeding the instantaneous filament emission rate
d. Exceeding the prescribed SID
e. Successive high-intensity exposures

31. In the design of a rotating anode x-ray tube:
a. Dual-focus tubes require two high-voltage, step-up transformers.
b. Dual-focus tubes require two separate anodes.
c. Dual-focus tubes require two target materials.
d. Most anodes rotate at 3400 or 10,000 rpm.
e. The disk can be made thicker so that the rpm can be increased.

32. Regarding the tube rating charts on page 68:
a. "Heat units per second" refers to the fluoroscopic use of the x-ray tube.
b. The anode thermal characteristics chart is for fluoroscopic use only.
c. The filament chart is used to select exposure times.
d. The housing cooling chart can be applied only to fluoroscopy.
e. The maximum radiographic exposure time is shown on the anode cooling chart.

33. A fluoroscopic examination at 85 kVp and 4 mA, single phase, requires 4 minutes. The number of anode heat units produced would be approximately:
a. 1360
b. 1836
c. 40,800
d. 81,600
e. 96,400

Worksheet 7-1
Electron-Target Interactions
Characteristic Radiation

 In characteristic x-ray production, the projectile electron ionizes a target atom through the removal of a tightly bound inner-shell electron. The hole created in the inner-electron shell of the target atom is filled by an outer-shell electron or a free electron falling into the hole. This transition of an electron from an outer shell to an inner shell is accompanied by the emission of an x-ray of energy equal to the difference between the binding energies of the two electron shells involved.

Energy of characteristic x-rays equals the difference between the binding energy of the ejected inner electron, and the binding energy of the outer or free electron replacing it.

Approximate Electron Binding Energy, keV

Shell	Molybdenum (Mo)	Tungsten (W)
K	20.0	69.0
L	3.0	12.0
M	0.5	2.0
N	—	1.0
O	—	0.1

EXERCISES

1. If mass is expressed in kilograms and velocity in meters per second, kinetic energy will be expressed in:
   a. Coulombs
   b. Electron volts
   c. Ergs
   d. Joules
   e. Newtons

2. The kinetic energy of the projectile electron in an x-ray tube:
   a. Causes excitation in the vacuum of the x-ray tube
   b. Causes ionization in the vacuum of the x-ray tube
   c. Is about 1% efficient in the production of x-rays
   d. Is converted to mass
   e. Is totally converted to x-ray energy

3. The shift of the characteristic x-ray spectrum to higher energy occurs because of which of the following?
   a. A decrease in voltage ripple
   b. A decrease in kVp
   c. A higher atomic number filter
   d. An increase in kVp
   e. An increase in target atomic number

4. Useful characteristic x-rays are produced in tungsten:
   a. By excitation of a K-shell electron
   b. By removal of a K-shell electron
   c. By ionization of an L-shell electron
   d. When a valence electron is removed
   e. When the projectile electron interacts with an outer-shell electron

5. An L-shell electron (binding energy 26 keV) is removed from an atom that has M-shell binding energy of 4 keV and N-shell binding energy of 1 keV. If a free electron fills the vacancy in the L-shell, the characteristic x-ray produced will have energy of:
   a. 1 keV
   b. 4 keV
   c. 22 keV
   d. 25 keV
   e. 26 keV

6. What is produced when the projectile electron excites an outer-shell electron?
   a. Bremsstrahlung x-ray
   b. Characteristic x-ray
   c. Energy
   d. Heat
   e. Photoelectric x-ray

7. The energy of characteristic x-rays increases with increasing:
   a. Filtration
   b. Atomic mass of target material
   c. Atomic number of target material
   d. kVp
   e. Voltage waveform

8. X-rays are produced when:
   a. Electric current flows through the x-ray tube filament.
   b. Projectile electrons bounce off the cathode.
   c. Projectile electrons interact with target atoms.
   d. The target angle is sufficiently large.
   e. The x-ray tube filament is heated to thermionic emission.

9. Characteristic x-rays:
   a. Are characteristic of target Z
   b. Are characteristic of the filter material
   c. Are characteristic of the voltage waveform
   d. Have velocity varying from zero to the speed of light
   e. Vary in energy as kVp is varied

10. When a tungsten-targeted x-ray tube is operated at 68 kVp:
    a. K-shell characteristic x-rays can be produced.
    b. L-shell x-rays cannot be produced.
    c. One possible K-shell characteristic x-ray will have 12 keV of energy.
    d. Some projectile electrons may have 68 keV of energy.
    e. Some projectile electrons may have 75 keV of energy.

11. According to the table on page 71:
    a. The farther from the nucleus, the higher the electron binding energy.
    b. The K-shell characteristic x-rays of molybdenum are lower in energy than the L-shell characteristic x-rays of tungsten.
    c. The L-shell characteristic x-rays of molybdenum are of higher energy than the L-shell characteristic x-rays of tungsten.
    d. Tungsten obviously has a lower atomic number than molybdenum.
    e. Tungsten obviously has a greater number of electrons than molybdenum.

12. When characteristic x-rays are produced, the energy of the x-rays is characteristic of:
    a. The atomic number of the filter
    b. The atomic number of the target
    c. The outer-shell electron binding energy
    d. The mass of filtration
    e. The orientation of the target

13. Gold is sometimes used as target material in special types of radiation-producing systems. Its electron-binding energies are as follows: K-shell: 81 keV; L-shell: 14 keV; M-shell: 3 keV; and N-shell: 1 keV. Which of the following characteristic x-rays would be produced with operation at 90 kVp?
    a. 12 keV
    b. 67 keV
    c. 76 keV
    d. 87 keV
    e. 90 keV

14. The kinetic energy of a projectile electron can be measured in:
    a. Amperes
    b. Coulombs
    c. Joules
    d. Newtons
    e. Rads

15. The efficiency of x-ray production is:
    a. Approximately 5%
    b. Greater than that of heat production
    c. In excess of 5%
    d. Independent of tube current
    e. Independent of tube voltage

16. The joules (J) of energy generated by electron-target interactions is given by:
    a. $kV \times mA \times s$
    b. $kV \times mA \times ms$
    c. $kVp \times A \times s$
    d. $kVp \times mA \times s \times s$
    e. $kVp \times mA \times ms$

Worksheet 7-2
Electron-Target Interactions
Bremsstrahlung Radiation

Bremsstrahlung x-rays are produced when a projectile electron from the cathode passes close enough to the nucleus to be influenced by the nucleus. As the projectile electron passes the nucleus, the electron slows and its direction changes. Therefore, it leaves the electron with reduced kinetic energy.

The loss in kinetic energy reappears as an x-ray. These are bremsstrahlung x-rays. They can have energy ranging from zero to a maximum that is equal to the projectile electron energy. The most frequent bremsstrahlung x-ray energy is approximately one third of the maximum energy of the projectile electron. Most x-rays in a diagnostic x-ray beam are bremsstrahlung x-rays.

EXERCISES

1. In a tungsten-targeted x-ray tube operated at 90 kVp, the *most* abundant x-ray would be a:
   a. 10 keV characteristic x-ray
   b. 12 keV characteristic x-ray
   c. 30 keV bremsstrahlung x-ray
   d. 69 keV bremsstrahlung x-ray
   e. 90 keV bremsstrahlung x-ray

2. Which of the following electron transitions results in the *most* useful bremsstrahlung x-ray?
   a. L to K
   b. M to K
   c. M to L
   d. O to K
   e. None of the above

3. Bremsstrahlung radiation is produced by:
   a. Conversion of projectile electron kinetic energy to electromagnetic energy
   b. Conversion of target electron kinetic energy to electromagnetic energy
   c. Intrashell electron transitions
   d. Projectile electron–target electron interaction
   e. Target electron–nuclear interaction

4. When a bremsstrahlung x-ray is produced:
   a. A projectile electron is absorbed.
   b. A projectile electron loses energy.
   c. A target electron is displaced.
   d. A target electron is excited.
   e. A target electron is ionized.

5. In bremsstrahlung x-ray production:
   a. The projectile electron is bound to tungsten.
   b. The projectile electron is from the cathode.
   c. The target electron exists as a free electron.
   d. The target electron is from the cathode.
   e. The target electron is ionized.

6. If an average radiographic technique is used:
   a. Excitation of the target is approximately 50%.
   b. Ionization of the target is almost complete.
   c. Maximum-energy x-ray is the electron binding energy.
   d. Most x-rays are bremsstrahlung.
   e. Most x-rays are characteristic.

7. Bremsstrahlung x-rays are produced only at:
   a. Discrete energies
   b. Energies above characteristic x-rays
   c. Energies below characteristic x-rays
   d. Energies up to projectile electron energy
   e. Projectile electron kinetic energy

8. If radiographic technique is 74 kVp/80 mAs:
   a. Bremsstrahlung x-ray energy increases if the voltage is increased to 84 kVp.
   b. Bremsstrahlung x-rays are emitted at discrete energies.
   c. Bremsstrahlung x-rays have a maximum energy of 80 keV.
   d. Characteristic x-ray energy increases if the voltage is increased to 84 kVp.
   e. Characteristic x-rays are emitted only at 74 keV.

9. If radiographic technique in a tungsten target at 60 kVp/80 mAs is changed to 80 kVp/80 mAs:
   a. Additional filtration is required.
   b. Bremsstrahlung x-ray intensity remains unchanged.
   c. Characteristic x-ray intensity remains unchanged.
   d. The number of projectile electrons increases.
   e. The number of x-rays produced increases.

10. Bremsstrahlung x-rays produced in a tungsten-targeted x-ray tube:
    a. Are all diagnostically useful
    b. Are generally less useful than characteristic x-rays
    c. Are less intense than characteristic x-rays
    d. Are less intense than if produced in molybdenum
    e. Outnumber characteristic x-rays

11. When a bremsstrahlung x-ray is emitted:
    a. A projectile electron is absorbed.
    b. An inner-shell electron is removed from the target atom.
    c. An outer-shell electron is removed from the target atom.
    d. This results from the conversion of kinetic energy.
    e. The target atom is ionized.

12. The wavelength of an x-ray:
    a. Becomes longer as projectile electron kinetic energy is reduced
    b. Becomes longer with increasing projectile electron energy
    c. Is longer than that of ultraviolet light
    d. Is longest when the projectile electron loses all its kinetic energy
    e. Is proportional to its frequency

13. When projectile electron energy is increased:
    a. Characteristic x-ray energy decreases.
    b. Characteristic x-ray energy increases.
    c. More bremsstrahlung x-rays are produced.
    d. More bremsstrahlung x-rays are produced, but only at high energies.
    e. More bremsstrahlung x-rays are produced, but only at low energies.

14. The efficiency of bremsstrahlung x-ray production increases with increasing:
    a. Collimation
    b. Filtration
    c. mA
    d. SID
    e. Target atomic number

15. The output intensity of an x-ray tube:
    a. Increases when filtered
    b. Is limited by the K-shell binding energy
    c. Is monoenergetic
    d. Often is measured in curies (Becquerels)
    e. Is primarily due to bremsstrahlung x-rays

16. Which of the following projectile electron-target interactions results in x-ray emission?
    a. Excitation of inner-shell electron
    b. Excitation of outer-shell electron
    c. Removal of inner-shell electron
    d. Removal of nucleus
    e. Removal of outer-shell electron

17. When a projectile electron enters a target atom and interacts with the nuclear force field:
    a. It decreases in velocity
    b. It increases in velocity
    c. It ionizes the atom
    d. It ionizes the nucleus
    e. It removes an inner-shell electron

18. In a tungsten-targeted x-ray tube operated at 90 kVp, the most abundant x-ray would be a:
    a. 10 keV characteristic x-ray
    b. 12 keV characteristic x-ray
    c. 30 keV bremsstrahlung x-ray
    d. 69 keV bremsstrahlung x-ray
    e. 90 keV bremsstrahlung x-ray

Worksheet 7-3
X-Ray Emission Spectrum

 An x-ray emission spectrum is a graph of the relative number of x-rays plotted as a function of the energy of each x-ray.

The characteristic x-ray emission spectrum represents monoenergetic x-rays emitted after ionization of the target atom. It consists of vertical lines at fixed energies and is called a **discrete** x-ray emission spectrum.

The bremsstrahlung x-ray emission spectrum results from x-rays created by the bremsstrahlung process and has energy ranging from zero to the maximum projectile electron energy. This spectrum is the **continuous** emission spectrum, and its maximum amplitude occurs at an energy that is approximately one third of the maximum energy.

EXERCISES

1. The area under the curve of the x-ray emission spectrum represents:
   a. The average energy of the x-rays
   b. The average number of x-rays per unit of energy
   c. The total energy of the x-rays
   d. The total number of x-rays
   e. Total exposure (mGy_a)

2. Normally, the x-ray emission spectrum contains:
   a. Both characteristic and bremsstrahlung x-rays
   b. Both photoelectric and Compton x-rays
   c. Only bremsstrahlung x-rays
   d. Only characteristic x-rays
   e. Only discrete lines

3. The characteristic x-ray emission spectrum principally depends on which of the following?
   a. Filtration
   b. kVp
   c. mAs
   d. Projectile electron energy
   e. Target material

4. The continuous x-ray emission spectrum principally depends on which of the following?
   a. Exposure time
   b. Filtration
   c. mAs
   d. Projectile electron energy
   e. Target material

5. Which of the following factors explains the low number of x-rays emitted at low energy?
   a. Added filtration
   b. The glass envelope of the x-ray tube
   c. The kVp
   d. The mAs enclosing the x-ray tube
   e. The product of tube current and exposure time

6. The x-ray emission spectrum represents:
   a. Projectile electron energy
   b. Atomic mass and number of the target atom
   c. Electron binding energy of target material
   d. Total x-ray beam filtration
   e. X-rays emitted from the x-ray tube

7. Both the shape and the position of the characteristic x-ray emission spectrum:
   a. Are described by the number of projectile electrons
   b. Represent projectile electron energy
   c. Can be described as continuous
   d. Correspond to target electron binding energies
   e. Result from nuclear interaction

8. A diagnostic x-ray beam contains:
   a. Bremsstrahlung only
   b. Mostly bremsstrahlung x-rays, with some characteristic x-rays
   c. Mostly Compton x-rays, few bremsstrahlung x-rays, and some pair production x-rays
   d. Some Compton x-rays, some bremsstrahlung x-rays, and no pair production x-rays
   e. Some photoelectric x-rays

9. The x-ray emission spectrum is a plot of:
   a. mAs versus kVp
   b. The number of electrons versus energy
   c. The number of x-rays versus energy
   d. X-rays and electrons emitted from cathode atoms
   e. X-rays and electrons emitted from target atoms

10. The amplitude of the bremsstrahlung x-ray emission spectrum:
    a. Approaches maximum at an energy equal to the kVp
    b. Approaches maximum at zero energy
    c. Has maximum value at energy approximately one third of the kVp
    d. Has maximum value at energy equal to the kVp
    e. Is enhanced with filtration

11. If an x-ray emission spectrum represented operation at 85 kVp with a tungsten target:
    a. At 85 keV, the number of projectile electrons would be maximum.
    b. Bremsstrahlung x-rays would be most intense at 85 keV.
    c. The K-characteristic x-ray emission would occur at 69 keV.
    d. X-rays representing maximum frequency would occur at 69 keV.
    e. X-rays representing minimum wavelength would occur at 0 keV.

12. If an x-ray emission spectrum represented operation at 26 kVp with a molybdenum target:
    a. K-characteristic x-rays would not be produced.
    b. More characteristic bremsstrahlung x-rays would be emitted.
    c. The characteristic radiation would have an energy of approximately 19 keV.
    d. Maximum-frequency x-rays would have an energy of 17 keV.
    e. Minimum-wavelength x-rays would have an energy of 20 keV.

13. Which of the following factors principally accounts for the reduced x-ray intensity at low energy?
    a. Added filtration
    b. Beam collimation
    c. Atomic number of the target material
    d. Energy spectrum of the projectile electrons
    e. Voltage waveform

14. Characteristic x-radiation is related to the:
    a. Difference between K- and L-shell binding energy
    b. Energy required to eject K-shell electrons
    c. Energy to eject L-shell electrons
    d. Number of electrons
    e. Number of K-shell electrons

15. Molybdenum has a lower atomic number than tungsten; therefore, the molybdenum x-ray emission spectrum:
    a. Extends to higher energies
    b. Extends to lower energies
    c. Has higher amplitude
    d. Has higher energy characteristic x-rays
    e. Has lower amplitude

16. To construct an x-ray emission spectrum, one must know the:
    a. kVp and mAs
    b. mAs and x-ray frequency
    c. Number of x-rays at each energy interval
    d. Projectile electron number and energy interval
    e. Target element and filtration

Worksheet 7-4
X-Ray Emission Spectrum
Minimum Wavelength

X-ray emission sometimes is shown as a function of x-ray wavelength rather than energy. Because x-ray energy and wavelength are inversely proportional, the highest x-ray energy corresponds to the shortest x-ray wavelength, which is also called the **minimum wavelength.**

Planck equation is:

$$E = hv$$

where

$$v = c/l$$

Therefore:

$$E = \frac{hc}{\lambda}$$

$$E = \frac{(4.14 \times 10^{-15} \text{eVs}) (3 \times 10^8 \text{ m/s})}{\lambda}$$

$$E = \frac{12.4 \times 10^{-7} \text{ eV m}}{\lambda} \quad \frac{1 \text{ keV}}{10^3 \text{ eV}}$$

$$E = \frac{12.4 \times 10^{-10} \text{ keV m}}{\lambda}$$

This equation can be rearranged to solve for λ, which is the wavelength of an x-ray having energy E in keV:

$$\lambda = \frac{12.4 \times 10^{-10} \text{ keV m}}{E}$$

$$\lambda_{min} = \frac{12.4 \times 10^{-10} \text{ keV m}}{kVp}$$

$$\lambda_{min}(nm) = \frac{1.24}{kVp}$$

EXERCISES

1. Which characteristic is reduced as x-ray energy increases?
   a. Filtration
   b. Projectile electron energy
   c. Target electron energy
   d. X-ray frequency
   e. X-ray wavelength

2. The wavelength of an x-ray is:
   a. Determined by filter thickness
   b. Determined by the number of projectile electrons
   c. Determined by the number of target electrons
   d. Directly proportional to its energy
   e. Inversely proportional to its energy

3. The product of the Planck constant (h) and the velocity of light (c) has units of:
   a. Jm^2
   b. Jm
   c. J/m
   d. Js
   e. J/s

4. The product of the Planck constant (h) and the velocity of light (c) equals:
   a. 12.4 eVm
   b. 12.4 keVm
   c. 12.4×10^{-7} eVm
   d. 12.4×10^{-10} eVm
   e. 12.4×10^{-15} eVm

5. If one knows the minimum wavelength of a given x-ray beam, the kVp of operation can be determined if one also knows which of the following fixed values?
   a. The Planck constant
   b. That nothing more is needed
   c. The mA
   d. The mAs
   e. The voltage waveform

6. Indicate which of the following figures represents an x-ray emission spectrum:

(a)

(b)

(c)

(d)

7. The relationship of minimum wavelength to maximum x-ray energy is sometimes called the:
   a. Duane-Hunt law
   b. Faraday's law
   c. Haus-Hendrick law
   d. Hurter-Driffield curve
   e. Quantum theory of Planck

8. Minimum wavelength is related to:
   a. Nuclear charge
   b. The atomic number of the target material
   c. The degree of collimation of the x-ray beam
   d. The kinetic energy of the projectile electron
   e. The total filtration in the x-ray beam

9. That region of the x-ray emission spectrum associated with minimum wavelength is the:
   a. Highest energy bremsstrahlung x-ray
   b. Highest energy characteristic line
   c. Intersection of the two axes
   d. Lowest energy bremsstrahlung x-ray
   e. Lowest energy characteristic line

10. If one knows the minimum wavelength of an x-ray emission spectrum, one can calculate:
    a. Filter atomic number
    b. Filtration thickness
    c. mA
    d. mAs
    e. Maximum projectile electron energy

11. To calculate minimum x-ray wavelength, one must know the value of:
    a. Filtration
    b. kVp
    c. mA
    d. mAs
    e. Phase

12. At 80 kVp and 80 mAs, how would the total emission spectrum be affected by operation at 80 kVp/400 mA/100 ms? The relative position of the spectrum would:
    a. Remain the same
    b. Remain the same, but the amplitude would decrease
    c. Remain the same, but the amplitude would increase
    d. Shift to the left, and the amplitude would be lower
    e. Shift to the right

13. How would the emission spectrum be affected by the addition of 2 mm Al filtration? The relative position of the spectrum would:
    a. Remain the same
    b. Remain the same, but the amplitude would decrease
    c. Remain the same, but the amplitude would increase
    d. Shift to the left, and the amplitude would be lower
    e. Shift to the right, and the amplitude would be lower

14. How would the emission spectrum be affected if the power supply were changed from single phase to three phase? The relative position of the spectrum would:
    a. Not change, but the energy of the characteristic lines would increase
    b. Remain the same
    c. Remain the same, the amplitude would increase, and the characteristic lines would increase in height
    d. Shift to the left, the amplitude would increase, and the characteristic lines would increase in height
    e. Shift to the right, the amplitude would increase, and the characteristic lines would increase in height

Worksheet 7-5
X-Ray Emission Spectrum
Factors That Affect the X-Ray Emission Spectrum

The shape of the emission spectrum and its relative position vary with changes in kVp, mAs, filtration, target material, and voltage waveform. Higher amplitude in the emission spectrum represents greater x-ray intensity (beam quantity), whereas a shift of the spectrum to the right along the energy axis represents greater penetrability (beam quality).

In general, the following relationships apply:

- Increasing kVp increases the height of the x-ray emission spectrum and extends it to the right along the energy axis.
- Increasing mAs increases the height of the x-ray emission spectrum.
- Increasing filtration decreases the height of the x-ray emission spectrum and shifts the shape to the right along the energy axis.
- Changing to a higher atomic number x-ray target increases the x-ray emission spectrum amplitude, shifts the spectrum to the right, and results in higher-energy characteristic lines.
- Changing from half-wave to full-wave rectification doubles the height of the spectrum.
- Changing from single-phase to three-phase power results in greater amplitude and a shift to the right on the energy axis.

EXERCISES

1. Which of the following statements applies to the x-ray emission spectrum?
   a. Adding filtration affects characteristic x-ray energy.
   b. Adding filtration affects minimum wavelength.
   c. Adding filtration increases entrance skin exposure.
   d. The target material affects the amplitude of bremsstrahlung x-rays.
   e. The target material affects the minimum wavelength.

2. An increase in mAs results in an increase in:
   a. Average x-ray energy.
   b. Both characteristic and bremsstrahlung x-rays
   c. Minimum wavelength
   d. Only the bremsstrahlung x-rays
   e. Only the characteristic x-rays

3. An increase in kVp results in an increase in:
   a. Characteristic x-ray energy.
   b. Only the bremsstrahlung x-ray emission spectrum
   c. Only the characteristic x-ray emission spectrum
   d. Radiation quality
   e. Minimum wavelength

4. The intensity of x-ray exposure is best represented by:
   a. The amplitude of the bremsstrahlung x-ray emission spectrum
   b. The amplitude of the characteristic x-ray emission spectrum
   c. The amplitude of the highest emission spectrum
   d. The area under the emission spectrum
   e. The energy range of the emission spectrum

79

Examine the following figure, and answer questions 5 through 7.

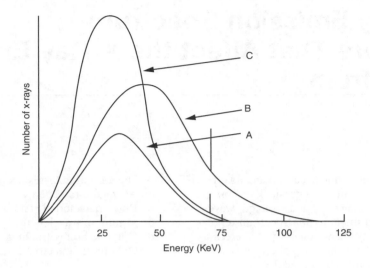

5. Which of these curves have equal minimum wavelength and equal maximum energy?
   a. A, B, and C
   b. A and B
   c. A and C
   d. B and C
   e. None of the above

6. Of the three curves represented:
   a. A and B represent two different targets.
   b. A and C were produced at the same kVp.
   c. A and C were produced at the same mAs.
   d. A is single phase and C is three phase.
   e. C and B represent two different targets.

7. Of the three spectra:
   a. A is more penetrating than B.
   b. A is more penetrating than C.
   c. B is more penetrating than C.
   d. C is more penetrating than A.
   e. C is more penetrating than B.

8. Which of the following factors primarily affects the low-energy side of the x-ray emission spectrum?
   a. Exposure time
   b. Filtration
   c. Tube current
   d. Tube voltage
   e. Voltage waveform

9. In general, when changes are made that affect the x-ray emission spectrum and the:
   a. Amplitude increases, the radiation quantity decreases
   b. Line spectrum moves, voltage waveform has changed
   c. Spectrum shifts to the left, a higher quality beam is emitted
   d. Spectrum shifts to the left, more filtration was used
   e. Spectrum shifts to the right, a more penetrating beam is emitted

Answer the remaining questions about an emission spectrum that represents a diagnostic imaging system operated at 80 kVp/200 mA/100 ms with a tungsten target.

10. How would the bremsstrahlung spectrum change if operation at 80 kVp/200 mA/100 ms were changed to 64 kVp/200 mA/100 ms?
    a. It would remain the same, but the amplitude would decrease.
    b. It would remain the same, but the amplitude would increase.
    c. It would shift to the left, and the amplitude would be lower.
    d. It would shift to the left, and the amplitude would be higher.
    e. It would shift to the right, and the amplitude would be higher.

11. How would the characteristic spectrum change if operation were at 64 kVp/200 mA/20 ms? The characteristic x-ray spectrum would:
    a. Decrease in height
    b. Disappear
    c. Increase in height
    d. Shift slightly to the left
    e. Shift slightly to the right

Worksheet 8-1
X-Ray Emission
X-Ray Quantity

 The intensity of x-rays in the useful beam is measured in roentgens (R) or mGy_a and milliroentgens (mR), and is referred to as *x-ray quantity*. At 70 kVp, the output intensity (or quantity) of a radiographic tube ranges from about 3 to 10 mR/mAs at a 100 cm source-to-image receptor distance (SID). This wide range of x-ray quantity exists because of differences in tube design, filtration, and voltage generation.

Three adjustable factors affect x-ray quantity:

1. mAs: X-ray quantity is directly proportional to milliampere-seconds (mAs)

$$\frac{I_1}{I_2} = \frac{mAs_1}{mAs_2}$$

2. kVp: X-ray quantity varies approximately as the square of the change in kilovolt peak (kVp):

$$\frac{I_1}{I_2} = (kVp_1/kVp_2)^2$$

3. Distance: X-ray quantity varies inversely with the square of the distance from the target (the inverse square law):

$$I_1/I_2 = (d_2/d_1)^2$$

When these factors are viewed collectively, x-ray exposure of a patient can be estimated at a reasonable approximation with the use of the following equation:

$$\text{X-ray quantity (mR)} = \frac{k\ (mAs)\ (kVp)^2}{d^2}$$

where *d* is the source-to-skin distance (SSD) in centimeters. The constant *k* will vary from approximately 10 to 30, depending on many factors, including voltage, voltage ripple, filtration, and field size.

EXERCISES

1. When the mAs is increased, x-ray quantity:
   a. Decreases as the square of the mAs
   b. Decreases proportionately
   c. Increases as the square of the mAs
   d. Increases proportionately
   e. Remains the same

2. When the kVp is increased, x-ray quantity:
   a. Decreases in proportion to kVp^2
   b. Decreases proportionately
   c. Increases in proportion to kVp^2
   d. Increases proportionately
   e. Remains the same

3. When distance is increased, x-ray quantity at that distance:
   a. Decreases in proportion to distance squared
   b. Decreases proportionately
   c. Increases in proportion to distance squared
   d. Increases proportionately
   e. Remains the same

4. When x-ray tube filtration is increased, x-ray quantity:
   a. Decreases
   b. Decreases proportionately
   c. Increases
   d. Increases proportionately
   e. Remains the same

5. In general, x-ray quantity will increase with a/an:
   a. Decrease in exposure time
   b. Decrease in tube current
   c. Increase in distance
   d. Increase in filtration
   e. Increase in kVp

6. X-ray quantity usually is measured as which of the following?
   a. Absorbed dose in rad
   b. Absorbed dose in roentgens
   c. Dose equivalent in roentgens
   d. Exposure in rad
   e. Exposure in roentgens

7. A tungsten-targeted x-ray imaging system is operated at 66 kVp/150 mAs and has an output intensity of 6 mGy$_a$. Therefore:
   a. Characteristic x-rays will be prominent.
   b. If the mAs is increased to 200, the minimum wavelength will be increased.
   c. Most electron–target atom interactions will result in x-ray emission.
   d. No useful bremsstrahlung radiation will be produced.
   e. The most frequent x-ray emission will be in the 20 to 25 keV range.

8. X-ray quantity can be measured in which of the following?
   a. Bq
   b. Gy$_a$
   c. Gy$_t$
   d. Rem
   e. Sv

9. Another meaning of "x-ray quantity" is x-ray:
   a. Energy
   b. Filtration
   c. Intensity
   d. Penetrability
   e. Quality

10. Which of the following does *not* affect x-ray quantity?
    a. Filtration
    b. kVp
    c. mA
    d. Radioactivity
    e. Time

11. To maintain a constant optical density, what percentage increase in kVp should be accompanied by a reduction of one half in mAs?
    a. 5%
    b. 10%
    c. 15%
    d. 30%
    e. 50%

12. An extremity radiograph requires 5 mAs and results in an exposure of 180 uGy$_a$. What will be the exposure if the technique is changed to 7 mAs?
    a. 180 uGy$_a$
    b. 190 uGy$_a$
    c. 220 uGy$_a$
    d. 250 uGy$_a$
    e. 360 uGy$_a$

13. An abdominal view is taken at 82 kVp and results in a patient exposure of 1.3 mGy$_a$. To improve contrast and density, the kVp is reduced to 74 with no change in mAs. What is the new patient exposure?
    a. 1.1 mGy$_a$
    b. 1.2 mGy$_a$
    c. 1.3 mGy$_a$
    d. 1.5 mGy$_a$
    e. 1.6 mGy$_a$

14. A portable chest x-ray is taken at 90 cm SID, and the patient exposure is 280 uGy$_a$. What will the exposure be if the distance is increased to 180 cm and there is no accompanying technique change?
    a. 70 uGy$_a$
    b. 120 uGy$_a$
    c. 170 uGy$_a$
    d. 630 uGy$_a$
    e. 1420 uGy$_a$

15. The output intensity for an x-ray imaging system operated at 70 kVp/400 mA and 50 ms is 0.7 mGy$_a$. If the mA selector is changed to 600 mA and the exposure time is increased to 80 ms, what will be the output intensity?
    a. 1.05 mGy$_a$
    b. 1.12 mGy$_a$
    c. 1.68 mGy$_a$
    d. 2.10 mGy$_a$
    e. 2.34 mGy$_a$

Worksheet 8-2
X-Ray Emission
X-Ray Quality

 An x-ray beam that easily penetrates soft tissue and bone is said to be of high quality, whereas a beam that is easily absorbed is of low quality. X-ray quality therefore is a measure of the penetrating ability of an x-ray beam or the energy of the x-ray beam.

- As the voltage of operation is increased, the energy of the x-ray beam is increased; therefore, penetrating ability and quality also increase.
- When filtration is added to the beam, it becomes lower quantity, higher energy, and more penetrating, and therefore of greater quality.
- Tube current (mA), exposure time (s), and distance (SID) do not influence the quality of an x-ray beam.
- X-ray beam quality usually is measured by the half-value layer (HVL).
- The HVL is that thickness of an absorber that will reduce the x-ray intensity to one half of its original value.

EXERCISES

1. Which of the following is the *most* appropriate measure of x-ray beam quality?
   a. Added filtration
   b. HVL
   c. kVp
   d. mAs
   e. Total filtration

2. The quality of an x-ray beam is principally a function of which of the following?
   a. Field size
   b. Filtration
   c. kVp
   d. mAs
   e. SID

3. The HVL is affected principally by a change in which of the following?
   a. Filter thickness
   b. kVp
   c. mAs
   d. SID
   e. X-ray intensity

4. When filtration is added to an x-ray tube, which of the following increases?
   a. Radiation output
   b. Radiation quality
   c. Radiation quantity
   d. SID
   e. SSD

5. Which of the following is the probable HVL of a radiographic x-ray beam at 70 kVp?
   a. 0.5 cm Al
   b. 5.0 cm Al
   c. 0.5 cm of soft tissue
   d. 5.0 cm of soft tissue
   e. 10 cm of soft tissue

6. As filtration is added to an x-ray beam:
   a. All x-rays are removed about equally from the useful beam.
   b. High-energy x-rays are removed more readily than low-energy x-rays.
   c. Low-energy x-rays are removed more readily than high-energy x-rays.
   d. No x-rays are removed, but their average energy is increased.
   e. No x-rays are removed, but their average energy is reduced.

7. An increase in mAs will increase which of the following?
   a. Exposure time
   b. HVL
   c. Total filtration
   d. X-ray quality
   e. X-ray quantity

8. It is often stated that mAs controls quantity and kVp controls:
   a. Collimation
   b. Filtration
   c. Output
   d. Quality
   e. SID

9. However, it should be clear that mAs controls quantity and kVp controls:
   a. Filtration and quality
   b. Output and filtration
   c. Quality and quantity
   d. SID and quality
   e. SID and SSD

10. If the mA during fluoroscopy is increased by 25%:
    a. kVp should be reduced by 4.
    b. The effective energy of the beam is increased.
    c. The scatter exposure to the operator is increased by 25%.
    d. The scatter exposure to the operator is reduced by 25%.
    e. The x-ray output is reduced by 25%.

11. A minimum HVL is required for diagnostic x-ray beams because:
    a. A greater HVL would mean lower than average x-ray energy.
    b. A higher HVL would result in an increased absorbed dose to the patient with no improvement in image quality.
    c. A lower HVL would result in an increased absorbed dose to the patient with no improvement in image quality.
    d. A lower HVL would result in reduced subject contrast.
    e. It protects the operator from excessive scatter.

12. An x-ray beam can be made to have higher effective energy if which of the following occurs?
    a. Filtration is added.
    b. Filtration is removed.
    c. mAs is increased.
    d. SID is increased.
    e. SSD is increased.

13. According to the data below, which were obtained at 26 kVp, which of the following is closest to the HVL?

mm Al	0	0.2	0.4	0.6	1.0
mR	94	69	52	39	30

    a. 0.1 mm Al
    b. 0.2 mm Al
    c. 0.3 mm Al
    d. 0.5 mm Al
    e. 1.0 mm Al

14. Which of the following will enhance x-ray beam quality?
    a. Collimation
    b. Filtration
    c. mA
    d. mAs
    e. SID

15. Reducing kVp will do which of the following?
    a. Harden the x-ray beam
    b. Increase the x-ray quality
    c. Increase the x-ray quantity
    d. Require removal of filtration
    e. Soften the x-ray beam

16. Adding filtration to an x-ray beam will do which of the following?
    a. Decrease x-ray quality
    b. Increase inherent filtration
    c. Increase x-ray quality
    d. Increase x-ray quantity
    e. Reduce scatter radiation

17. A radiographic tube has 0.5 mm Al inherent filtration, 1.0 mm Al added filtration, and 1.0 mm Al filtration in the light-localizing collimator. Therefore, the total filtration is:
    a. 0.5 mm Al
    b. 1.0 mm Al
    c. 2.0 mm Al
    d. 2.5 mm Al
    e. 4.0 mm Al

Worksheet 8-3
X-Ray Emission
Half-Value Layer

Attenuation is the reduction in x-ray beam intensity resulting from photoelectric absorption and Compton scattering of x-rays. The degree of attenuation affects the penetrability of the x-ray beam. Penetrability is one descriptor of the ability of an x-ray beam to pass through tissue and therefore x-ray beam quality. A better descriptor is half-value layer (HVL). The HVL of an x-ray beam is the thickness of absorbing material necessary to reduce the x-ray intensity to half its original value.

The approximate HVL for a diagnostic x-ray beam is:

0.3 mm Pb

3.0 mm Al

3 cm of soft tissue

EXERCISES

1. A representative radiographic tube has 0.5 mm Al inherent filtration and 2.0 mm Al added filtration. Therefore:
   a. An additional 1.0 mm Al filtration will harden the x-ray beam.
   b. An additional 1.0 mm Al will increase the x-ray quantity.
   c. An additional 1.0 mm Al will increase total filtration to 3.0 mm Al.
   d. An additional 1.0 mm Al will reduce scatter radiation.
   e. The total filtration is 1.5 mm Al.

2. Which of the following is the softest radiation?
   a. Diagnostic x-rays
   b. Grenz rays
   c. Megavoltage x-rays
   d. Orthovoltage x-rays
   e. Supervoltage x-rays

3. The HVL is defined as:
   a. A thickness of attenuator that will double x-ray quantity
   b. A thickness of attenuator that will halve x-ray quantity
   c. Half the required shielding
   d. The mAs value required to double quantity
   e. Twice the required shielding

4. To measure HVL, which of the following is required?
   a. A collimator
   b. A densitometer
   c. A penetrameter
   d. A sensitometer
   e. Aluminum absorbers

5. As the HVL of a beam increases, its penetrability:
   a. Decreases
   b. Decreases as Z^2
   c. Increases
   d. Increases as Z^2
   e. Is unchanged

6. If increasing the kVp increases the HVL, x-ray quantity will:
   a. Decrease
   b. Decrease by kVp^2
   c. Increase
   d. Increase by kVp^2
   e. Not change

7. If the HVL is increased by the addition of 1 mm Al, x-ray quantity will:
   a. Decrease
   b. Decrease by $(mm Al)^2$
   c. Increase
   d. Increase by $(mm Al)^2$
   e. Not change

8. At 70 kVp, the x-ray beam is attenuated in soft tissue approximately:
   a. 0.05%/cm
   b. 0.5%/cm
   c. 5%/cm
   d. 25%/cm
   e. 50%/cm

Examine the following illustration and answer Exercises 9 and 10:

9. The approximate HVL of curve A is closest to:
   a. 1 mm Al
   b. 2 mm Al
   c. 3 mm Al
   d. 4 mm Al
   e. 6 mm Al

10. The approximate HVL of curve B is closest to:
   a. 1 mm Al
   b. 2 mm Al
   c. 3 mm Al
   d. 4 mm Al
   e. 6 mm Al

11. There is a 75% chance that an x-ray will be attenuated by 2 mm of lead. The HVL is:
   a. 0.5 mm Pb
   b. 1.0 mm Pb
   c. 1.5 mm Pb
   d. 2.0 mm Pb
   e. 4.0 mm Pb

12. What occurs when the small rather than the large cathode coil is energized?
   a. Increased cathode heating
   b. Increased x-ray quality
   c. Longer exposures needed
   d. Lower HVL
   e. Smaller effective focal spot

13. Added filtration affects the x-ray beam in what way?
   a. Higher beam quantity
   b. Higher patient dose
   c. Increased beam hardening
   d. Poorer beam quality
   e. Reduced kVp

14. An aluminum filter:
   a. Decreases the intensity of all energies of the x-ray beam
   b. Increases skin dose
   c. Is not necessary below 50 kVp
   d. Of at least 1 cm is required
   e. Reduces the effective energy of the beam

15. If patient thickness is 6 HVLs, what is the approximate intensity at the midline of the patient?
   a. 1%
   b. 5%
   c. 12%
   d. 50%
   e. 75%

16. A diagnostic x-ray beam has an HVL of approximately 3 cm of soft tissue. What percentage of the beam is absorbed by a 21-cm abdomen?
   a. 0 to 10
   b. 10 to 20
   c. 20 to 60
   d. 60 to 90
   e. >90

17. Which is reduced as x-ray energy increases?
   a. Filtration
   b. Projectile-electron energy
   c. Target-electron energy
   d. X-ray frequency
   e. X-ray wavelength

18. An increase in kVp results in an increase in:
   a. Characteristic x-ray energy
   b. Only the bremsstrahlung x-ray emission spectrum
   c. Only the characteristic x-ray emission spectrum
   d. Radiation quality
   e. The maximum x-ray wavelength

19. An x-ray beam HVL can be increased by increasing which of the following?
   a. Filtration
   b. mA
   c. mAs
   d. SID
   e. SSD

20. The HVL is affected most by a change in:
   a. Added filtration
   b. kVp
   c. mAs
   d. SID
   e. X-ray intensity

21. The added filtration in a conventional light-localizing variable aperture collimator is:
   a. 0 mm Al
   b. 0.5 mm Al
   c. 1.0 mm Al
   d. 3.0 mm Al
   e. 10 mm Al

Worksheet 8-3 **X-Ray Emission**

Worksheet 8-4
X-Ray Emission
Filtration

 Three types of x-ray beam filtration exist:

- **Inherent filtration**—This results from the glass or metal envelope of the x-ray tube and the window in the x-ray tube housing. It is usually equivalent to approximately 0.5 mm Al.
- **Added filtration**—This is the result of placing an absorber in the path of the x-ray beam. The absorber, usually 1 to 3 mm Al, is positioned between the collimator and the tube housing.
- **Compensating filtration**—This has nothing to do with patient dose; compensating filters are used specifically for shaping the x-ray intensity over the beam area, so that radiation that reaches the image receptor is more uniform and produces more uniform optical density.

EXERCISES

1. The inherent filtration in a general purpose radiographic x-ray tube is usually equivalent to:
   a. 0 mm Al
   b. 0.1 mm Al
   c. 0.5 mm Al
   d. 1.0 mm Al
   e. 2.5 mm Al

2. The equivalent added filtration provided by a conventional light-localizing, variable-aperture collimator is closest to:
   a. 0 mm Al
   b. 0.5 mm Al
   c. 1.0 mm Al
   d. 2.0 mm Al
   e. 2.5 mm Al

3. The purpose of a wedge filter in diagnostic radiology is to produce:
   a. A harder beam
   b. A softer beam
   c. A uniform x-ray beam intensity at the image receptor
   d. A uniform x-ray beam intensity at the patient
   e. An x-ray beam to fit the image receptor

4. The primary purpose of adding filtration to an x-ray beam is to:
   a. Cause high-energy x-rays to Compton scatter
   b. Protect the film from low-energy x-rays
   c. Remove low-energy electrons
   d. Remove low-energy x-rays
   e. Remove penetrating x-rays

5. An x-ray beam filter has the *greatest* effect on dose reduction to the:
   a. Gonads
   b. Lens
   c. Skin
   d. Thyroid
   e. Whole body

6. X-rays of higher maximum energy can be obtained by doing which of the following?
   a. Increasing filtration
   b. Increasing kVp
   c. Increasing mAs
   d. Reducing inherent filtration
   e. Using a higher Z target

7. The light-localizing, variable-aperture collimator contributes:
   a. No filtration when its light is off
   b. No filtration when its light is on
   c. Scatter x-rays
   d. To added filtration
   e. To inherent filtration

8. If 5 mm Al filtration is added to the x-ray tube:
   a. Contrast resolution will improve.
   b. Motion unsharpness will decrease.
   c. Optical density will decrease.
   d. Patient dose will increase.
   e. Radiographic contrast will increase.

9. An x-ray beam can be made harder by increasing which of the following?
   a. Filtration
   b. mA
   c. mAs
   d. SID
   e. SSD

10. When filtration is added to a normally filtered x-ray beam, the x-ray emission spectrum will:
    a. Decrease in amplitude
    b. Have higher energy discrete lines
    c. Have lower energy discrete lines
    d. Increase in amplitude
    e. Shift to the left

11. Added filtration:
    a. Increases x-ray quantity
    b. Is expensive
    c. Is usually thinner than inherent filtration
    d. Protects the patient from unnecessary radiation exposure
    e. Reduces x-ray quality

12. Inherent filtration:
    a. Consists of sheets of aluminum
    b. Helps harden the x-ray beam
    c. Is approximately 2.0 mm Al
    d. Is mainly due to the light localizer
    e. Tends to decrease with tube age

13. To produce low inherent filtration in an x-ray beam:
    a. A thin section of glass is used.
    b. Insulating oil is placed around the tube.
    c. kVp should be reduced.
    d. The collimator should be removed.
    e. Windows made of copper are used.

14. Wedge filters are:
    a. Always better than uniform filters because they attenuate a greater number of x-rays
    b. Used for lateral skull examinations
    c. Used to image a knee
    d. Used to match the image receptor
    e. Used to obtain uniform optical density

15. During mammography:
    a. Added filtration is removed to enhance x-ray quality.
    b. Aluminum is the usual filter.
    c. Low total filtration is desirable.
    d. No filtration is required.
    e. The total filtration should be between 2 and 3 mm Al.

16. When added filtration is increased:
    a. kVp must be reduced.
    b. mAs must be reduced.
    c. Effective x-ray energy is reduced.
    d. X-ray quality is enhanced.
    e. X-ray quantity is increased.

17. If a radiographic tube has 0.5 mm Al inherent filtration and 2.0 mm Al added filtration, which of the following is *true?*
    a. Adding 1.0 mm Al will harden the x-ray beam.
    b. Adding 1.0 mm Al will increase the total filtration to 2.5 mm Al.
    c. Adding 1.0 mm Al will increase the x-ray quantity.
    d. Removing 1.0 mm Al will increase HVL.
    e. The total filtration is 1.5 mm Al.

18. Inherent filtration is:
    a. Dependent on the type of aluminum used
    b. Increased when kVp is raised
    c. Increased with patient thickness
    d. Increased with tube age
    e. Produced by slowing down electrons

19. An x-ray tube has a total filtration of 3.0 mm Al and an HVL of 2.5 mm Al, and emits 1.8 mGy_a. Therefore:
    a. The addition of 1.0 mm Al filtration will increase the quantity of the beam.
    b. The addition of 1.0 mm Al will enhance the quality of the beam.
    c. The addition of 2.5 mm Al will reduce the output intensity to 1 mGy_a.
    d. The addition of 2.5 mm Al will reduce the output intensity to 1.35 mGy_a.
    e. The output is also 0.07 mGy_a/mAs.

Worksheet 9-1
X-Ray Interaction with Matter
Compton Effect

X-ray interaction with loosely bound electrons of tissue atoms is responsible for scatter radiation. The incident x-ray interacts with an outer-shell electron of a tissue atom and transfers some of its energy to the electron. After the interaction, the electron is ejected from the atom (the atom is ionized) and the x-ray is scattered. Because the incident x-ray imparts some of its energy to the Compton electron, it loses energy.

The probability that an x-ray will undergo a Compton interaction decreases with increasing x-ray energy. The occurrence of the Compton effect is independent of the atomic number of the absorber. In conventional radiography, more than 70% of the incident x-rays undergo Compton interactions; this interaction contributes to the radiographic noise that reduces contrast.

EXERCISES

1. Which of the following is *not* one of the five basic x-ray interactions with matter?
   a. Bremsstrahlung
   b. Classical scattering
   c. Compton scattering
   d. Photodisintegration
   e. Photoelectric effect

2. Which of the following x-rays would be *most* likely to undergo classical scattering?
   a. 5 keV
   b. 15 keV
   c. 35 keV
   d. 66 keV
   e. 85 keV

3. Which of the following interactions contributes to image noise?
   a. Bremsstrahlung
   b. Characteristic
   c. Compton scattering
   d. Photodisintegration
   e. Photoelectric effect

4. Which of the following occurs in a Compton interaction?
   a. An atom is excited.
   b. An atom is ionized.
   c. The secondary electron has kinetic energy equal to the difference between the energy of the incident x-ray and the electron binding energy.
   d. The secondary electron has kinetic energy equal to the incident x-ray.
   e. The secondary photon has wavelength equal to the primary x-ray.

5. If Ei = incident x-ray energy, E_s = scattered x-ray energy, E_b = electron binding energy, and E_{KE} = secondary electron kinetic energy, then which of the following is *true*?
   a. $E_i = E_s + E_b + E_{KE}$
   b. $E_i = E_s - E_b - E_{KE}$
   c. $E_i = E_s - E_b + E_{KE}$
   d. $E_i = E_s + (E_b - E_{KE})$
   e. $E_i + E_{KE} - (E_b + E_s)$

6. If E_i = incident x-ray energy, E_s = scattered x-ray energy, E_b = electron binding energy, and E_{KE} = secondary electron kinetic energy, then which of the following is *true*?
   a. $E_s = E_b + E_{KE} + E_i$
   b. $E_s = E_b - (E_{KE} + E_i)$
   c. $E_s = E_{KE} - (E_b + E_i)$
   d. $E_s = E_i - (E_b + E_{KE})$
   e. $E_s = E_{KE} + E_i - E_b$

7. During the Compton effect, *most* of the incident x-ray energy is given to which of the following?
   a. Characteristic radiation
   b. Excitation
   c. Electron binding energy
   d. Electron mass
   e. Scattered x-ray

8. After Compton scattering, the scattered x-ray has:
   a. Higher energy
   b. Higher frequency
   c. Less mass
   d. Longer wavelength
   e. Lower velocity

9. Compton interaction affects the image by increasing which of the following?
   a. Contrast resolution
   b. Latitude
   c. Noise (fog)
   d. Spatial resolution
   e. Speed

10. The probability that an x-ray will interact with an outer-shell electron is influenced principally by:
    a. The atomic number of the absorber
    b. The binding energy of the electron
    c. The energy of the incident x-ray
    d. The kinetic energy of the electron
    e. The x-ray production mode

11. The Compton effect is:
    a. Independent of Z
    b. Inversely proportional to Z
    c. Proportional to E
    d. Proportional to Z
    e. Proportional to Z^2

12. The Compton effect is:
    a. Also called classical scattering
    b. The principal source of image noise (fog)
    c. The same as Rayleigh scattering
    d. The same as the Thomson effect
    e. The source of static marks on film

13. If a 45 keV x-ray interacts with the K-shell electron in an atom of molybdenum (E_b = 20 keV) and ejects it with 8 keV energy, what will be the energy of the scattered x-ray?
    a. 12 keV
    b. 17 keV
    c. 25 keV
    d. 37 keV
    e. 45 keV

14. The probability that an x-ray will undergo Compton interaction:
    a. Decreases with increasing x-ray energy
    b. Increases with decreasing electron energy
    c. Increases with increasing electron energy
    d. Increases with increasing x-ray energy
    e. Increases with increasing Z of the target atom

15. The Compton interaction involves so-called unbound electrons because:
    a. Excitation occurs
    b. Free electrons are ejected
    c. Ionization occurs
    d. K-shell electrons are not involved
    e. They have a very low binding energy

16. Which of the following is the x-ray interaction that does *not* cause ionization?
    a. Classical scattering
    b. Compton scattering
    c. Pair production
    d. Photodisintegration
    e. Photoelectric effect

17. Compton-scattered x-rays:
    a. Are helpful in diagnostic radiology
    b. Have lower energy than the incident x-ray
    c. Improve contrast resolution
    d. Produce image artifacts
    e. Result from bremsstrahlung

90

Worksheet 9-2
X-Ray Interaction with Matter
Photoelectric Effect

 The photoelectric effect occurs when an incident x-ray imparts all its energy to an orbital electron of a tissue atom, usually a K-shell electron. The x-ray disappears, and the orbital electron is ejected from the atom. This electron is a **photoelectron,** and it escapes with kinetic energy equal to the difference between the incident x-ray energy and its binding energy.

The probability that a given x-ray will undergo a photoelectric interaction is **inversely** proportional to the third power of the photon energy ($1/E^3$) and **directly** proportional to the third power of the atomic number (Z^3) of the absorber.

Photoelectric effect results in image contrast. Contrast a gent studies incorporating barium or iodine are successful because the atomic number of these atoms is much higher than that of the atoms of surrounding tissue.

EXERCISES

1. If E_i = incident x-ray energy, E_s = scattered x-ray energy, E_b = electron binding energy, and E_{KE} = photoelectric kinetic energy, then which of the following is *true?*
   a. $E_i = E_s + E_b + E_{KE}$
   b. $E_i = E_s - (E_b + E_{KE})$
   c. $E_i = E_b + E_{KE}$
   d. $E_i = E_b - E_{KE}$
   e. $E_i = E_{KE} - E_b$

2. If E_i = incident x-ray energy, E_s = scattered x-ray energy, E_b = electron binding energy, and E_{KE} = photoelectric kinetic energy, then which of the following is *true?*
   a. $E_{KE} = E_i - E_b$
   b. $E_{KE} = E_i/E_b$
   c. $E_s = E_i - (E_b + E_{KE})$
   d. $E_s = (E_b + E_{KE}) E_i$
   e. $E_i = E_s + E_b + E_{KE}$

3. The photoelectric effect is principally associated with which of the following?
   a. Absorption of an x-ray
   b. Bremsstrahlung x-ray production
   c. Characteristic x-ray production
   d. Electron excitation
   e. Scattering of an x-ray

4. A 50 keV x-ray has a 0.02 chance of photoelectric interaction with muscle (Z = 7.4). What is its chance of interacting with bone (Z = 13.8)?
   a. 0.01
   b. 0.04
   c. 0.07
   d. 0.14
   e. 0.37

5. Which of the following has the lowest effective atomic number?
   a. Air
   b. Bone
   c. Fat
   d. Lung
   e. Muscle

6. Photoelectric interaction with soft tissue is *most* likely with which of the following x-rays?
   a. 0.3 keV
   b. 3.0 keV
   c. 30 keV
   d. 300 keV
   e. 3000 keV

7. During photoelectric interaction:
   a. An electron is emitted from the atom.
   b. An x-ray is emitted from the atom.
   c. Electron excitation results.
   d. The atom is made radioactive.
   e. The incident x-ray reappears with reduced energy.

8. During operation at 80 kVp, which of the following photoelectric interactions is *most* probable?
   a. 30 keV x-ray and bone
   b. 30 keV x-ray and fat
   c. 50 keV x-ray and lung
   d. 70 keV x-ray and bone
   e. 70 keV x-ray and fat

9. The radiographic image is formed principally by which of the following?
   a. Classical scattering
   b. Compton scattering
   c. Off-focus radiation
   d. Photoelectric interactions
   e. Uniform distribution of remnant x-rays

10. A 35 keV x-ray *most* likely will undergo K-shell photoelectric interaction with which of the following?
   a. Barium (E_b = 37 keV)
   b. Calcium (E_b = 4 keV)
   c. Iodine (E_b = 33 keV)
   d. Muscle (E_b <1 keV)
   e. Tungsten (E_b = 69 keV)

11. The probability of photoelectric effect varies as what function of x-ray energy (E)?
   a. E^{-3}
   b. E^{-2}
   c. E
   d. E^2
   e. E^3

12. As a result of photoelectric interaction:
   a. An electron is absorbed.
   b. An electron leaves the atom.
   c. The incident x-ray is scattered.
   d. The incident x-ray leaves the atom with more energy.
   e. The incident x-ray leaves the atom with reduced energy.

13. The photoelectric effect is:
   a. A partially exciting event
   b. A partially ionizing event
   c. A radiation-scattering event
   d. The complete absorption of an electron with the subsequent emission of an x-ray
   e. The complete absorption of an x-ray with the subsequent emission of an electron

14. Lead has a K-shell electron binding energy of 88 keV. Therefore:
   a. An 84 keV x-ray can undergo photoelectric interaction with the K-shell electron.
   b. An 84 keV x-ray can undergo photoelectric interaction with the L-shell electron.
   c. An 87 keV x-ray is more likely to undergo photoelectric interaction with a K-shell electron than is an 84 keV x-ray.
   d. An 87 keV x-ray is more likely to undergo photoelectric interaction with an L-shell electron than is an 84 keV x-ray.
   e. An 87 keV x-ray will be replaced by a 1 keV electron.

15. A 39 keV x-ray interacts through photoelectric effect with a K-shell electron of barium (binding energy 37 keV). Therefore:
   a. The photoelectron will have 2 keV energy.
   b. The photoelectron will have 37 keV energy.
   c. The photoelectron will have 39 keV energy.
   d. The scattered x-ray will have 2 keV energy.
   e. The scattered x-ray will have 37 keV energy.

16. The probability of photoelectric effect varies as what function of target atomic number (Z)?
   a. Z^{-3}
   b. Z^{-2}
   c. Z
   d. Z^2
   e. Z^3

Worksheet 9-3
X-Ray Interaction with Matter
Differential Absorption/Atomic Number

 ■ Only two interactions of the incident x-ray are important to diagnostic x-ray imaging: Compton scattering and the photoelectric effect. The photoelectric effect predominates when low-energy x-rays interact with atoms that have a high atomic number.

■ Compton scattering predominates at high voltage, where it accounts for most of the interactions between x-rays and tissue.

■ Both interactions are equally proportional to mass density.

■ However, the ratio of Compton scattering to photoelectric effect increases with increasing x-ray energy.

■ The pattern of absorption and scatter of the incident x-ray beam caused by atomic number, mass density, and thickness of tissue is called **differential absorption.**

EXERCISES

1. Anatomic structures that readily transmit x-rays:
   a. Are called *radiolucent*
   b. Are called *radiopaque*
   c. Have a high effective atomic number
   d. Have a high probability for photoelectric effect
   e. Usually have high mass density

2. Differential absorption, although a complicated process, is basically the result of differences between:
   a. Compton scattering and photoelectric effect
   b. Compton scattering and transmission
   c. High-E and low-E x-rays
   d. High-Z and low-Z tissue
   e. Photoelectric effect and transmission

3. When a radiograph is taken:
   a. High kVp is preferred for maximum differential absorption.
   b. Low kVp is necessary when soft tissue is imaged because it leads to high Compton effect.
   c. Low kVp is necessary when soft tissue is imaged because it leads to high photoelectric effect.
   d. The most probable interaction is no interaction.
   e. With increasing kVp, differential absorption increases.

4. At what approximate x-ray energy is the probability of a photoelectric interaction in soft tissue equal to the probability of a Compton interaction?
   a. 10 keV
   b. 20 keV
   c. 40 keV
   d. 80 keV
   e. 120 keV

5. Which of the following has the greatest mass density?
   a. Blood
   b. Bone
   c. Fat
   d. Lung
   e. Muscle

6. The colon is imaged during a barium enema examination principally because of differences in:
   a. Beam energy
   b. Beam intensity
   c. Subject atomic number
   d. Subject mass density
   e. Subject mass number

7. Air-contrast studies such as a colon examination are successful principally for which of the following reasons?
   a. High-kVp technique is used.
   b. Low-kVp technique is used.
   c. There are differences in effective x-ray energy.
   d. There are differences in mass density.
   e. X-rays are produced with a continuous-energy spectrum.

8. To optimize x-ray mammography:
   a. High kVp is required to minimize the Compton effect.
   b. High kVp should be used with adequate filtration.
   c. Low kVp is necessary to take advantage of the Compton effect.
   d. Low kVp is required because of the high Z of microcalcifications.
   e. The main x-ray interaction should be the photoelectric effect.

9. Differential absorption between bone and soft tissue occurs principally for which of the following reasons?
   a. There is a difference in effective atomic number.
   b. There is a difference in mass density.
   c. There is a difference in reflectance.
   d. The x-ray beam is monoenergetic.
   e. The x-ray beam is polyenergetic.

10. Angiography with iodinated compounds:
    a. Requires high kVp for high contrast
    b. Works because of Compton effect
    c. Works principally because of differences in effective atomic number
    d. Works principally because of differences in mass density
    e. Would not be possible with monoenergetic x-rays

11. Differential absorption is:
    a. Better with increasing Compton interaction
    b. Better with increasing kVp
    c. Better with thicker anatomy
    d. The difference between those x-rays that are absorbed and those that are reflected
    e. The difference between those x-rays that are absorbed and those that are transmitted

12. As kVp increases, the relative number of x-rays:
    a. That are reflected decreases
    b. That are transmitted decreases
    c. That interact by way of Compton effect increases
    d. That interact by way of the photoelectric effect increases
    e. That interact with tissue decreases

13. In which of the following tissues does differential absorption *most* depend on differences in mass density?
    a. Fat and bone
    b. Lung and bone
    c. Lung and fat
    d. Muscle and bone
    e. Muscle and fat

14. The SI unit of mass density is which of the following?
    a. m^3/g
    b. g/m^3
    c. kg/m^3
    d. Joule
    e. Newton

15. How is photoelectric interaction with tissue related to the mass density (ρ) of the tissue?
    a. It is inversely proportional.
    b. It is inversely proportional to ρ^3.
    c. It is proportional.
    d. It is proportional to ρ^3.
    e. It is unrelated.

16. Lungs are imaged on a chest radiograph principally because of differences in which of the following?
    a. Beam energy
    b. Beam intensity
    c. Tissue atomic number
    d. Tissue mass density
    e. Tissue mass number

Worksheet 9-4
X-Ray Interaction with Matter
Differential Absorption/Mass Density

Differential absorption occurs because of differences in photoelectric absorption and Compton scattering, both of which attenuate the x-ray beam. Image-forming x-rays consist of those transmitted through the patient and the Compton scattered x-rays.

Differential absorption is less with increasing x-ray beam energy. However, the interaction of x-rays with tissue is proportional to the mass density of the tissue regardless of x-ray quantity, quality, or the type of interaction.

EXERCISES

1. Differential absorption between lung and soft tissue occurs principally because of which of the following?
   a. The difference in effective atomic numbers (Z)
   b. The difference in mass density
   c. The x-ray beam is filtered.
   d. The x-ray beam is homogeneous.
   e. The x-ray beam is polyenergetic.

2. The reduction in intensity of an x-ray beam after it passes through tissue is called:
   a. Absorption
   b. Attenuation
   c. Exponential
   d. Interaction
   e. Scattering

3. X-ray transmission decreases exponentially, which also means that:
   a. Beam intensity is reduced abruptly.
   b. The number of x-rays is never reduced to zero.
   c. The x-ray beam becomes more penetrating.
   d. There is a finite thickness for 100% absorption.
   e. X-ray scattering increases.

4. Which of the following plots represents x-ray attenuation in matter?

5. Which process contributes *most* to the radiographic image?
   a. Classical scattering
   b. Compton scattering
   c. Pair production
   d. Photodisintegration
   e. Photoelectric effect

6. High kVp in chest radiography will:
   a. Increase contrast
   b. Increase patient dose
   c. Increase penumbra
   d. Reduce patient dose
   e. Reduce shadowing from rib

7. Increasing kVp in x-ray imaging will:
   a. Increase contrast
   b. Increase filtration
   c. Reduce screen sensitivity
   d. Reduce SID
   e. Reduce skin dose

8. In high-kVp chest radiography, contrast depends *most* upon:
   a. Atomic number
   b. mAs
   c. Mass density
   d. Mass number
   e. SID

9. Microcalcifications are imaged on mammograms principally because of:
   a. Atomic number
   b. Atomic mass
   c. Electron density
   d. Mass density
   e. Optical density

10. More contrast is present from a barium examination than from an iodine examination because:
    a. Barium has a higher atomic number.
    b. Barium has a higher concentration.
    c. Barium has a higher mass attenuation coefficient.
    d. The K edge of Ba is higher.
    e. The luminal size is greater for colon than for ureter.

11. Photoelectric effect is proportional to:
    a. $E^{-1/2}$
    b. $E^{1/2}$
    c. E^3
    d. $Z^{1/2}$
    e. Z^3

12. What will increase the energy of bremsstrahlung radiation?
    a. Filament current
    b. Exposure time
    c. SID
    d. Target material
    e. X-ray tube voltage

13. What is the ideal kVp for a given K edge?
    a. Approximately three times the K edge
    b. Much higher than the K edge
    c. Much lower than the K edge
    d. Slightly higher than the K edge
    e. Slightly lower than the K edge

14. Compton interaction occurs with outer-shell electrons and results in:
    a. Auger electron + photon of lower energy
    b. Conversion electron + photon of lower energy
    c. Electron capture + characteristic x-ray
    d. Recoil electron + photon of higher energy
    e. Reduced grayscale

15. At 60 keV in soft tissue, what predominates?
    a. Classical scattering
    b. Compton scattering
    c. Pair production
    d. Photodisintegration
    e. Photoelectric effect

16. Compton interaction affects the image by increasing which of the following?
    a. Contrast resolution
    b. Latitude
    c. Noise
    d. Spatial resolution
    e. Speed

17. Differential absorption in which of the following tissues is most dependent on differences in mass density?
    a. Fat and bone
    b. Lung and bone
    c. Lung and fat
    d. Muscle and bone
    e. Muscle and fat

18. Fat has a higher concentration of hydrogen than soft tissue, therefore which of the following is higher in fat than soft tissue?
    a. Mass density
    b. Effective atomic number
    c. Electron density
    d. X-ray absorption above 100 keV
    e. X-ray absorption below 30 keV

19. Differential absorption:
    a. Increases with increasing Compton scatter
    b. Increases with increasing kVp
    c. Is the difference between absorbed x-rays and reflected x-rays
    d. Is the difference between absorbed x-rays and transmitted x-rays
    e. Is improved with higher mAs

96

Worksheet 10-1
Film Factors

The characteristic curve, sometimes called an **H & D curve,** describes the relationship between **optical density** and **radiation intensity.** The characteristic curve is helpful in predicting a number of image receptor factors, such as optical density (OD), contrast, speed, and latitude. OD describes the degree of blackening on a film. It is related to the fraction of light transmitted through the exposed and processed film.

Image contrast is the difference between light and dark areas on a radiograph. High-contrast radiographs are nearly white-on-black, whereas low-contrast radiographs are very gray. Latitude is the reciprocal of contrast and describes the range of exposure techniques that will result in an acceptable image.

EXERCISES

1. Which of the following is not necessary for constructing a characteristic curve?
   a. Densitometer
   b. Processor
   c. Sensitometer
   d. Slit camera
   e. Step wedge

2. The diagnostically useful portion of a characteristic curve most often includes which of the following?
   a. The base density
   b. The base density plus fog
   c. The shoulder
   d. The straight-line portion
   e. The toe

3. If the OD of a radiograph is such that only 1% of incident light is transmitted, the OD has a value of:
   a. 0.01
   b. 0.1
   c. 1.0
   d. 2.0
   e. 3.0

4. The generally accepted range of useful ODs on a radiograph is:
   a. 0.1 to 0.25
   b. 0.25 to 2.5
   c. 1.0 to 3.0
   d. 1.5 to 4.0
   e. 3.0 to 5.0

5. Which of the following radiographic techniques should result in the widest exposure latitude?
   a. High kVp, contrast film, high grid ratio
   b. High kVp, direct exposure, high grid ratio
   c. High kVp, latitude film, low grid ratio
   d. Low kVp, direct exposure, high grid ratio
   e. Low kVp, screen film, low grid ratio

6. As the time of film development is increased beyond the manufacturer's recommendations:
   a. Contrast increases
   b. Fog increases
   c. Latitude narrows
   d. Spatial resolution is reduced
   e. Speed decreases

7. An exposure of 100 mR is equal to a log relative exposure of:
   a. 0.2
   b. 0.3
   c. 2.0
   d. 3.0
   e. 4.0

8. When one increases the exposure by four times, that is an increase in log relative exposure of:
   a. 0.1
   b. 0.3
   c. 0.6
   d. 2.0
   e. 4.0

9. Base density refers to which of the following?
   a. A log relative exposure of 0.25
   b. A log relative exposure of 0.5
   c. The fog of the base
   d. The optical density of the base
   e. The physical density of the film

10. Which of the following is the main component of radiographic noise?
    a. Graininess
    b. Quantum mottle
    c. Random mottle
    d. Structure mottle
    e. Uniform mottle

11. An optical density of 3.0 on a radiograph:
    a. Indicates good technique
    b. Indicates higher radiopacity than a density of 4
    c. Indicates underexposure
    d. Is usually on the toe of the characteristic curve
    e. Must be viewed with a hot light

12. Unexposed but processed film may appear cloudy
    and dull because of which of the following?
    a. Average gradient
    b. Base density
    c. Contrast
    d. Latitude
    e. Scatter radiation

Exercises 13 and 14 refer to the following illustration:

13. Which characteristic curve best represents a screen-
    film combination?
    a. A
    b. B
    c. C
    d. D
    e. E

14. Which characteristic curve best represents digital
    x-ray imaging?
    a. A
    b. B
    c. C
    d. D
    e. E

Worksheet 10-2
Geometric Factors

 To obtain a high-quality radiograph, an understanding of geometry is necessary. The x-ray source, the anatomic object, and the image receptor all lie in different planes; therefore, the image will always be larger than the object—a condition called magnification. Under some circumstances (e.g., cerebral angiography, mammography), magnification is desired and planned. Normally, however, it is preferable to have as little magnification as possible.

The degree of magnification is identified by the magnification factor (MF).

$$MF = \frac{\text{Image size}}{\text{Object size}} = \frac{SID}{SOD}$$

The size of the object is rarely accessible for measurement; consequently, the MF usually is determined by the ratio of SID to SOD. SOD usually can be estimated accurately.

Image **distortion** occurs when the object is not positioned in a plane that is parallel to the plane of the image receptor. This situation occurs frequently in clinical practice and is one of the principal reasons why precise patient positioning is necessary.

EXERCISES

1. Image magnification increases with increasing:
   a. Image size
   b. Object size
   c. OID
   d. SID
   e. SOD

2. Distortion primarily occurs:
   a. Because subject anatomy is inclined
   b. Because subject anatomy is thick rather than thin
   c. When improper kVp was selected
   d. When subject anatomy is flat
   e. When subject anatomy lies parallel to the image receptor

3. Distortion:
   a. Can be corrected by proper patient positioning
   b. Is controlled by focal-spot size
   c. Never accompanies magnification
   d. Occurs only lateral to the central axis of the x-ray beam
   e. Occurs only when the image is inclined

4. To reduce magnification, one should do which of the following?
   a. Reduce OID
   b. Reduce SID
   c. Reduce SSD
   d. Use the small focal spot
   e. Use tighter collimation

5. If the SID is 100 cm and an object is placed 20 cm from the image receptor, what is the magnification factor (MF)?
   a. 0.8
   b. 1.0
   c. 1.25
   d. 1.4
   e. 1.6

6. In a particular radiographic examination, the SID is 100 cm and the SOD is 86 cm. The image size-to-object size ratio is approximately:
   a. 0.86:1
   b. 1.12:1
   c. 1.16:1
   d. 2.14:1
   e. 3:1

7. Distortion of an x-ray image results from unequal:
   a. Exposure of the object
   b. Focal spot
   c. Heel effect
   d. Magnification
   e. SID

8. In magnification radiography, when the object is placed equidistant between the source and the image receptor, the size of the image will be:
   a. 1.33 times object size
   b. 2.0 times object size
   c. Four times object size
   d. One-half the object size
   e. The same size as the object

9. A 20 cm object is radiographed at 40 cm from the focal spot, and the SID is 60 cm. The size of the image will be:
   a. 30 cm
   b. 40 cm
   c. 50 cm
   d. 60 cm
   e. 70 cm

99

10. When an object is present to one side of the central axis of the x-ray beam:
    a. Distortion will disappear.
    b. Subject contrast will remain unchanged.
    c. The magnification factor will be larger.
    d. The magnification factor will be smaller.
    e. The magnification factor will remain unchanged.

11. To obtain minimum magnification, one should do which of the following?
    a. Make sure the object is positioned on the central axis.
    b. Position the anatomy close to the image receptor.
    c. Select a short SID.
    d. Select a short SSD.
    e. Use maximum collimation.

12. Which of the following conditions contributes least to image distortion?
    a. A thick object at a short SID
    b. A thin object at a long SID
    c. Angling of the central ray
    d. Object position
    e. Off-axis imaging

13. To minimize magnification, one should do which of the following?
    a. Position the object as close to the image receptor as is practical.
    b. Position the x-ray tube as close to the patient as is practical.
    c. Use high kVp, low mAs.
    d. Use the large focal spot.
    e. Use the small focal spot.

14. A foreshortened image:
    a. Can be corrected by increasing kVp and reducing mAs
    b. Can be corrected by reducing kVp and increasing mAs
    c. Can be corrected by reducing SID
    d. Can never be smaller than the object
    e. Results from an inclined object

15. Image magnification can be reduced with the use of which of the following?
    a. A cone
    b. Increased filtration
    c. Shorter OID
    d. Shorter SID
    e. Shorter SSD

16. Which of the following is not one of the geometric factors that affect radiographic quality?
    a. Collimation
    b. Distortion
    c. Focal-spot size
    d. Magnification
    e. SID

17. The magnification factor is not dependent on:
    a. Focal-spot size
    b. OID
    c. SOD
    d. SSD
    e. SID

18. The magnification factor increases with increasing:
    a. Focal-spot size
    b. OID
    c. SID
    d. SOD
    e. SSD

Worksheet 10-3
Focal-Spot Blur

 The smaller the focal-spot size, the sharper the image. Conversely, the larger the focal-spot size, the greater the image blur and the loss of image detail. This blur is called **focal-spot blur (FSB)** because the focal spot is more of an area than a point.

Focal-spot size is the principal parameter that controls spatial resolution.

The extent of FSB is also affected by the spatial relationships among source, object, and image receptor in a way similar to the relationships that influence magnification and distortion.

Mathematically, the FSB can be calculated as follows:

$$FSB = \text{Effective focal spot} \times \frac{OID}{SOD}$$

Although measurements of FSB usually are made on the central axis, it should be apparent that FSB off of the central axis varies. FSB on the cathode side is larger than that on the anode side. This phenomenon is a consequence of the line-focus principle.

EXERCISES

1. In mammography, which of the following conditions would be most effective in improving the sharpness of detail of microcalcifications near the chest wall?
   a. Positioning the anode on the same side as the chest wall
   b. Positioning the cathode on the same side as the chest wall
   c. Using a long OID
   d. Using a short SID
   e. Using a short SSD

2. Which of the following is most responsible for radiographic spatial resolution?
   a. Film graininess
   b. Focal-spot size
   c. Screen mottle
   d. SID
   e. Use of a grid

3. The sharpness of detail in a radiograph is best increased by the use of which of the following?
   a. High-speed screens
   b. Large focal spot
   c. Long SID
   d. Medium-speed screens
   e. Small focal spot

4. A radiograph that shows a relative lack of FSB would be:
   a. High in contrast
   b. Low in distortion
   c. Low in optical density
   d. Magnified
   e. Sharp in detail

5. An intravenous pyelogram (IVP) is routinely conducted with an anteroposterior projection to:
   a. Improve contrast resolution
   b. Maximize the effect of the contrast medium
   c. Minimize the FSB of the kidneys
   d. Reduce the dose
   e. Use the lowest kVp possible

6. Geometric blur is controlled principally by which imaging system characteristic?
   a. Contrast resolution
   b. Focal-spot size
   c. Noise
   d. Sensitivity
   e. Spatial resolution

7. The best way to minimize FSB without affecting optical density is to use a very:
   a. High-contrast image receptor
   b. Long OID
   c. Long SSD
   d. Short SID
   e. Small focal spot

8. Another term for FSB is:
   a. Actual focal spot
   b. Disumbra
   c. Effective focal spot
   d. Penumbra
   e. Umbra

9. A radiograph of the abdomen is taken at 100 cm SID with a 2.0 mm effective focal spot. If the OID is 10 cm, what is the FSB?
   a. 0.1 mm
   b. 0.2 mm
   c. 0.3 mm
   d. 0.1 cm
   e. 0.2 cm

10. When one images an object lateral to the central axis of the x-ray beam, the FSB will be:
    a. Larger on the anode side
    b. Larger on the cathode side
    c. Magnified
    d. Reduced
    e. The same as on the central axis

11. Increasing which of the following is effective in reducing FSB?
    a. Focal-spot size
    b. kVp
    c. Object size
    d. OID
    e. SID

12. When the focal spot is switched from large to small:
    a. FSB will be greater on the anode side.
    b. kVp must be increased for the same optical density.
    c. mAs must be increased for the same optical density.
    d. Motion blur will be enhanced.
    e. Penumbra will be reduced.

13. FSB can be reduced by:
    a. Increasing focal-spot size
    b. Increasing processing time or temperature
    c. Reducing OID
    d. Reducing SID
    e. Reducing SSD

14. Image contrast is the product of image receptor contrast and:
    a. Focal-spot contrast
    b. Grid contrast
    c. Resolution
    d. Screen contrast
    e. Subject contrast

15. Spatial resolution is principally affected by which of the following?
    a. Film speed
    b. Focal-spot size
    c. kVp
    d. mAs
    e. Screen speed

16. When proper radiographic detail cannot be obtained because of a large OID, what change in technique may be used to improve the detail?
    a. Increase image receptor speed
    b. Increase SID
    c. Increase time
    d. kVp
    e. Reduce mAs

17. For a radiograph with magnification of 2, which of the following focal-spot sizes will limit the FSB to 0.4 mm or less?
    a. 0.2 mm
    b. 0.3 mm
    c. 0.4 mm
    d. 0.5 mm
    e. 0.6 mm

Worksheet 10-4
Subject Factors

Maximizing radiographic contrast and image detail within the limitations of the examination is a principal objective of the radiologic technologist. Radiographic contrast is the product of the film contrast and the subject contrast.

Subject contrast varies with tissue thickness, mass, density, and atomic number. The greater the difference in each of these factors for various tissues, the greater will be the subject contrast. Subject shape also affects subject contrast.

Two factors controlled by the radiologic technologist are kVp and motion. In general, as kVp increases, subject contrast decreases. Blur caused by motion of the patient, tube, or image receptor is called **motion blur** and results in a loss of contrast resolution and spatial resolution.

EXERCISES

1. Which of the following radiographic techniques is likely to produce the best visualization of low subject contrast structures?
   a. 72 kVp, 100 mA, 100 ms
   b. 84 kVp, 200 mA, 100 ms
   c. 93 kVp, 400 mA, 50 ms
   d. 100 kVp, 200 mA, 100 ms
   e. 107 kVp, 800 mA, 25 ms

2. Short exposure times are recommended for radiography of the stomach to do which of the following?
   a. Enhance contrast
   b. Improve spatial resolution
   c. Minimize geometric blur
   d. Reduce magnification
   e. Reduce motion blur

3. An upper gastrointestinal image demonstrates motion blur. To increase image detail, the radiologic technologist could do which of the following?
   a. Increase grid ratio
   b. Increase kVp and reduce exposure time
   c. Increase mA and exposure time
   d. Reduce OID
   e. Reduce SID

4. Certain areas in a radiograph appear blurred while others are sharp. The radiologic technologist probably can adjust for this by doing which of the following?
   a. Increasing SID
   b. Reducing mAs and increasing kVp
   c. Reducing OID
   d. Using a different cassette
   e. Using a smaller focal spot

5. Absorption blur can be reduced by which of the following?
   a. Increasing OID
   b. Increasing kVp
   c. Patient compression
   d. Decreasing SID
   e. Use of contrast media

6. Motion blur gets worse with increasing:
   a. Field size
   b. Grid ratio
   c. Image receptor speed
   d. kVp
   e. Patient movement

7. Subject contrast is:
   a. Film contrast minus radiographic contrast
   b. Radiographic contrast divided by film contrast
   c. Radiographic contrast minus film contrast
   d. Radiographic contrast times film contrast
   e. The sum of radiographic contrast and film contrast

8. Which of the following does not affect subject contrast?
   a. Grid ratio
   b. kVp
   c. mAs
   d. Object shape
   e. Object size

9. Which of the following factors most often affects subject contrast with imaging microcalcifications during mammography?
   a. Atomic number of the microcalcification
   b. Breast mass density
   c. Breast shape
   d. Breast thickness
   e. Mass density of the microcalcification

10. Which of the following anatomic structures should exhibit the greatest subject contrast with muscle?
    a. Bladder
    b. Heart
    c. Kidney
    d. Liver
    e. Lung

11. Absorption blur is most closely related to which of the following?
    a. Film blur
    b. Focal-spot blur
    c. Geometric blur
    d. Object shape
    e. Screen blur

12. Extremity x-ray examination results in which of the following?
    a. High distortion
    b. High noise
    c. High patient dose
    d. Long-scale contrast
    e. Short-scale contrast

13. Subject contrast is enhanced with the use of contrast media because:
    a. Absorption blur is reduced
    b. Compton effect is increased
    c. Focal-spot blur is reduced
    d. Mass density is increased
    e. Photoelectric interaction is increased

14. The principal cause of motion blur is movement of which of the following?
    a. The Bucky mechanism
    b. The image receptor
    c. The patient
    d. The table
    e. The x-ray tube

15. Which of the following will reduce motion blur?
    a. Long exposure time
    b. Short SID
    c. Increased kVp
    d. Increased mAs
    e. Proper patient instructions

16. To improve bony detail in a radiograph, the radiologic technologist could do which of the following?
    a. Decrease kVp and mAs
    b. Decrease kVp and SID
    c. Decrease SID and mAs
    d. Use a faster screen
    e. Use a smaller focal spot

17. Which factor most often reduces the visualization of low-contrast structures on a properly exposed radiograph?
    a. Focal-spot size
    b. Grid ratio
    c. Patient motion
    d. Type of film
    e. Type of screens

18. Sharpness of detail on a radiograph is principally improved by which of the following?
    a. Increasing kVp
    b. Increasing scatter radiation
    c. Reducing image noise
    d. Reducing patient motion
    e. Reducing radiation dose

19. Radiographic spatial resolution is improved by the use of which of the following?
    a. A grid
    b. A larger focal spot
    c. Reduced kVp
    d. Reduced mAs
    e. Slower radiographic intensifying screens

Worksheet 10-5
Improving Radiographic Quality

 The radiologic technologist has many decisions to make before performing a patient examination, each of which will influence the quality of the resultant radiographic image. These decisions relate to choice of equipment, patient preparation and positioning, and selection of radiographic factors from the operating console. In general, a change in the selection of one factor will influence the selection of other factors; however, this is not always the case.

EXERCISES

1. Magnification is reduced by which of the following?
   a. Increasing kVp
   b. Increasing screen speed
   c. Increasing SID and OID
   d. Increasing SID and reducing OID
   e. Reducing focal-spot size

2. Focal-spot blur can be reduced by which of the following?
   a. Increasing kVp
   b. Increasing mAs
   c. Increasing OID
   d. Reducing SOD
   e. Using the small focal spot

3. When radiographic technique factors are adjusted to provide an acceptable image and then filtration is added to the x-ray tube, which of the following will increase?
   a. Average energy of the x-ray beam
   b. Optical density
   c. Patient dose
   d. Radiographic contrast
   e. Spatial resolution

4. Ensuring good screen-film contact also ensures reduced:
   a. Blur
   b. Contrast resolution
   c. Magnification
   d. Patient dose
   e. Radiographic noise

5. Use of contrast media principally affects which of the following?
   a. Blur
   b. Contrast resolution
   c. Mass density
   d. Optical density
   e. Speed

6. Reducing field size through proper collimation usually results in improved:
   a. Blur
   b. Contrast resolution
   c. Magnification
   d. Patient dose
   e. Spatial resolution

7. Which of the following is most often influenced by focal-spot size?
   a. Absorption blur
   b. Contrast resolution
   c. Geometric blur
   d. Motion blur
   e. Patient dose

8. In a radiographic examination of the lumbar spine, which of the following techniques would result in greatest exposure to the patient?
   a. 70 kVp/200 mAs
   b. 80 kVp/100 mAs
   c. 95 kVp/50 mAs
   d. 110 kVp/25 mAs
   e. 120 kVp/25 mAs

9. Which of the following does not affect image blur?
   a. Focal-spot size
   b. kVp
   c. OID
   d. SID
   e. SOD

10. Which of the following is the principal reason for using direct-exposure radiography?
    a. Better resolution of low-contrast tissues
    b. Better spatial resolution
    c. Higher contrast
    d. Less motion blur
    e. Lower patient dose

11. If other factors remain constant, which of the following would result in the highest optical density?
    a. 100 mA, 750 ms, 90 cm SID
    b. 200 mA, 500 ms, 90 cm SID
    c. 300 mA, 300 ms, 100 cm SID
    d. 400 mA, 200 ms, 100 cm SID
    e. 500 mA, 100 ms, 100 cm SID

12. An anteroposterior examination of the abdomen is taken at 80 kVp, 50 mAs, and 100 cm SID. If the scale of contrast is to be shortened, the radiologic technologist must do which of the following?
    a. Increase both mAs and kVp
    b. Reduce both mAs and kVp
    c. Reduce kVp and increase mAs
    d. Reduce mAs and increase kVp
    e. Shorten the SID

13. Assume that the usual exposure time for a lateral cervical spine radiograph at 100 cm SID is 100 ms. At an SID of 90 cm, all other factors remaining the same, the correct exposure time would be:
    a. 10 ms
    b. 25 ms
    c. 50 ms
    d. 80 ms
    e. 180 ms

14. When radiographic technique factors are adjusted to obtain an acceptable image, patient dose will increase as which of the following increases?
    a. Film speed
    b. Grid ratio
    c. SID
    d. SOD
    e. SSD

15. Geometric blur can be reduced by which of the following?
    a. Improving film-screen contact
    b. Increasing processing time or temperature
    c. Increasing SID and OID
    d. Increasing SSD and OID
    e. Reducing focal-spot size

16. When technique factors are adjusted to obtain an acceptable image, motion blur will increase with which of the following?
    a. Increase in focal-spot size
    b. Increased field size
    c. Low-ratio grid (compared with high-ratio grid)
    d. Reduced total filtration
    e. Slow radiographic intensifying screens (compared with fast screens)

17. With other factors constant, optical density will increase with increasing:
    a. Focal-spot size
    b. Grid ratio
    c. mAs
    d. SID
    e. SSD

18. Radiographic contrast is increased by which of the following?
    a. Increasing grid ratio
    b. Raising kVp
    c. Reducing the air gap
    d. Reducing the heel effect
    e. Using a slower film

19. When the mAs is adjusted to provide constant optical density after an increase in kVp:
    a. Absorption blur is reduced
    b. Geometric blur is reduced
    c. Latitude is reduced
    d. Motion blur is reduced if the same mA is used
    e. Spatial resolution will improve

Worksheet 10-6
Patient Factors

 The radiologic technologist has control over the following: exposure technique factors, patient factors, and image quality factors.

Radiographic technique is the selection of the proper x-ray exposure factors with the x-ray imaging system necessary to produce a high-quality radiograph.

The two principal patient factors are the thickness of the body part that is being examined and its composition. In general, the thicker and more dense the part is, the higher the settings should be for voltage and milliampere-seconds.

EXERCISES

1. The chest represents high-contrast anatomy (high subject contrast). Therefore, which of the following is most appropriate?
   a. High kVp
   b. High mAs
   c. Long SID
   d. Low kVp
   e. Low mAs

2. The anatomic part to be examined must be measured because:
   a. A change of focal spots may be required.
   b. A different image receptor may be required.
   c. The mass density of the part is determined by thickness.
   d. The selected radiographic technique depends on anatomy thickness.
   e. The SSD changes with anatomy thickness.

3. When fixed kVp technique is used for various anatomic thicknesses, a change will be required in which of the following?
   a. Added filtration
   b. kVp
   c. mAs
   d. SID
   e. SSD

4. The anatomic part must be measured for variable kVp technique because a change will be required in which of the following?
   a. Added filtration
   b. kVp
   c. mAs
   d. SID
   e. SSD

5. In the diagnostic x-ray range, the smallest change in kVp that can be perceived on the radiographic image is approximately:
   a. 2 kVp
   b. 4 kVp
   c. 6 kVp
   d. 8 kVp
   e. 12 kVp

6. In general, a chest radiograph should be taken with:
   a. A generalization about this is not possible; decisions are dependent on thickness.
   b. High kVp and high mAs
   c. High kVp and low mAs
   d. Low kVp and high mAs
   e. Low kVp and low mAs

7. What is the approximate mass density of lung tissue?
   a. $0.32 \ g/cm^3$
   b. $0.85 \ g/cm^3$
   c. $1.0 \ g/cm^3$
   d. $1.85 \ g/cm^3$
   e. $4.0 \ g/cm^3$

8. In general, a mammogram should be taken with:
   a. A generalization about this is not possible; decisions are dependent on thickness.
   b. High kVp and high mAs
   c. High kVp and low mAs
   d. Low kVp and high mAs
   e. Low kVp and low mAs

9. What is the effective atomic number of fat?
   a. 6.3
   b. 7.4
   c. 7.6
   d. 10.5
   e. 13.8

10. What is the approximate mass density of bone?
    a. $0.001 \ g/cm^3$
    b. $0.85 \ g/cm^3$
    c. $1.0 \ g/cm^3$
    d. $1.85 \ g/cm^3$
    e. $4.0 \ g/cm^3$

11. What is the effective atomic number of lung tissue?
    a. 6.3
    b. 7.4
    c. 7.6
    d. 10.5
    e. 13.8

12. What is the effective atomic number of soft tissue?
    a. 6.3
    b. 7.4
    c. 7.6
    d. 10.5
    e. 13.8

13. What is the approximate mass density of fat?
    a. 0.001 g/cm^3
    b. 0.91 g/cm^3
    c. 1.0 g/cm^3
    d. 1.85 g/cm^3
    e. 4.0 g/cm^3

14. What is the effective atomic number of bone?
    a. 6.3
    b. 7.4
    c. 7.6
    d. 10.5
    e. 13.8

15. For a given anatomic part, the smallest change in mAs that can be perceived on the radiographic image is approximately:
    a. 5%
    b. 15%
    c. 30%
    d. 50%
    e. 70%

16. What is the mass density of soft tissue?
    a. 0.001 g/cm^3
    b. 0.85 g/cm^3
    c. 1.0 g/cm^3
    d. 1.85 g/cm^3
    e. 4.0 g/cm^3

17. Which of the following tissue characteristics is most important when photoelectric interaction prevails, as in mammography?
    a. Effective atomic number
    b. Electron density
    c. Mass density
    d. Optical density
    e. Tissue shape

18. Which of the following tissue characteristics is most important when Compton interaction prevails, as in computed tomography?
    a. Effective atomic number
    b. Electron density
    c. Mass density
    d. Optical density
    e. Tissue shape

Worksheet 10-7
Image Quality Factors

 Radiographic technique factors set by the radiologic technologist consist of current, exposure time (ms), voltage, and SID (cm). These factors influence the radiographic exposure to the patient. The selected combination of these factors determines the quality of the radiograph. **Image quality factors** refers to terms used to evaluate the characteristics of a radiographic image. The principal terms are **optical density, contrast, definition,** and **distortion.**

The radiologic technologist selects a combination of exposure technique factors to produce a radiograph with an acceptable scale of contrast; the correct optical density and spatial and contrast resolution; and a minimum distortion of the image.

EXERCISES

1. If a radiographic technique calling for 100 mA at 100 ms is changed to 50 mA at 2000 ms:
   a. Grayscale contrast will become longer.
   b. Grayscale contrast will become shorter.
   c. There will be no change in grayscale contrast.
   d. There will be no change in exposed time.
   e. There will be no change in x-ray tube capacity.

2. A longer grayscale on a radiograph can be obtained by doing which of the following?
   a. Increasing kVp
   b. Increasing mAs
   c. Reducing kVp
   d. Reducing mAs
   e. Using a larger focal spot

3. For a mobile abdominal radiographic examination, radiographic contrast can be increased by doing which of the following?
   a. Increasing the kVp and decreasing the mAs
   b. Increasing the OID
   c. Increasing the SID
   d. Using a faster image receptor
   e. Using a high-ratio grid

4. A radiograph that exhibits a long grayscale contrast has which of the following features?
   a. Few shades of gray that have great differences
   b. Few shades of gray that have minimal differences
   c. Good spatial resolution
   d. Many shades of gray that have great differences
   e. Many shades of gray that have minimal differences

5. From the following set of exposure technique factors, select the set that is most likely to produce a radiograph with the best spatial resolution:
   a. A
   b. B
   c. C
   d. D
   e. E

	mAs	kVp	OID	SID	Focal Spot	Image Receptor
A	10	60	8 cm	90 cm	2.0 mm	High speed
B	20	68	10 cm	90 cm	2.0 mm	High speed
C	25	72	5 cm	180 cm	1.0 mm	Medium speed
D	30	86	5 cm	90 cm	1.0 mm	Medium speed
E	50	94	4 cm	100 cm	100 cm	Medium speed

6. Which of the preceding exposure technique factors would result in the worst spatial resolution?
   a. A
   b. B
   c. C
   d. D
   e. E

7. If a radiographic technique designed for an 8:1 grid is changed to accommodate a 10:1 grid:
   a. Grayscale contrast will become longer.
   b. Grayscale contrast will become shorter.
   c. There will be no change in contrast resolution.
   d. There will be no change in grayscale contrast.
   e. There will be no change in x-ray tube capacity.

8. Which of the following is the function of optimizing contrast?
   a. To control detail sharpness
   b. To control quantum mottle
   c. To determine optical density
   d. To improve spatial resolution
   e. To make detail visible

9. A radiographic technique that would ensure visibility of detail for a cervical spine is:
   a. Increasing the OID
   b. Reducing the SID
   c. Reducing the SSD
   d. Selecting the large focal spot
   e. Using a beam restriction device

10. A radiograph was made using these factors: 200 mA, 300 ms, 70 kVp, 100 cm SID. A mobile radiograph is then conducted at 80 cm. To maintain the same optical density, approximately what mAs should be selected?
    a. 15 mAs
    b. 20 mAs
    c. 28 mAs
    d. 38 mAs
    e. 48 mAs

Exercises 11 through 14 refer to the following exposure technique factors:
   a. 100 mA, 500 ms, 60 kVp, no grid
   b. 200 mA, 750 ms, 50 kVp, 16:1 grid
   c. 400 mA, 100 ms, 60 kVp, no grid
   d. 600 mA, 700 ms, 70 kVp, 8:1 grid
   e. 800 mA, 200 ms, 80 kVp, 8:1 grid

11. Which technique factors should result in the greatest latitude?
    a. A
    b. B
    c. C
    d. D
    e. E

12. Which technique factors should result in the highest contrast?
    a. A
    b. B
    c. C
    d. D
    e. E

13. Which technique factors should result in the highest optical density?
    a. A
    b. B
    c. C
    d. D
    e. E

14. Which technique factors should result in the highest patient dose?
    a. A
    b. B
    c. C
    d. D
    e. E

Worksheet 10-8
Radiographic Technique Charts

 Radiographic technique charts are guides that are prepared for specific x-ray imaging systems for the purpose of assisting radiologic technologists in selecting exposure factors for each radiographic procedure.

There are four types of radiographic technique charts: variable kilovoltage, fixed kilovoltage, high kilovoltage, and automatic exposure.

For the variable-kilovoltage chart, voltage is adjusted for different tissue thickness. The fixed-kilovoltage chart uses an optimum voltage selection for each body part, and the milliampere-seconds setting is the variable used to accommodate for differences in tissue thickness.

High kilovoltage means that the voltage selection is in excess of 100 kVp. Radiographic technique charts of this type are used primarily for barium studies and chest radiography. The automatic exposure chart serves as a guide for control panel selections when automatic exposure control systems are used.

EXERCISES

1. Which of the following technique charts provides the least amount of patient radiation exposure?
   a. Anatomically programmed radiography (APR)
   b. Automatic exposure
   c. Fixed kilovoltage
   d. High kilovoltage
   e. Variable kilovoltage

2. Accuracy in positioning the patient is most critical with which of the following?
   a. APR
   b. Automatic exposure
   c. Fixed-kilovoltage technique chart
   d. High-kilovoltage technique chart
   e. Variable-kilovoltage technique chart

3. Before a radiographic technique chart is prepared, which of the following would be most important?
   a. Calculating the mAs distance rule
   b. Calibrating the x-ray imaging system
   c. Marking all kVp stations on the control panel
   d. Marking each image receptor
   e. Measuring the part size with calipers

4. Which of the following is a basic characteristic of the variable-kilovoltage chart?
   a. Large focal spot
   b. Long scale of contrast
   c. Low mAs selection
   d. Short exposure time
   e. Short scale of contrast

5. Which of the following is the procedure for selection of the kVp for a body part when the variable-kilovoltage chart is used?
   a. Measure the part, multiply by 2, and then add 30.
   b. Measure the part, multiply by 5, and then add 30.
   c. Preselect the kVp, and multiply the mAs by 2.
   d. Preselect the kVp, multiply by 2, and then add 20.
   e. Preselect the kVp, multiply by 2, and then add 30.

6. Which of the following will increase exposure latitude?
   a. Automatic exposure
   b. Faster image receptor
   c. Fixed-kilovoltage chart
   d. High-kilovoltage chart
   e. Variable-kilovoltage chart

7. The optical density present on the radiograph can best be controlled by which of the following?
   a. Collimation
   b. Focal-spot size
   c. kVp
   d. mAs
   e. Measurement of the part

8. Penetration of the anatomic part by the x-ray beam can best be controlled by which of the following?
   a. Calibration of the equipment
   b. kVp
   c. mAs
   d. Measurement of the part
   e. Tissue thickness

9. Which of the following procedures would make best use of a high-kilovoltage chart?
   a. Barium enema
   b. Chest
   c. Knee
   d. Mammography
   e. Pelvis

10. Which of the following technique charts requires accurate measurement?
    a. Automatic exposure control
    b. Combination fixed and variable
    c. Fixed kilovoltage
    d. High kilovoltage
    e. Variable kilovoltage

11. Which of the following technique charts requires higher patient radiation dose?
    a. Automatic exposure control
    b. Combination fixed and variable kilovoltage
    c. Fixed kilovoltage
    d. High kilovoltage
    e. Variable kilovoltage

12. Which of the following technique charts has the shortest scale of contrast?
    a. Automatic exposure control
    b. Combination fixed and variable kilovoltage
    c. Fixed kilovoltage
    d. High kilovoltage
    e. Variable kilovoltage

13. Which of the following technique charts has the least exposure latitude?
    a. Automatic exposure control
    b. Combination fixed and variable kilovoltage
    c. Fixed kilovoltage
    d. High kilovoltage
    e. Variable kilovoltage

14. Which of the following technique charts requires accurate patient positioning?
    a. Automatic exposure control
    b. Combination fixed and variable kilovoltage
    c. Fixed kilovoltage
    d. High kilovoltage
    e. Variable kilovoltage

15. Which of the following technique charts recommends a 2 kVp change for each centimeter of thickness?
    a. Automatic exposure control
    b. Combination fixed and variable kilovoltage
    c. Fixed kilovoltage
    d. High kilovoltage
    e. Variable kilovoltage

16. Which of the following technique charts requires no specific mAs selection?
    a. Automatic exposure control
    b. Combination fixed and variable kilovoltage
    c. Fixed kilovoltage
    d. High kilovoltage
    e. Variable kilovoltage

17. Which of the following technique charts results in higher contrast?
    a. Automatic exposure control
    b. Combination fixed and variable kilovoltage
    c. Fixed kilovoltage
    d. High kilovoltage
    e. Variable kilovoltage

Worksheet 11-1
Production of Scatter Radiation

Scatter radiation results from Compton interaction with patient tissue and reduces image contrast. Three principal factors influence the quantity of scatter radiation. Two of these can be manipulated by the radiologic technologist.

- **Kilovoltage (kVp):** Increasing kVp also increases the proportion of scatter radiation because the Compton effect predominates at higher energies.
- **Field size:** Scatter radiation increases with increasing field size because more tissue is exposed.
- **Patient thickness:** Scatter radiation increases as patient thickness increases. X-ray beam collimation and tissue compression reduce scatter radiation and therefore improve image contrast.

EXERCISES

1. Remnant x-rays are those that:
   a. Are absorbed within the patient
   b. Do not interact with the patient or the image receptor
   c. Exit the patient
   d. Interact with the patient and are scattered away
   e. Scatter back toward the source

2. Which of the following factors that affect scatter radiation can be controlled by the radiologic technologist?
   a. Added filtration
   b. Field size
   c. Inherent filtration
   d. mAs
   e. Patient thickness

3. As kVp increases, scatter radiation production will:
   a. Decrease because of less Compton interaction
   b. Decrease because of less photoelectric interaction
   c. Increase because of more Compton interaction
   d. Increase because of more photoelectric interaction
   e. Remain unchanged

4. What is the approximate percentage of x-rays that are transmitted through a patient?
   a. 0.1%
   b. 1%
   c. 5%
   d. 10%
   e. 20%

5. At high kVp (e.g., 125 kVp), most x-rays are:
   a. Backscattered
   b. Not transmitted through the body
   c. Remnant x-rays
   d. Transmitted through the body with interaction
   e. Transmitted through the body without interaction

6. When kVp is increased with a compensating reduction in mAs, which of the following is reduced?
   a. Optical density
   b. Patient dose
   c. Remnant radiation
   d. Scatter proportion
   e. Spatial resolution

7. If a constant optical density is maintained while kVp is increased:
   a. Collimation should be enlarged.
   b. Collimation should be reduced.
   c. Contrast resolution will improve.
   d. Patient dose will decrease.
   e. Patient dose will increase.

8. As field size is increased, scatter radiation:
   a. Increases
   b. Is reduced
   c. Is removed
   d. Is reversed
   e. Remains constant

9. Which of the following is not a device designed to reduce the level of scatter radiation that reaches the image receptor?
   a. A beam restrictor
   b. A collimator
   c. A compression device
   d. A diaphragm
   e. A test pattern

10. Scatter radiation reduces radiographic quality by changing:
    a. Blurring
    b. Contrast
    c. Distortion
    d. Mass density
    e. Optical density

11. X-rays that the technologist would like to have interact with the image receptor are those that are:
    a. Absorbed in the body
    b. Attenuated in the body
    c. High energy
    d. Scattered in the body
    e. Transmitted in the body

12. As kVp is increased from 70 to 80 reaching the IR:
    a. Contrast resolution will improve.
    b. The mAs must be increased.
    c. The SID must be increased.
    d. There will be a higher proportion of scatter radiation.
    e. There will be a lower proportion of scatter radiation.

13. Image-forming x-rays consist of which following type that emerge from the patient in the direction of the image receptor?
    a. Absorbed x-rays
    b. Backscattered x-rays
    c. Emitted x-rays
    d. Intercepted x-rays
    e. Transmitted x-rays

14. As kVp increases from 70 to 90, if all other factors remain constant:
    a. Contrast resolution will improve.
    b. The number of absorbed x-rays will decrease.
    c. The number of transmitted x-rays will decrease.
    d. The ratio of absorbed to transmitted x-rays will increase.
    e. The ratio of scattered to transmitted x-rays will increase.

15. What increases as the field size of the x-ray beam increases?
    a. Heel effect
    b. kVp
    c. mAs
    d. Scatter radiation
    e. Total filtration

16. In general, as the thickness of the anatomy for which radiographs are made increases:
    a. Contrast resolution improves.
    b. kVp is increased.
    c. mAs is increased.
    d. Patient exposure is unaffected.
    e. Total filtration is increased.

17. Which of the following processes is most responsible for the production of scatter radiation?
    a. Bremsstrahlung interaction
    b. Characteristic interaction
    c. Compton effect
    d. Photoelectric effect
    e. Transmission

Worksheet 11-2
Control of Scatter Radiation

 Beam-restricting devices are used in radiology to limit the volume of tissue irradiated to reduce patient dose and scatter radiation. Three types of beam-restricting devices exist:

- **Aperture diaphragm:** A fixed-aperture device that consists of a lead or lead-lined metal diaphragm attached to the head of the x-ray tube.
- **Cones and cylinders:** Fixed-aperture devices that consist of an extended metal structure attached to the x-ray tube head.
- **Variable-aperture collimator:** A device that consists of two or more pairs of lead shutters that are independently adjustable. Square or rectangular fields are possible, and the x-ray field can be illuminated by a coincidence light field. **Positive-beam–limiting (PBL)** devices automatically collimate to the image receptor size.

EXERCISES

1. Which of the following is not a beam-restricting device?
   a. A cone
   b. A PBL device
   c. A variable-aperture collimator
   d. Added filtration

2. An aperture diaphragm should allow x-rays to expose an area:
   a. Equal to the image receptor
   b. Just larger than the image receptor
   c. Just smaller than the image receptor
   d. That varies according to patient size
   e. That varies according to technique

3. When an aperture diaphragm is used:
   a. A PBL device is required.
   b. Added filtration should be increased.
   c. Grid cutoff can occur if the diaphragm is not properly positioned.
   d. Technique should be enhanced.
   e. X-ray field cutoff can occur if the diaphragm is not properly positioned.

4. In a light-localizing, variable-aperture collimator:
   a. Added filtration is required.
   b. Equipped with a PBL device, light field illumination is unnecessary.
   c. If the lightbulb burns out, the graduated scale on the adjusting mechanism can be used.
   d. It is not necessary to center the crosshairs in the light beam.
   e. Periodic checks of x-ray beam and light field coincidence are necessary.

5. Which of the following is the simplest of all beam-restricting devices?
   a. A fluoroscopic collimator
   b. A radiographic cone
   c. An aluminum filter
   d. An aperture diaphragm
   e. PBL

6. Which of the following devices is normally designed to limit off-focus radiation?
   a. Added filtration
   b. First-stage shutters of a variable-aperture collimator
   c. Fixed-aperture circular diaphragms
   d. Fixed-aperture rectangular diaphragms
   e. Second-stage shutters of a variable-aperture collimator

7. Off-focus radiation:
   a. Consists of scattered electrons
   b. Consists of scattered electrons and x-rays
   c. Improves image quality
   d. Increases patient dose
   e. Results when projectile electrons do not strike the focal spot

8. Which of the following is a beam-restricting device?
   a. 2.5 mm Al added filtration
   b. A cone without an integral diaphragm
   c. A rectangular film mask on a viewbox
   d. A fluoroscopic spot-film device
   e. PBL

9. Cone cutting:
   a. Is useful in high-kVp examinations
   b. Is useful in low-kVp examinations
   c. Occurs when the axis of the cone, tube, and image receptor are not aligned
   d. Occurs when the edge of the cone intercepts the scattered x-ray beam
   e. Occurs when the tip of the cone is too close to the patient

10. If a fixed-aperture, rectangular, beam-restricting device is used:
    a. Added filtration is unnecessary.
    b. An unexposed border should be visible on all four sides of the radiograph.
    c. An unexposed border should be visible on at least two sides of the radiograph.
    d. PBL must be used.
    e. The central axis of the aperture diaphragm must be centered somewhere on the image receptor.

11. A properly designed, light-localizing, variable-aperture collimator:
    a. Concentrates off-focus radiation onto the image receptor
    b. Is designed to enhance off-focus radiation
    c. Needs no added filtration
    d. Requires light field/x-ray beam coincidence
    e. Will have field-defining shutters of aluminum

12. Radiographic cones and cylinders are used principally to reduce which of the following?
    a. Beam quality
    b. Off-focus radiation
    c. Scatter radiation
    d. The need for added filtration
    e. The required radiographic technique

13. Which of the following are the two general types of devices designed to control scatter radiation?
    a. Filtration and beam restrictors
    b. Filtration and image masks
    c. Grids and beam restrictors
    d. Grids and filtration
    e. Image masks and beam restrictors

14. When a diaphragm is used:
    a. A 1-cm unexposed border should be visible on all sides.
    b. A 1-cm unexposed border should be visible on two sides.
    c. A 3-cm unexposed border should be visible on at least three sides.
    d. Added filtration must be increased.
    e. An unexposed border is not necessary.

15. PBL stands for which of the following?
    a. Photon beam level
    b. Photon beam limitation
    c. Photon border level
    d. Positive beam level
    e. Positive beam limitation

16. A diaphragm is machined to just match image receptor size. If an unexposed border is required on the radiograph, the diaphragm opening will:
    a. Have to be enlarged
    b. Have to be reduced
    c. More information is required before a change can be determined
    d. Remain the same
    e. Require additional filtration

17. An aperture diaphragm is designed for 25-cm × 30-cm film. If the SID is 100 cm and the source-to-diaphragm distance is 10 cm, what size should the opening of the diaphragm be?
    a. 2.0 cm × 2.5 cm
    b. 2.0 cm × 3.0 cm
    c. 2.5 cm × 3.0 cm
    d. 2.5 cm × 3.5 cm
    e. 3.0 cm × 3.5 cm

Worksheet 11-3
Characteristics of Grid Construction

X-rays that leave a patient and are incident on the image receptor are called image-forming radiation. There are two basic components of image-forming radiation: (1) those x-rays that have passed directly through the patient without interaction, and (2) those x-rays that have been scattered within the patient. Only the x-rays that are not significantly scattered carry useful diagnostic information to the image receptor.

Scattered x-rays are the result of Compton interaction. Because the image receptor is not capable of distinguishing primary x-rays from scattered x-rays, it will image a scattered x-ray as having come directly from the x-ray source, when, in fact, its direction was from the tissue from which it was scattered. This scattered radiation reduces image contrast.

The main device used to intercept scattered radiation is the grid. There are two principal characteristics of grid construction: (1) grid ratio is the thickness of the grid (the height of the grid strip) divided by the width of the interspace material; and (2) grid frequency is the number of grid strips per inch or per centimeter.

EXERCISES

1. The principal reason for using a grid is to:
   a. Enhance differential absorption
   b. Improve image contrast
   c. Improve spatial resolution
   d. Reduce patient dose
   e. Remove remnant radiation

2. Which of the following materials would be most radiolucent?
   a. Aluminum
   b. Carbon fiber
   c. Copper
   d. Iodine
   e. Lead

3. Which of the following is the most important grid characteristic?
   a. Grid frequency
   b. Grid height
   c. Grid mass
   d. Grid ratio
   e. Grid weight

4. In a grid that has lead strips 0.5 mm apart and 4 mm high, the grid ratio is:
   a. 4:1
   b. 6:1
   c. 8:1
   d. 12:1
   e. 16:1

5. A grid has the following characteristics: grid ratio = 10:1; grid height = 4.5 mm; grid strip width = 40 µm; and interspace width = 450 µm. What is the grid frequency?
   a. 20 lines/cm
   b. 22 lines/cm
   c. 40 lines/cm
   d. 45 lines/cm
   e. 60 lines/cm

6. If only scatter radiation reached the image receptor:
   a. Image contrast would be very high.
   b. Image contrast would be very low.
   c. Image receptor speed would be very high.
   d. Image receptor speed would be very low.
   e. Spatial resolution would be improved.

7. In the design of a radiographic grid, which of the following must be true?
   a. The added filtration must be aluminum.
   b. The grid strips are radiolucent.
   c. The grid strips are radiotransparent.
   d. The interspace material is radiolucent.
   e. The interspace material is radiopaque.

8. Grids are principally effective in attenuating which of the following?
   a. All remnant radiation
   b. Photoelectrons
   c. Transmitted x-rays
   d. X-rays after Compton interaction
   e. X-rays after photoelectric interaction

9. If the interspace dimension is constant, increasing the grid ratio will:
   a. Make the grid lighter
   b. Make the grid thicker
   c. Reduce grid mass
   d. Require less grid strip material
   e. Require less interspace material

10. As grid frequency increases, (choose all that apply):
    a. Grid mass is usually decreased.
    b. The grid ratio is reduced if the thickness of the grid remains constant.
    c. The interspace width becomes thinner if the width of the grid strip remains constant.
    d. The number of grid strips per centimeter increases.
    e. The patient dose is reduced.

11. Which of the following would be the most acceptable grid strip material from the standpoint of x-ray attenuation?
    a. Barium
    b. Copper
    c. Iodine
    d. Tungsten
    e. Uranium

12. Which of the following will not improve image contrast?
    a. A decrease in kVp
    b. Collimating the x-ray beam
    c. The use of a grid
    d. The use of added filtration
    e. The use of positive-beam limitation (PBL)

13. Grids with a high ratio are:
    a. Easier to manufacture than those with a low ratio
    b. More effective than those with a low ratio
    c. Most effective at low kVp
    d. Produced by increasing grid strip width
    e. Produced by increasing interspace width

14. The efficiency of a grid for reducing scatter radiation is related principally to which of the following?
    a. Grid frequency
    b. Grid interspace
    c. Grid mass
    d. Grid radius
    e. Grid ratio

15. Radiographic grids:
    a. Can be placed anywhere between the source and the image receptor
    b. Can be placed between the patient and the image receptor
    c. Can be placed between the source and the patient
    d. Must be placed between the patient and the image receptor
    e. Must be placed between the source and the patient

16. The construction of a radiographic grid:
    a. Has an aluminum cover for filtration
    b. Has an aluminum cover to reduce scatter radiation
    c. Incorporates aluminum or copper as the grid strip material
    d. Incorporates high Z interspace material
    e. Is easier to achieve with an aluminum interspace than with plastic fiber

17. Use of which of the following will reduce radiographic contrast?
    a. Collimators
    b. Filtration
    c. Grids
    d. Intensifying screens
    e. PBL

Worksheet 11-4
Measuring Grid Performance

 The principal function of a radiographic grid is to absorb scattered radiation from the image-forming x-ray beam before it reaches the image receptor. If scattered radiation does reach the image receptor, image contrast is reduced. The function of radiographic grids is to increase image contrast.

The higher the grid ratio and the higher the grid frequency, the greater will be the image contrast. The principal measure of grid performance is the contrast improvement factor, k:

$$K = \frac{\text{Radiographic contrast with a grid}}{\text{Radiographic contrast without a grid}}$$

Another measure of grid performance is selectivity:

$$\text{Selectivity} = \frac{\text{Transmitted primary x-rays}}{\text{Transmitted scattered x-rays}}$$

Both the contrast improvement factor and selectivity depend on the characteristics of the x-ray beam and the characteristics of the grid. However, the contrast improvement factor depends more on the characteristics of the x-ray beam, whereas selectivity depends more on the construction of the grid.

EXERCISES

1. Which of the following is the least important indicator of grid performance?
   a. Contrast improvement factor
   b. Grid frequency
   c. Grid mass
   d. Grid strip height
   e. Grid ratio

2. The contrast improvement factor is defined as the radiographic contrast obtained:
   a. At a density of 1
   b. At a density of 1.0 above base plus fog
   c. With a grid compared with that obtained without a grid
   d. With a collimator compared with that obtained without a collimator
   e. With a screen compared with that obtained without a screen

3. As the grid ratio increases, there is also an increase in which of the following?
   a. Contrast improvement factor
   b. Intensification factor
   c. Spatial resolution
   d. System speed
   e. Width of interspace material

4. In general, the selectivity of a grid depends principally on which of the following?
   a. Contrast improvement factor
   b. Focal length
   c. Grid frequency
   d. Grid mass
   e. Grid radius

5. Radiographic grids with high contrast improvement usually:
   a. Are low-ratio grids
   b. Improve contrast resolution
   c. Improve spatial resolution
   d. Reduce patient dose
   e. Transmit more scatter radiation

6. A radiograph is made at 76 kVp and 25 mAs without a grid. If an 8:1 ratio grid is added, the mAs required would be approximately:
   a. 25 mAs
   b. 50 mAs
   c. 100 mAs
   d. 150 mAs
   e. 300 mAs

7. Which of the following is the simplest type of grid?
   a. Crossed grid
   b. Focused grid
   c. High-ratio grid
   d. Linear grid
   e. Zero frequency grid

8. The undesirable absorption of image-forming x-rays by a grid is called:
   a. Anode heel effect
   b. Grid cutoff
   c. Malpositioned grid
   d. Primary beam scatter
   e. Upside-down grid

9. Which of the following would be included in the three major classifications of moving grids?
   a. Crossed grid
   b. Focused grid
   c. Linear grid
   d. Reciprocating grid
   e. Zero frequency grid

10. If one had two grids whose characteristics were unknown but grid B weighed twice as much as grid A, one might conclude that grid B would have:
   a. A higher contrast improvement factor
   b. A greater mass effect
   c. A lower grid frequency
   d. A lower grid ratio
   e. A lower selectivity

11. Focused grids:
   a. Cut off the four edges of an image if placed too close to the source
   b. Cut off two edges of an image if placed too far from the tube
   c. Do not move
   d. Reduce the amount of scatter radiation that reaches the image receptor
   e. Reduce the radiation exposure to the patient compared with no grid

12. One factor that does not affect the percentage of scatter radiation that reaches the image receptor is:
   a. Grid mass
   b. Grid ratio
   c. kVp
   d. mAs
   e. Patient thickness

13. The significance of the Bucky factor increases with which of the following?
   a. Decreasing contrast improvement factor
   b. Decreasing grid ratio
   c. Increasing interspace width
   d. Increasing x-ray quality
   e. Increasing x-ray quantity

14. Which of the following would principally reduce the production of scatter radiation?
   a. A decrease in field size
   b. A decrease in SID
   c. An increase in SSD
   d. Use of a filter
   e. Use of a grid

15. Radiographic grids:
   a. Have reduced selectivity as the mass is increased
   b. May have aluminum step wedges incorporated into them
   c. Must include a filter
   d. Usually have contrast improvement factors from 0 to 1.0
   e. Usually have grid ratios between 5:1 and 16:1

16. A crossed radiographic grid:
   a. Allows considerable positioning latitude compared with linear grids
   b. Has a contrast improvement factor equal to a linear grid of equal ratio
   c. Is said to have a grid ratio of 10:1; therefore, it consists of two 5:1 linear grids
   d. Must be used for tomography
   e. Reduces scatter radiation along two axes

17. Which of the following is a disadvantage of moving grids?
   a. They may produce motion blur.
   b. They may result in decreased magnification.
   c. They require higher grid frequency.
   d. They require higher grid ratio.
   e. They require thinner strips.

Worksheet 11-5
Types of Grids
Use of Grids
Grid Selection

If the construction and performance characteristics of a grid are known and understood, grid selection and use will be more accurate. Selection of a grid usually requires that one specify the type of grid (parallel, crossed, focused, or moving), the ratio of the grid, and the grid frequency.

Such selection is made on the basis of the types of radiographic examination to be performed. If grid lines are objectionable, moving grids should be used.

Cerebral angiography often requires crossed grids, so that contrast is maximized for imaging small-vessel details. Low-kVp techniques usually demand low-ratio grids, and high-kVp techniques usually require high-ratio grids. For general purpose radiographic rooms, focused grids with ratios of approximately 8:1 to 12:1 usually are used.

Focused grids normally are preferred to parallel grids because with parallel grids, grid cutoff can occur.

$$\text{Distance to grid cutoff} = \frac{\text{Source-to-image receptor distance}}{\text{Grid ratio}}$$

EXERCISES

1. Which of the following is not a grid positioning error?
   a. Air-gap grid
   b. Lateral decentering
   c. Off-center grid
   d. Off-focus grid
   e. Off-level grid

2. In the design of radiographic techniques, the most common practice is to use which of the following?
   a. A crossed grid
   b. A focused moving grid
   c. A focused stationary grid
   d. A parallel moving grid
   e. A parallel stationary grid

3. Which of the following techniques will result in the highest patient dose if mAs is changed to maintain optical density?
   a. 5:1 crossed grid; 70 kVp
   b. 5:1 crossed grid; 90 kVp
   c. 10:1 focused grid; 70 kVp
   d. 10:1 focused grid; 90 kVp
   e. 12:1 parallel grid; 70 kVp

4. Grids generally:
   a. Must be cleaned on schedule
   b. Require faster image receptors
   c. Require less mAs
   d. Require periodic replacement because of radiation fatigue
   e. Result in increased patient dose

5. When comparable radiographs are produced, which of the following combinations will result in the lowest patient dose?
   a. High kVp and high-ratio grids
   b. High kVp and low-ratio grids
   c. High kVp and no grid
   d. Low kVp and high-ratio grids
   e. Low kVp and low-ratio grids

6. Grid cutoff:
   a. Is measured by the Bucky factor
   b. Is more pronounced with high-ratio grids
   c. Is more pronounced with low-ratio grids
   d. Never occurs with focused grids
   e. Occurs only with focused grids

7. Air-gap technique:
   a. Increases the Bucky factor
   b. Reduces contrast by absorption of scattered radiation in the air
   c. Requires that the grid and the film must be separated by at least 30 cm
   d. Results in approximately the same patient dose as nongrid techniques
   e. Results in image magnification

121

8. If radiographic grids are used and the technique is compensated, patient exposure:
   a. Increases with increasing grid ratio
   b. Increases with increasing kVp
   c. Is independent of grid frequency
   d. Is independent of grid mass
   e. Remains unchanged from that with nongrid techniques

9. Bedside examinations require a wide range of SIDs. Which of the following parallel grids would be most likely to produce grid cutoff?
   a. 5:1
   b. 6:1
   c. 8:1
   d. 12:1
   e. 16:1

10. In general, which of the following has the greatest contrast improvement factor?
    a. Crossed grids
    b. Focused grids
    c. Moving grids
    d. Parallel grids
    e. Zero grids

11. Which of the following is an undesirable characteristic of linear grids compared with focused grids?
    a. Higher Bucky factor
    b. Increased patient dose
    c. Lower grid frequencies
    d. Lower grid ratios
    e. More grid cutoff

12. What is the result of replacing an 8:1 grid with a 12:1 grid?
    a. Greater positioning latitude
    b. Higher patient dose
    c. Less contrast
    d. Less spatial resolution
    e. Lower patient dose

13. When air-gap radiography is performed:
    a. A high-ratio grid must be used
    b. A low-ratio grid must be used
    c. Contrast resolution is improved
    d. Patient dose is increased
    e. The heel effect is accentuated

14. As grid frequency increases:
    a. Grid mass is usually reduced.
    b. The grid ratio will be reduced if the thickness of the grid remains constant.
    c. The interspace width becomes thinner if the width of the grid strip remains constant.
    d. The number of grid strips per centimeter increases.
    e. The patient dose is reduced.

15. As the grid ratio increases, there is also an increase in which of the following?
    a. Contrast improvement factor
    b. Intensification factor
    c. Spatial resolution
    d. System speed
    e. Width of interspace material

16. Radiographic grids:
    a. Have reduced selectivity as the mass is increased
    b. May have aluminum step wedges incorporated into them
    c. Must also include a filter
    d. Usually have contrast improvement factors from 0 to 1.0
    e. Usually have grid ratios between 5:1 and 16:1

17. Bedside examinations require a wide range of SIDs. Which of the following linear grids would be most likely to produce grid cutoff?
    a. 5:1
    b. 6:1
    c. 8:1
    d. 12:1
    e. 16:1

Worksheet 12-1
Film Construction

The physical characteristics of radiographic film make it perhaps the strongest link in the radiographic imaging system. Radiographic film consists of two principal parts: the base and the emulsion. The manufacture of each is precisely controlled.

The base is made of polyester and is somewhat rigid—not flexible, like photographic film. This rigidity allows a radiograph to be easily handled and positioned on a viewbox. This property of the base is known as *dimensional stability*.

The emulsion is a homogenous mixture of gelatin and silver halide crystals. The silver halide is the ingredient that is sensitive to x-ray or light exposure. The concentration and crystal size distribution give the emulsion speed and contrast characteristics.

EXERCISES

1. An easily observable difference between x-ray film and photographic film is:
   a. The archival quality
   b. The processing requirements
   c. The speed of the film
   d. The thickness and rigidity of the base
   e. The thickness of the emulsion

2. The principal characteristic of the emulsion that makes it particularly x-ray sensitive is its:
   a. Atomic mass
   b. Atomic number
   c. Mass density
   d. Optical density
   e. Sensitivity center

3. Average silver halide crystal surface size in radiographic film is approximately:
   a. 0.1 μm
   b. 1.0 μm
   c. 10 μm
   d. 100 μm
   e. 1000 μm

4. The radiographic film base appears blue:
   a. Because of added hardeners
   b. Because of the sensitivity centers
   c. Because of the silver halide crystals
   d. So that image viewing is more comfortable
   e. To match the light emitted by intensifying screens

5. Which of the following has been used as a radiographic film base? (choose all that apply)
   a. Cellulose nitrate
   b. Cellulose triacetate
   c. Gadolinium oxysulfide
   d. Gelatin
   e. Silver halide

6. The emulsion that is commonly used in x-ray film consists of which of the following?
   a. Cellulose acetate and silver halide
   b. Gelatin and cellulose acetate
   c. Gelatin and silver nitrate
   d. Silver halide and gelatin
   e. Silver nitrate and cellulose acetate

7. A common base of contemporary x-ray film is:
   a. Polyester
   b. Polyethylene
   c. Polyurethane
   d. Silver bromide
   e. Silver nitrate

8. In the manufacture of radiographic film:
   a. Direct-exposure film contains a thicker emulsion layer with a greater number of silver halide crystals.
   b. Screen film is made before direct-exposure film.
   c. Single-emulsion type is most frequently produced.
   d. The emulsion layer is thicker than the base.
   e. X-ray interaction accounts for approximately one half of the latent-image centers in screen-film exposure.

9. The adhesive layer of radiographic film:
   a. Ensures uniform adhesion of the emulsion to the base
   b. Ensures uniform adhesion of the protective layer to the emulsion
   c. Is approximately 200 μm thick
   d. Is between 5 and 25 μm thick
   e. Serves as the protective layer

10. Which of the following are the two basic parts of radiographic film?
    a. Base and emulsion
    b. Emulsion and phosphor
    c. Emulsion and supercoating
    d. Phosphor and base
    e. Phosphor and density

11. The overcoat usually consists of which of the following?
    a. Cellulose
    b. Gelatin
    c. Phosphor
    d. Polyester
    e. Silver halide

12. Dimensional stability is the property of maintaining the size and shape of which of the following?
    a. Base
    b. Emulsion
    c. Image
    d. Phosphor
    e. Supercoiling

13. When polyester is compared with cellulose triacetate as a base, which of the following does not apply to polyester?
    a. Better dimensional stability
    b. Less warping with age
    c. Nonflammable
    d. Stronger
    e. Thicker

14. The principal purpose of gelatin in the emulsion is to:
    a. Facilitate image processing
    b. Produce film that is lucent
    c. Provide dimensional stability to the film
    d. Provide for easier roller transport
    e. Support the silver halide crystals uniformly

15. Which of the following properties of silver halide is most important in the production of a latent image?
    a. Atomic number
    b. Dimensional stability
    c. Mass
    d. Mass density
    e. Optical density

16. X-ray film is sensitive to which of the following?
    a. All x-rays and gamma rays, visible light, and radio waves
    b. Only electromagnetic radiation
    c. Only x-rays and gamma rays
    d. Only x-rays, gamma rays, and visible light
    e. Only x-rays

17. X-ray film used with radiographic intensifying screens usually has which of the following?
    a. A base made of cellulose nitrate
    b. A clear base
    c. A phosphor coat on the surface
    d. A treatment to make the film especially sensitive to x-rays
    e. An emulsion coat on both sides of the base

18. Which of the following is usually thinner than 5 µm?
    a. Base
    b. Emulsion
    c. Film
    d. Overcoat
    e. Phosphor

19. Which of the following is a principal component of the emulsion?
    a. Bromine nitrate
    b. Cellulose nitrate
    c. Cellulose triacetate
    d. Silver bromide
    e. Silver nitrate

Worksheet 12-2
Formation of Latent Image

 The interaction of electromagnetic radiation (light or x-rays) with the radiographic film emulsion results in a latent image. The latent image is the invisible change in the silver halide crystals of the emulsion.

The latent image is made visible by processing. Six steps are necessary for processing a radiograph: (1) wetting, (2) development, (3) stop bath, (4) fixation, (5) washing, and (6) drying. All are important, but the two most critical steps are development and fixation. During development, the latent image is made visible. During fixation, that visibility is made permanent (archival quality).

EXERCISES

1. The latent image actually is formed in the:
   a. Base
   b. Bromine atom
   c. Gelatin
   d. Protective layer
   e. Silver halide crystal

2. During the photographic process, metallic silver accumulates at the:
   a. Base
   b. Bromine ion
   c. Gelatin contaminant
   d. Secondary electron
   e. Sensitivity center

3. The latent image at the crystal level:
   a. Is a collection of bromine atoms
   b. Is a collection of silver atoms
   c. Is present regardless of whether that crystal was irradiated
   d. Is visible with a microscope
   e. Requires x-ray interaction

4. The term latent image actually refers to which of the following?
   a. A processed image
   b. An unprocessed image
   c. Film inertia
   d. Image intensification
   e. Reciprocity law failure

5. The sensitivity center is usually silver:
   a. Atoms
   b. Bromide
   c. Iodide
   d. Ions
   e. Sulfide

6. In the manufacture of the emulsion, which of the following molecules is particularly sensitive to visible light?
   a. $AgBr$
   b. $AgNO_3$
   c. $CaWO_4$
   d. KBr
   e. KNO_3

7. When the latent image is processed, what type of image does it become?
   a. Crystal
   b. Dimensional
   c. Excited
   d. Induced
   e. Manifest

8. What do we call the radiation exiting the patient that is responsible for latent image formation?
   a. Image-forming
   b. Leakage
   c. Remnant
   d. Scatter
   e. Useful beam

9. When x-rays interact directly with film, which of the following most likely is involved?
   a. Bromine
   b. Gelatin
   c. Iodine
   d. Silver
   e. Tungsten

10. An ion is an atom:
    a. That has electric charge
    b. That is neutral
    c. That is radioactive
    d. With a sensitivity center
    e. With too many nucleons

125

11. The interstitial atoms in a crystal of silver halide include which of the following?
    a. Bromine, iodine, and gelatin
    b. Gelatin, silver, and bromine
    c. Iodine, gelatin, and silver
    d. Silver, bromine, and iodine
    e. Silver, sulfide, and gelatin

12. X-ray interaction with silver halide can result in formation of all except which of the following?
    a. A charged electron
    b. A latent-image center
    c. A radioactive atom
    d. A secondary electron
    e. An ion

13. After irradiation, a secondary electron most likely will interact with a silver ion to form:
    a. A positive ion
    b. A sensitivity center
    c. A silver atom
    d. A silver bromide crystal
    e. A silver halide crystal

14. In a silver halide crystal, which of the following is missing an electron?
    a. Bromine
    b. Gelatin
    c. Iodine
    d. Silver
    e. Sulfide

15. Which of the following statements about processing is true?
    a. It includes AgBr formation.
    b. It includes gelatin ionization.
    c. It includes neutral silver migration.
    d. It is required for latent-image formation.
    e. It is required for manifest-image formation.

16. The latent-image center:
    a. Consists of halide crystals
    b. Consists of migrating electrons
    c. Consists of silver ions
    d. Forms at the sensitivity center
    e. Forms on the surface of a crystal

17. The formation of a latent image follows which interaction with the emulsion?
    a. Classical scattering
    b. Pair production
    c. Photodisintegration
    d. Photoelectric effect
    e. Thomson scattering

18. If one observes a film immediately after exposure, what is seen?
    a. A distributed image
    b. A latent image
    c. A manifest image
    d. A visible image
    e. Nothing

19. Which of the following theories best explains the photographic effect?
    a. Duane-Hunt
    b. Gurney-Mott
    c. Haus-Hendrick
    d. Hurter-Driffield
    e. Planck-Bohr

Worksheet 12-3
Types of Film
Handling and Storage of Film

Radiologic imaging has advanced so far techno-logically that it is imperative that the radiologic technologist be aware of the various image receptors available and the bases for differences among radio-graphic films.

- Contrast, speed, and spectral characteristics are three exceedingly important parameters by which a radiologic technologist should select film.
- Proper matching of film emulsion with screen phosphor is also essential.
- Proper darkroom safelight protection is absolutely essential.
- Storage in a climate-controlled environment is necessary for the ultimate production of acceptable images.

EXERCISES

1. The most commonly used radiographic image receptor is which of the following?
   a. Direct-exposure film
   b. Electrostatic plate
   c. Nonscreen film
   d. Screen film
   e. Single-emulsion film

2. Which of the following is not a characteristic the radiographer should consider when selecting film?
   a. Contrast
   b. Latitude
   c. Light absorption
   d. Light emission
   e. Sensitivity

3. The contrast of radiographic film is:
   a. Directly proportional to dose
   b. Directly proportional to its sensitivity
   c. Highest at high dose
   d. Important to archival quality
   e. Inversely proportional to its latitude

4. High-contrast film has:
   a. A thinner base
   b. A wide range of grain size
   c. Larger grain size
   d. Less silver halide
   e. Uniform grain size

5. The difference between fast film and slow film is silver halide crystal:
   a. Charge
   b. Concentration
   c. Shape
   d. Size
   e. Size distribution

6. The spectral response of an emulsion refers to:
   a. Its ability to detect x-rays
   b. Its absorption of visible light
   c. Its emission of visible light
   d. Its sensitivity to x-rays
   e. Its transmission of viewbox light

7. Calcium tungstate screens emit which of the following?
   a. Blue light
   b. Green light
   c. Infrared light
   d. Red light
   e. Yellow light

8. Which of the following will not fog film?
   a. A darkroom light leak
   b. Background radiation
   c. Fringe magnetic fields from an MRI
   d. Gamma radiation from an adjacent nuclear medicine laboratory
   e. X-radiation from the adjacent x-ray room

9. Orthochromatic film is sensitive to which of the following?
   a. Green light
   b. Infrared light
   c. Red light
   d. Visible light
   e. Yellow light

10. Which of the following is the principal result of using rare earth screens with green-sensitive film?
   a. Darkroom fog
   b. Fewer artifacts
   c. Higher contrast
   d. Increased patient dose
   e. Reduced patient dose

127

11. When rare earth screens are in use, what type of safelights are required?
    a. Amber
    b. Blue
    c. Green
    d. None
    e. Red

12. Mammography film:
    a. Has a thick emulsion
    b. Has a thin base
    c. Is coarse-grain, double-emulsion
    d. Is used with a screen
    e. Must be viewed in the dark

13. When comparing 35-mm cine film with 16-mm film, the 35-mm film can be seen to have:
    a. Better resolution
    b. Four times the area
    c. Higher contrast
    d. Less patient dose
    e. Twice the area

14. Most rare earth screens emit which of the following?
    a. Blue light
    b. Green light
    c. Infrared light
    d. Ultraviolet light
    e. Violet light

15. If film is stored near steam pipes, the most likely result will be which of the following?
    a. Artifacts
    b. Loss of contrast
    c. Loss of latitude
    d. Loss of speed
    e. The appearance of radiopaque artifacts

16. Which of the following is most likely to fog film?
    a. 0.2 mR
    b. An improper safelight filter
    c. High humidity
    d. High temperature
    e. Storage of film for longer than 1 month

17. Which of the following are acceptable storage conditions for film?
    a. 16°C and 10% humidity
    b. 20°C and 90% humidity
    c. 32°C and 50% humidity
    d. 36°C and 60% humidity
    e. 50°C and 50% humidity

18. Which of the following darkroom conditions is not acceptable?
    a. Blue-sensitive film, amber safelight
    b. Green-sensitive film, amber safelight
    c. Orthochromatic film, red safelight
    d. Silver halide emulsion, amber safelight
    e. Silver halide emulsion, red safelight

19. Which of the following is the least important characteristic of screen film?
    a. Contrast
    b. Cost
    c. Light absorption
    d. Light emission
    e. Sensitivity

20. Which of the following would be considered an image artifact?
    a. A pressure mark
    b. A smudge mark on the viewbox diffuser
    c. An unexposed but processed film
    d. Developer depletion
    e. Film identification mark

21. If other factors are equal, which of the following emulsions is fastest?
    a. Blue sensitive
    b. Green sensitive
    c. Large grain
    d. Small grain
    e. Uniform grain size

Worksheet 12-4
Screen Construction
Luminescence
Screen Characteristics

 ■ Radiographic intensifying screens are used principally to reduce patient radiation dose.

■ The radiographic intensifying screen is constructed by pasting a phosphor on a base material with a reflective layer in between.

■ The intensification factor (IF) gives us an idea about how much dose reduction we can achieve by comparing radiographic screen exposure with non-screen exposure and is computed as follows:

$$IF = \frac{\text{Exposure required without screen}}{\text{Exposure required with screen}}$$

EXERCISES

1. Radiographic intensifying screen speed increases with increasing:
   a. Atomic mass
   b. Base thickness
   c. mAs
   d. Optical density
   e. Phosphor thickness

2. Direct-exposure, nonscreen technique:
   a. Produces less noise
   b. Reduces scatter radiation
   c. Results in better contrast resolution
   d. Results in better spatial resolution
   e. Results in less motion blur

3. Afterglow is a property of intensifying screens that:
   a. Enhances resolution
   b. Improves contrast
   c. Is enhanced at high kVp
   d. Reduces screen speed
   e. Results in image blur

4. The resolution achievable with radiographic intensifying screens is approximately:
   a. 1 lp/mm
   b. 2 lp/mm
   c. 5 lp/mm
   d. 15 lp/mm
   e. 20 lp/mm

5. Which of the following factors controlled by the radiologic technologist affects radiographic screen speed the most?
   a. Exposure time
   b. kVp
   c. mAs
   d. Processor temperature
   e. Room temperature

6. When screen film is the image receptor, image quality is a trade-off among speed, spatial resolution, and noise. In general:
   a. As noise increases, spatial resolution improves.
   b. As quantum mottle increases, spatial resolution improves.
   c. As speed increases, so does noise.
   d. As speed increases, spatial resolution improves.
   e. Low-noise systems have fewer artifacts.

7. At x-ray energies below the K-shell electron binding energy:
   a. Another rapid reduction in photoelectric absorption occurs with increasing x-ray energy.
   b. The incident photon does not have sufficient energy to ionize K-shell electrons.
   c. The two K-shell electrons become available for photoelectric interaction.
   d. There is an abrupt increase in the probability of photoelectric absorption.
   e. None of the above

8. The intensification factor:
   a. Decreases with increasing kVp
   b. Increases with increasing temperature
   c. Is greater for detail screens than for par speed screens
   d. Is greater for rare earth screens than for calcium tungstate screens
   e. Is less at high mAs

9. A phosphor currently used in radiographic intensifying screens is:
   a. Barium fluorochloride
   b. Barium platinocyanide
   c. Cadmium tungstate
   d. Calcium sulfate
   e. Cesium iodide

10. Screen blur:
    a. Is greater with detail screens than with par speed screens
    b. Is less with rare earth screens
    c. Is reduced with fast screens
    d. Is the loss of sharpness of an image when screens are used
    e. Occurs because the light emitted is not properly focused on the film

11. With regard to luminescence, which of the following statements is true?
    a. Fluorescence lasts longer than phosphorescence.
    b. Luminous watch dials that fade in the dark are fluorescent devices.
    c. Materials that luminesce are called lumenites.
    d. Phosphorescence occurs only when a stimulus is applied.
    e. There are two types: fluorescence and phosphorescence.

12. Radiographic intensifying screens are used with radiographic film principally to:
    a. Allow for shorter exposures
    b. Improve contrast resolution
    c. Improve spatial resolution
    d. Increase radiographic latitude
    e. Reduce patient radiation exposure

13. Radiographic intensifying screens are used with radiographic film to:
    a. Increase the latitude of the imaging system
    b. Increase the spatial resolution of the imaging system
    c. Lower the necessary kVp
    d. Reduce image noise
    e. Reduce motion blur

14. Which of the following properties principally determines screen blur?
    a. Antihalation dye
    b. Phosphor concentration
    c. Phosphor crystal size
    d. Reflective layer
    e. Type of phosphor

15. Luminescence is a process that:
    a. Absorbs light
    b. Always requires x-ray absorption
    c. Always requires x-ray attenuation
    d. Involves inner-shell electrons
    e. Involves outer-shell electrons

16. Because x-ray interaction with a phosphor produces light isotropically:
    a. A base is required.
    b. A protective layer is required.
    c. The light is focused.
    d. The light is parallel.
    e. The light spreads out.

17. Mammography conducted with detail screens results in entrance skin exposures (ESE) as low as 300 mR (3 mGy$_a$). The intensification factor for these screens is about 30. If such an examination were conducted as a nonscreen procedure, what would be the ESE?
    a. 100 mR
    b. 900 mR
    c. 1000 mR
    d. 9000 mR
    e. 1200 mR

Worksheet 12-5
Screen-Film Combinations
Screen Care
Fluoroscopic Screens

 Most radiographic intensifying screens are described as rare earth because the phosphors are compounds that incorporate the rare earth elements gadolinium (Gd), lanthanum (La), and yttrium (Y).

The principal advantage of rare earth screens is speed. They are much faster than an earlier standard: calcium tungstate screens. **The principal disadvantage is quantum mottle, a source of image noise.** Rare earth screens have spatial resolution equal to that of calcium tungstate screens.

The increased speed of rare earth screens results from their ability to absorb a greater number of x-rays and to convert more of the x-ray energy to light.

EXERCISES

1. Which of the following is a rare earth element?
   a. Gadolinium
   b. Nobelium
   c. Thallium
   d. Thulium
   e. Palladium

2. In the formula La2O2S:Tb, the Tb:
   a. Improves contrast resolution
   b. Improves luminescence
   c. Improves spatial resolution
   d. Reduces noise
   e. Stands for tungsten bromide

3. The principal advantage of rare earth screens over calcium tungstate screens is:
   a. Better contrast resolution
   b. Better spatial resolution
   c. Faster speed
   d. Lower cost
   e. Reduced noise

4. Rare earth screens exhibit higher x-ray absorption than calcium tungstate screens:
   a. Because of their thickness
   b. Only at high x-ray energy
   c. Only at low x-ray energy
   d. Only over an intermediate x-ray energy range
   e. Regardless of the x-ray energy

5. Which of the following elements has the highest atomic number?
   a. Gadolinium
   b. Lanthanum
   c. Molybdenum
   d. Tungsten
   e. Yttrium

6. Which of the following principally contributes to the increased speed of rare earth screens?
   a. Conversion efficiency
   b. Higher atomic number
   c. Longer wavelength emission
   d. Phosphor thickness
   e. Screen-film contact

7. Which of the following spectra is discrete?
   a. Bremsstrahlung
   b. Calcium tungstate emission
   c. Orthochromatic absorption
   d. Panchromatic absorption
   e. Rare earth emission

8. Compared with calcium tungstate, rare earth screens:
   a. Are faster because of scatter radiation
   b. Have better spatial resolution
   c. Have higher rates of absorption for x-rays greater than 80 keV
   d. Have higher rates of absorption for x-rays less than 25 keV
   e. Have higher rates of x-ray absorption in the diagnostic range

9. When diagnostic x-rays interact with rare earth phosphors:
   a. K-shell interaction will not occur at energies less than 70 keV.
   b. Light is not emitted isotropically.
   c. The lower the x-ray energy, the more probable is photoelectric absorption.
   d. The number of x-rays absorbed is approximately the same as that for calcium tungstate.
   e. With increasing x-ray energy, an abrupt decrease in x-ray absorption will occur.

131

10. When rare earth intensifying screens are used:
    a. All rare earth elements have higher K-shell electron binding energy than tungsten.
    b. As x-ray energy increases up to the K-shell binding energy, absorption also increases.
    c. Contrast resolution is improved.
    d. There is an abrupt increase in absorption at an energy equal to the K-shell binding energy.
    e. There is an abrupt reduction in x-ray absorption at an energy equal to the K-shell binding energy.

11. Compared with calcium tungstate, when an x-ray is absorbed in a rare earth screen:
    a. It will be absorbed, never scattered.
    b. More energy will be transferred.
    c. More light will be emitted.
    d. Shorter-wavelength light will be emitted.
    e. The ratio of visible light emitted to x-ray energy absorbed will be less.

12. Compared with calcium tungstate screens, rare earth screens:
    a. Absorb one to two times as many x-rays
    b. Absorb three to five times as many x-rays
    c. Emit higher-energy light
    d. Emit shorter-wavelength light
    e. Have less internal absorption

13. Compared with calcium tungstate screens, rare earth screens:
    a. Do not need grids
    b. Emit light in the blue-violet region
    c. Emit more intense light per x-ray interaction
    d. May require a new darkroom
    e. Should be used with blue-sensitive radiographic film

14. Compared with calcium tungstate screens, rare earth radiographic intensifying screens:
    a. Have better spatial resolution
    b. Have less noise
    c. Have less quantum mottle
    d. Require less screen-film contact
    e. Result in lower patient dose

15. Which of the following statements about radiographic intensifying screens is true?
    a. All screens have conversion efficiencies greater than one.
    b. Calcium tungstate screens emit green-yellow light.
    c. Par speed screens emit green light.
    d. Rare earth screens must be used in carbon fiber cassettes.
    e. They are used to reduce patient dose.

16. What is the principal limitation of the rare earth radiographic intensifying screen?
    a. Increased exposure factor
    b. Increased quantum mottle
    c. Patient dose
    d. Reduced contrast resolution
    e. Reduced spatial resolution

17. In the proper design and use of a radiographic cassette:
    a. Scratches on the front cover indicate that replacement is necessary.
    b. The back cover should be made of high Z material so that it can function as a primary barrier for personnel protection.
    c. The back cover should be made of high Z material to reduce scatter radiation.
    d. The back cover should be made of low Z material to protect unexposed film while it is in the passbox.
    e. The front cover should be made of low Z material to minimize x-ray attenuation.

Worksheet 12-6
Processing Chemistry

Automatic processing uses three principal chemistries, each contained in a separate tank of the processor.

- The **developer** contains developing agents, activators, hardeners, preservatives, and water.
- The **fixer** contains clearing agents, activators, preservatives, and hardeners.
- The third chemistry is **water,** which is used in copious amounts at high flow rates to wash the film clear of unused chemistries.

EXERCISES

1. At what stage in automatic processing is the latent image made visible?
   a. Developing
   b. Drying
   c. Fixation
   d. Stop bath
   e. Wetting

2. Which of the following is the component of the developer that helps to keep unexposed crystals from the developing agent?
   a. Hydroquinone (developing agent)
   b. Phenidone (developing agent)
   c. Potassium bromide (restrainer)
   d. Silver halide (crystal)
   e. Sodium carbonate (buffer)

3. What stage of processing involves a synergistic reaction?
   a. Development
   b. Drying
   c. Fixation
   d. Washing
   e. Wetting

4. Aerial oxidation is controlled by which of the following?
   a. The activator
   b. The concentrator
   c. The fixer
   d. The preservative
   e. The restrainer

5. The hardeners in a fixer:
   a. Cause swelling and softening of the emulsion
   b. Cause the emulsion to swell
   c. Clean the rollers of the transport system
   d. Ensure archival quality
   e. Remove excess hypo from the emulsion

6. Which of the following is the most common result of inadequate washing?
   a. A damp film
   b. Excess hypo retention
   c. Incomplete development
   d. Incomplete fixing
   e. Loss of archival quality

7. Conversion of the latent image to a visible image occurs:
   a. In less than 10 seconds
   b. In the developer
   c. In the fixer
   d. In the gelatin portion of the emulsion
   e. When silver bromide is cleared

8. Which of the following ingredients of the developer is responsible for producing the blackest parts of a radiograph?
   a. Glutaraldehyde
   b. Hydroquinone
   c. Phenidone
   d. Potassium bromide
   e. Sodium sulfite

9. During development, silver:
   a. Atoms are changed to ions.
   b. Atoms are ionized.
   c. Ions are changed to atoms.
   d. Ions are oxidized.
   e. Is removed

10. The archival quality of a radiograph is principally:
    a. Controlled by developer concentration
    b. Controlled by the activator
    c. Controlled by the developing agent
    d. Established during development
    e. Established during fixing

133

11. Which of the following terms does not belong?
    a. Clearing agent
    b. Fixer
    c. Hypo
    d. Stop bath
    e. Thiosulfate

12. Which of the following is not a separate stage in automatic processing?
    a. Development
    b. Drying
    c. Fixation
    d. Washing
    e. Wetting

13. Which of the following is the preservative normally used in both the developer and the fixer?
    a. Glutaraldehyde
    b. Potassium alum
    c. Silver sulfide
    d. Sodium carbonate
    e. Sodium sulfite

14. Which of the following is a reducing agent?
    a. Hydroquinone
    b. Glutaraldehyde
    c. Potassium bromide
    d. Silver sulfite
    e. Sodium sulfite

15. Which of the following ingredients in the fixer functions as a stop bath?
    a. The activator
    b. The clearing agent
    c. The hardener
    d. The preservative
    e. The silver sulfide

16. Hypo retention refers to which of the following?
    a. Improved archival quality
    b. Replenishment of a clearing agent
    c. The formation of silver sulfide
    d. The formation of sodium sulfite
    e. Thiosulfate left in the emulsion

17. Development fog will increase when which of the following is abnormally low in the developer?
    a. Glutaraldehyde
    b. Hydroquinone
    c. Potassium bromide
    d. Silver sulfide
    e. Sodium sulfite

18. Which of the following is the component of the developer that is most responsible for archival quality?
    a. Glutaraldehyde
    b. Hydroquinone
    c. Silver sulfide
    d. Sodium carbonate
    e. Sodium sulfite

19. The wetting agent used in automatic processors is usually which of the following?
    a. Acetic acid
    b. Glutaraldehyde
    c. Silver halide
    d. Silver sulfite
    e. Water

20. The temperature of the wash water should be approximately:
    a. 5°C below the developer
    b. 5°C below the fixer
    c. 5°F below the developer
    d. 5°F below the fixer
    e. The same temperature as the fixer

21. Which of the following is sometimes used as a developing agent?
    a. Glutaraldehyde
    b. Phenidone
    c. Silver sulfide
    d. Sodium sulfite
    e. Water

Worksheet 12-7
Automatic Processing

The time from insertion of the exposed radiograph into the processor to the appearance of the processed radiograph in the receiving bin—the dry-to-drop time—is 90 seconds. This type of automatic processor is an electromechanical device that consists of four main systems: (1) the transport system, (2) the circulation system, (3) the replenishment system, and (4) the dryer system.

The transport system is a series of rollers, racks, and drive chains that takes the exposed radiograph and automatically feeds it through the four stations of the processor: (1) the developing tank, (2) the fixing tank, (3) the wash tank, and (4) the drying chamber.

The circulation system is powered by pumps that continuously circulate the chemistries in each tank to ensure complete chemistry mixing and uniform temperature of the solution. The circulation system in the developing tank and the fixing tank is a closed loop, whereas the wash tank is a single-pass, flow-through system.

The replenishment system consists of a small pump, tubing, and a microswitch control. As the film is fed into the receiving tray of the automatic processor, the microswitch activates the pump to feed a measured amount of developer into the developing tank and fixer into the fixing tank.

EXERCISES

1. Which of the following is an assembly that consists of one master roller, several planetary rollers, and two guide shoes?
   a. A crossover rack
   b. A detector assembly
   c. A roller subassembly
   d. A transport rack
   e. A turnaround assembly

2. Replenishment of which tank in the processing system is most important?
   a. Developer
   b. Dryer
   c. Fixer
   d. Wash
   e. Wetter

3. When a film is inserted into an automatic processor:
   a. A microswitch grips it.
   b. Guide shoes grip it.
   c. It should be centered on the feed tray.
   d. The long dimension should be against the rail.
   e. The short dimension should be against the rail.

4. Adequate drying is necessary to:
   a. Complete development
   b. Complete fixation
   c. Obtain adequate contrast
   d. Reduce artifacts
   e. Strengthen the base

5. The fastest automatic processors can process a film in:
   a. 30 seconds
   b. 90 seconds
   c. 180 seconds
   d. 5 minutes
   e. 7 minutes

6. Between the fixing tank and the wash tank, the film passes through a:
   a. Crossover rack
   b. Drying chamber
   c. Receiving bin
   d. Transportation rack
   e. Turnaround rack

7. Which of the following is not one of the major systems of an automatic processor?
   a. The development system
   b. The drying system
   c. The electrical system
   d. The replenishment system
   e. The transport system

8. The principal purpose of the circulation system is to:
   a. Agitate the chemistry
   b. Agitate the film
   c. Control chemistry concentration
   d. Control chemistry temperature
   e. Replenish the chemistry

135

9. Which segment of the circulation system is most important to archival quality?
   a. Developing
   b. Drying
   c. Fixation
   d. Washing
   e. Wetting

10. Underreplenishment of the developer will result in:
    a. A decrease in contrast
    b. A reduction in spatial resolution
    c. An improvement in spatial resolution
    d. An increase in contrast
    e. No change in contrast

11. Replenishment tanks should have close-fitting floating lids primarily:
    a. For control of replenishment rate
    b. For control of temperature
    c. To control aerial oxidation
    d. To easily monitor fluid level
    e. To reduce splash hazard

12. Dry-to-drop time refers to:
    a. Development time
    b. Exposure-to-viewbox time
    c. Passbox-to-receiving bin time
    d. Time from feed tray to receiving bin
    e. Time in the passbox

13. The segment of the circulation system that is most likely to contain a filter is the:
    a. Developer
    b. Dryer
    c. Fixer
    d. Wash cycle
    e. Wetting cycle

14. If the power of the drive motor is transferred through a chain, the connecting device is usually a:
    a. Gear
    b. Pulley
    c. Roller
    d. Spring
    e. Sprocket

15. Control of the replenishment system is accomplished by a:
    a. Drive motor
    b. Float valve
    c. Microswitch
    d. Timer
    e. Transport rack

16. The approximate developer conditions in a 90-second processor are:
    a. 85°C, 22 s
    b. 85°C, 45 s
    c. 85°F, 45 s
    d. 95°C, 25 s
    e. 95°F, 22 s

17. The transport system includes all except which of the following?
    a. Drive motor
    b. Drying chamber
    c. Guide shoes
    d. Rollers
    e. Transport racks

18. The 3-inch master roller is a part of a:
    a. Guide shoe
    b. Microswitch
    c. Planetary roller
    d. Replenishment system
    e. Turnaround assembly

Worksheet 12-8
Quality Control
Artifacts

An unwanted optical density on a radiograph is an artifact. Artifacts are undesirable because they may obscure a meaningful optical density and thereby reduce diagnostic accuracy.

Artifacts are identified according to three general classifications: (1) processing artifacts, (2) exposure artifacts, and (3) handling and storage artifacts.

To minimize the generation of artifacts, a program of quality control must be implemented.

EXERCISES

1. Which of the following artifacts is associated with inadequate processing?
   a. A kink
   b. A smudge
   c. Crown static
   d. Grid lines
   e. Pi lines

2. If a radiograph turns yellow during storage, this is *most* likely the result of which of the following?
   a. Developer retention
   b. Incomplete washing
   c. Presence of sodium sulfite
   d. Radiation fog
   e. Wet pressure sensitization

3. A radiographic image shows the central region exposed and the sides unexposed. The probable cause is:
   a. A laterally positioned grid
   b. An off-center grid
   c. An upside-down grid
   d. Improper SID
   e. Patient motion

4. Which of the following *best* describes an example of preventive maintenance?
   a. Changing motor oil every 3000 miles
   b. Quitting smoking
   c. Repairing a flat tire
   d. Rotating intensifying screens
   e. Using gonadal shields in radiology

5. What is the limiting factor when an extremely fast image receptor is used?
   a. Contrast resolution
   b. Noise
   c. Screen blur
   d. Screen-film contact
   e. Spatial resolution

6. Which of the following artifacts is *most* likely to occur before processing?
   a. A small blur on an otherwise sharp radiograph
   b. Chemical fog
   c. Dichroic stain
   d. Image yellowing
   e. Wet pressure sensitization

7. What is the likely result of excessively high developer temperature?
   a. Increased base density
   b. Increased fog density
   c. Increased graininess
   d. Reduced quantum mottle
   e. Reduced speed

8. In a 90-second processor, immersion time in the developer is approximately:
   a. 10 s
   b. 20 s
   c. 30 s
   d. 40 s
   e. 60 s

9. Most facilities would be sure that the automatic processor was:
   a. Cleaned weekly
   b. Maintained annually
   c. Monitored hourly
   d. Replaced biannually
   e. Replenished daily

10. The classification of artifacts includes all of the following, *except:*
    a. Exposure artifacts
    b. Handling artifacts
    c. Location artifacts
    d. Processing artifacts
    e. Storage artifacts

11. Which of the following would be identified as a handling artifact?
    a. Curtain effect
    b. Double exposure
    c. Kink marks
    d. Motion
    e. Radiation fog

12. Motion blur is usually caused by too:
    a. High a kVp
    b. Long an SID
    c. Long an exposure time
    d. Short an SID
    e. Short an exposure time

13. Processor cleaning:
    a. Does not require disassembly
    b. Is unnecessary unless artifacts appear
    c. Should be done monthly
    d. Should be scheduled for a 4-hour interval
    e. Takes no longer than a few minutes

14. Which of the following would be considered a storage artifact?
    a. Pi lines
    b. Radiation fog
    c. Tree static
    d. Warped cassette
    e. Wrong screen-film match

15. Failure of a system or subsystem of an automatic processor will result in which of the following?
    a. Equipment replacement
    b. High retake rate
    c. Nonscheduled maintenance
    d. Preventive maintenance
    e. Scheduled maintenance

16. Pi lines are so called because they have which of the following characteristics?
    a. They look like a slice of pie.
    b. They look like parallel lines.
    c. They occur at 3.1416-inch intervals.
    d. They occur at intervals of p times the roller diameter.
    e. They occur at principal intervals.

17. Which of the following artifacts is the *most* distinctive and identifiable?
    a. Chemical fog
    b. Light leaks
    c. Pi lines
    d. Poor screen-film contact
    e. Radiation fog

18. Artifacts caused by wet pressure sensitization usually occur:
    a. After drying
    b. Before processing
    c. In the developing tank
    d. In the drying chamber
    e. In the fixing tank

19. Where will guide shoe artifacts be found on a radiograph?
    a. Center
    b. Leading and trailing edges
    c. Leading edge
    d. Side
    e. Trailing edge

20. Archival quality is a term that refers to
    a. Long-term storage of film
    b. Organization of the film file room
    c. The lucency of unexposed film
    d. The range of optical densities on an image
    e. Unintended radiation exposure

Worksheet 13-1
Fifteen Percent Rule

The mathematical problems that each radiologic technologist faces in daily practice include (1) mentally applying the 15% rule for kVp to adjust radiographic technique, (2) having a desired total mAs in mind and trying mentally to determine an mA/time combination that will yield that total, and (3) mentally applying the inverse square law for distance changes.

The following exercises will give you an idea of how well you are able to solve applications of the 15% rule in your head.

To obtain the greatest benefit from the following problems, solve them mentally, without a calculator or pencil and paper. If you have trouble with any of these, turn to Part II of the Math Tutor section of this workbook for review. Remember that application of the 15% rule must be done in "steps" for accuracy. For example, to quadruple the optical density starting at 80 kVp, do not simply increase kVp by 30%. Rather, think of the change as two doublings of the optical density (OD), or two steps of 15%. The first doubling is accomplished with an increase of 12 kVp (15% of 80), but the second doubling must be obtained with an increase of 14 kVp (15% of 92), for a total of 106 kVp.

EXERCISES

1. What is 5% of 70?
   a. 0.5
   b. 1.5
   c. 2.5
   d. 3.5
   e. 4.5

2. What is 5% of 90?
   a. 0.5
   b. 1.5
   c. 2.5
   d. 3.5
   e. 4.5

3. What is 15% of 80?
   a. 8
   b. 12
   c. 16
   d. 20
   e. 22

4. What is 15% of 100?
   a. 10
   b. 15
   c. 20
   d. 25
   e. 30

5. What is one half of 15% of 60?
   a. 4.5
   b. 10.5
   c. 12.5
   d. 15
   e. 17

6. What is one half of 15% of 80?
   a. 4
   b. 5
   c. 6
   d. 10
   e. 14

7. Starting at 60 kVp, what new kVp would result in an optical density that is one half that of the original?
   a. 48 kVp
   b. 51 kVp
   c. 54 kVp
   d. 66 kVp
   e. 69 kVp

8. Original technique: 100 mA, 500 ms, 60 kVp; new technique: 200 mA, 125 ms, _____.
   a. 69 kVp
   b. 70 kVp
   c. 74 kVp
   d. 78 kVp
   e. 80 kVp

9. Original technique: 300 mA, 20 ms, 120 kVp; new technique: 400 mA, 120 kVp, _____.
   a. 5 ms
   b. 10 ms
   c. 15 ms
   d. 25 ms
   e. 30 ms

10. Original technique: 400 mA, 8 ms, 40 kVp; new technique: 50 mA, 90 ms, _____.
    a. 37 kVp
    b. 44 kVp
    c. 46 kVp
    d. 48 kVp
    e. 52 kVp

11. Original technique: 400 mA, 33 ms, 80 kVp; new technique: 300 mA, 33 ms, _____.
    a. 83 kVp
    b. 86 kVp
    c. 90 kVp
    d. 92 kVp
    e. 98 kVp

12. Original technique: 300 mA, 23 ms, 70 kVp; new technique: 150 mA, 100 ms, _____.
    a. 60 kVp
    b. 64 kVp
    c. 77 kVp
    d. 80 kVp
    e. 84 kVp

13. Original technique: 400 mA, 8 ms, 40 kVp; new technique: 50 mA, 90 ms, _____.
    a. 37 kVp
    b. 44 kVp
    c. 46 kVp
    d. 48 kVp
    e. 52 kVp

14. If the required technique is 5 mAs and the mA station selected is 100 mA, what is the required exposure time?
    a. 5 ms
    b. 15 ms
    c. 25 ms
    d. 50 ms
    e. 100 ms

15. When radiographic technique is changed from 12.5 mAs, 100 cm SID, to 150 cm SID, what should be the new mAs?
    a. 18 mAs
    b. 20 mAs
    c. 22 mAs
    d. 28 mAs
    e. 32 mAs

16. If the required technique is 7.5 mAs and the mA station selected is 150 mA, what is the required exposure time?
    a. 10 ms
    b. 20 ms
    c. 30 ms
    d. 40 ms
    e. 50 ms

17. When radiographic technique is changed from 5 mAs, 100 cm SID, to 240 cm SID, what should be the new mAs?
    a. 14 mAs
    b. 19 mAs
    c. 24 mAs
    d. 29 mAs
    e. 36 mAs

Worksheet 13-2
Exposure Time

$$mAs = mA \times s$$

Therefore, exposure time $(s) = \dfrac{mAs}{mA}$

To get the greatest benefit from this worksheet, try to solve the problems mentally, without writing them down or using a calculator. If you need additional help with technique math, turn to the Math Tutor section of this workbook.

EXERCISES

1. If the required technique is 2.5 mAs and the mA station selected is 100 mA, what is the required exposure time?
   a. 10 ms
   b. 15 ms
   c. 25 ms
   d. 75 ms
   e. 125 ms

2. If the required technique is 7.5 mAs and the mA station selected is 150 mA, what is the required exposure time?
   a. 10 ms
   b. 20 ms
   c. 30 ms
   d. 40 ms
   e. 50 ms

3. If the required technique is 20 mAs and the mA station selected is 300 mA, what is the required exposure time?
   a. 15 ms
   b. 67 ms
   c. 87 ms
   d. 133 ms
   e. 140 ms

4. If the required technique is 80 mAs and the mA station selected is 400 mA, what is the required exposure time?
   a. 15 ms
   b. 50 ms
   c. 150 ms
   d. 200 ms
   e. 350 ms

5. If the required technique is 33 mAs and the mA station selected is 100 mA, what is the required exposure time?
   a. 17 ms
   b. 33 ms
   c. 170 ms
   d. 330 ms
   e. 670 ms

6. If the required technique is 20 mAs and the mA station selected is 400 mA, what is the required exposure time?
   a. 5 ms
   b. 10 ms
   c. 20 ms
   d. 33 ms
   e. 50 ms

7. If the required technique is 25 mAs and the mA station selected is 200 mA, what is the required exposure time?
   a. 125 ms
   b. 150 ms
   c. 225 ms
   d. 275 ms
   e. 325 ms

8. If the required technique is 60 mAs and the mA station selected is 300 mA, what is the required exposure time?
   a. 100 ms
   b. 200 ms
   c. 300 ms
   d. 400 ms
   e. 600 ms

9. If the required technique is 240 mAs and the mA station selected is 400 mA, what is the required exposure time?
   a. 600 ms
   b. 900 ms
   c. 1200 ms
   d. 1500 ms
   e. 1800 ms

10. If the required technique is 5 mAs and the mA station selected is 100 mA, what is the required exposure time?
    a. 5 ms
    b. 15 ms
    c. 25 ms
    d. 50 ms
    e. 100 ms

11. If the required technique is 40 mAs and the mA station selected is 200 mA, what is the required exposure time?
    a. 25 ms
    b. 50 ms
    c. 100 ms
    d. 150 ms
    e. 200 ms

12. If the required technique is 5 mAs and the mA station selected is 300 mA, what is the required exposure time?
    a. 10 ms
    b. 17 ms
    c. 34 ms
    d. 50 ms
    e. 67 ms

13. If the required technique is 1.6 mAs and the mA station selected is 100 mA, what is the required exposure time?
    a. 16 ms
    b. 17 ms
    c. 34 ms
    d. 40 ms
    e. 50 ms

14. If the required technique is 1.25 mAs and the mA station selected is 50 mA, what is the required exposure time?
    a. 10 ms
    b. 25 ms
    c. 75 ms
    d. 125 ms
    e. 250 ms

15. If the required technique is 15 mAs and the mA station selected is 100 mA, what is the required exposure time?
    a. 15 ms
    b. 25 ms
    c. 50 ms
    d. 150 ms
    e. 250 ms

16. If the required technique is 120 mAs and the mA station selected is 300 mA, what is the required exposure time?
    a. 100 ms
    b. 200 ms
    c. 300 ms
    d. 400 ms
    e. 500 ms

17. If the required technique is 1.25 mAs and the mA station selected is 100 mA, what is the required exposure time?
    a. 1.25 ms
    b. 12.5 ms
    c. 25 ms
    d. 40 ms
    e. 50 ms

18. If the required technique is 4 mAs and the mA station selected is 200 mA, what is the required exposure time?
    a. 2 ms
    b. 4 ms
    c. 10 ms
    d. 20 ms
    e. 40 ms

19. If the required technique is 12.5 mAs and the mA station selected is 100 mA, what is the required exposure time?
    a. 1.25 ms
    b. 5 ms
    c. 12.5 ms
    d. 25 ms
    e. 125 ms

Worksheet 13-3
Adjusting for Change in Distance

 Use the "square law" to find a new mAs that will compensate for a change in distance. Whereas the **inverse square law** is used to predict radiation intensity and therefore optical density, the square law is used to compensate radiographic technique so that optical density is maintained constant when SID changes.

The square law:

$$\frac{mAs_2}{mAs_1} = \frac{(SID_2)^2}{(SID_1)^2}$$

where mAs_1 is the original mAs used at SID_1 (the original SID), and mAs_2 is the new mAs needed to maintain equal optical density (OD) if the SID is changed to SID_2.

EXERCISES

1. When radiographic technique is changed from 30 mAs, 100 cm SID, to 75 cm SID, what should be the new mAs?
   a. 17 mAs
   b. 20 mAs
   c. 24 mAs
   d. 30 mAs
   e. 32 mAs

2. When radiographic technique is changed from 12.5 mAs, 100 cm SID, to 150 cm SID, what should be the new mAs?
   a. 18 mAs
   b. 20 mAs
   c. 22 mAs
   d. 28 mAs
   e. 32 mAs

3. When radiographic technique is changed from 10 mAs, 100 cm SID, to 180 cm SID, what should be the new mAs?
   a. 20 mAs
   b. 26 mAs
   c. 30 mAs
   d. 32 mAs
   e. 36 mAs

4. When radiographic technique is changed from 5 mAs, 100 cm SID, to 240 cm SID, what should be the new mAs?
   a. 14 mAs
   b. 19 mAs
   c. 24 mAs
   d. 29 mAs
   e. 36 mAs

5. When radiographic technique is changed from 48 mAs, 80 cm SID, to 90 cm SID, what should be the new mAs?
   a. 51 mAs
   b. 55 mAs
   c. 59 mAs
   d. 61 mAs
   e. 71 mAs

6. When radiographic technique is changed from 22.5 mAs, 100 cm SID, to 200 cm SID, what should be the new mAs?
   a. 50 mAs
   b. 70 mAs
   c. 78 mAs
   d. 84 mAs
   e. 90 mAs

7. When radiographic technique is changed from 36 mAs, 150 cm SID, to 113 cm SID, what should be the new mAs?
   a. 20 mAs
   b. 26 mAs
   c. 30 mAs
   d. 38 mAs
   e. 48 mAs

8. When radiographic technique is changed from 10 mAs, 150 cm SID, to 225 cm SID, what should be the new mAs?
   a. 17 mAs
   b. 22.5 mAs
   c. 27.5 mAs
   d. 32.5 mAs
   e. 36 mAs

9. When radiographic technique is changed from 60 mAs, 70 kVp, 150 cm SID, to 113 cm SID, what should be the new mAs?
   a. 34 mAs
   b. 86 mAs
   c. 96 mAs
   d. 102 mAs
   e. 116 mAs

10. A PA chest examination done at 100 cm SID tabletop technique requires 1.5 mAs. What is the required mAs when testing is conducted with a dedicated chest imaging system with a fixed 180 cm SID?
    a. 1 mAs
    b. 2 mAs
    c. 3 mAs
    d. 5 mAs
    e. 10 mAs

11. If the dedicated chest room in Question 10 was designed for a fixed SID of 300 cm, what would be the required mAs?
    a. 1 mAs
    b. 3 mAs
    c. 5 mAs
    d. 13.5 mAs
    e. 20 mAs

12. A dedicated mammography imaging system has a fixed SID of 55 cm and normal technique calls for 200 mAs. If this system is replaced by a 75-cm mammography imaging system, what will be the approximate new mAs?
    a. 200 mAs
    b. 275 mAs
    c. 325 mAs
    d. 375 mAs
    e. 500 mAs

13. In magnification radiography, when the object is placed equidistant between the source and the image receptor, the size of the image will be:
    a. 1.33 times object size
    b. 2.0 times object size
    c. 4 times object size
    d. One half the object size
    e. The same size as the object

14. A radiographic technique that would ensure visibility of detail for a cervical spine examination is:
    a. Increasing the OID
    b. Reducing the SID
    c. Reducing the SSD
    d. Selecting the large focal spot
    e. Using a beam restricting device

15. The major disadvantage to magnification radiography is increased
    a. Artifacts
    b. Blur
    c. Cost
    d. Noise
    e. Patient radiation dose

16. If source-to-image receptor distance (SID) is increased from 50 to 75 cm, what should happen to exposure time?
    a. Increase by $\frac{4}{9}$
    b. Increase by $\frac{2}{3}$
    c. No change
    d. Increase by $\frac{3}{2}$
    e. Increase by $\frac{3}{4}$

17. An x-ray field that is 25×30 cm at 100 cm SID is projected at 180 cm SID. The area of the projected field is:
    a. 750 cm^2
    b. 1350 cm^2
    c. 2430 cm^2
    d. 13,500 cm^2
    e. 22,600 cm^2

Worksheet 13-4
Characteristics of the Imaging System

Proper radiographic exposure must take into account several variable characteristics of the x-ray imaging system. Perhaps the most important characteristic is the type of high-voltage generator incorporated into the imaging system. In general, compared with single-phase generators, full-wave–rectified and more complex waveform generators require a lower kVp and less mAs to produce acceptable radiographs. The radiologic technologist has no control over this characteristic.

Essentially all x-ray imaging systems now have selectable added filtration. The choices of added filtration available to the radiologic technologist usually range from 0 to 4 mm Al, resulting in total filtration of 1.5 to 5.5 mm Al. In general, when one increases added filtration, a reduction in kVp and an increase in mAs are required to maintain constant optical density.

EXERCISES

1. Which of the following is a popular focal-spot combination (small/large) for a dedicated mammography imaging system?
   a. 0.05 mm/0.2 mm
   b. 0.1 mm/0.3 mm
   c. 0.1 mm/3 mm
   d. 0.3 mm/1.0 mm
   e. 0.3 m/1.2 mm

2. The approximate filtration of the x-ray beam contributed by the light-localizing collimator is:
   a. 0.1 mm Al
   b. 0.5 mm Al
   c. 1.0 mm Al
   d. 2.0 mm Al
   e. 3.0 mm Al

3. The radiologic technologist cannot change the type of high-voltage generator used because:
   a. A change can be made only by the medical physicist.
   b. It is fixed at the time of purchase.
   c. Only the radiologic engineer can make that change.
   d. Only the radiologist can make that change.
   e. The service engineer determines this at installation.

4. Compared with half-wave rectification for a fixed exposure time:
   a. Full-wave rectification will have four times the number of pulses.
   b. High-frequency will have six times the number of pulses.
   c. Three-phase will have at least six times the number of pulses.
   d. Three-phase will have at least 12 times the number of pulses.
   e. Three-phase will have four times the number of pulses.

5. The principal advantage of a large focal spot compared with a small focal spot is:
   a. Spatial resolution is enhanced.
   b. Contrast resolution is improved.
   c. Faster image receptors can be used.
   d. Voltage ripple is reduced.
   e. A greater number of x-rays can be produced.

6. An acceptable radiograph is made with the large focal spot. If the examination were repeated with the small focal spot using the same technique:
   a. Patient dose would be lower.
   b. The image would be darker.
   c. The image would be lighter.
   d. The image would be sharper.
   e. The image would have better contrast.

7. General purpose x-ray tubes usually have inherent filtration of:
   a. 0.1 mm Al
   b. 0.5 mm Al
   c. 1.0 mm Al
   d. 2.0 mm Al
   e. 3.0 mm Al

8. Which of the following has the least voltage ripple?
   a. High-frequency
   b. Single-phase, full-wave
   c. Single-phase, half-wave
   d. Three-phase, six-pulse
   e. Three-phase, 12-pulse

145

9. Three-phase–rectified power has which of the following?
   a. Three pulses per cycle
   b. Six pulses per cycle
   c. Nine pulses per cycle
   d. Fifteen pulses per cycle
   e. Eighteen pulses per cycle

10. An acceptable radiograph is made with the large focal spot. If the examination were repeated with the small focal spot:
    a. kVp should be reduced.
    b. mAs and kVp should be increased.
    c. mAs and kVp should be reduced.
    d. mAs should be reduced.
    e. No technique change is required.

11. The principal advantage of a small focal spot compared with a large focal spot is:
    a. Better detail
    b. Use of faster image receptors
    c. Higher heat capacity
    d. Reduced voltage ripple
    e. Production of a greater number of x-rays

12. An acceptable radiograph is made with 1.0 mm Al added filtration and the small focal spot. If the examination were repeated with 3.0 mm Al added filtration, what would be the most likely technique change? (choose all that apply)
    a. Increase kVp
    b. Increase kVp and mAs
    c. Increase mAs
    d. Increase SID
    e. Use the larger focal-spot size

13. An acceptable radiograph is produced with a half-wave–rectified x-ray imaging system. If the examination is repeated on a full-wave imaging system, what should be changed?
    a. Exposure time
    b. kVp
    c. mAs
    d. Object-to-image receptor distance (OID)
    e. SID

14. An acceptable radiograph is made with 1.0 mm Al added filtration. If the examination were repeated with 3.0 mm Al added filtration and appropriate technique changes made:
    a. Image blur would be reduced.
    b. Image contrast would improve.
    c. Patient dose would be reduced.
    d. Spatial resolution would improve.
    e. Such an exposure would not be possible.

15. An acceptable radiograph is made with a single-phase generator. If a repeat examination is performed with a three-phase generator, what technique change should be made?
    a. Increase kVp and mAs
    b. Increase mAs
    c. No change is required
    d. Reduce kVp
    e. Reduce kVp and mAs

16. What is the principal advantage of high-frequency generators?
    a. Better spatial resolution
    b. Enhanced radiation quality
    c. Increased radiation quantity and quality
    d. Reduced radiation quantity
    e. Reduced radiation quantity and quality

Worksheet 13-5 /15-5
Tomography
Magnification Radiography

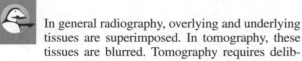 In general radiography, overlying and underlying tissues are superimposed. In tomography, these tissues are blurred. Tomography requires deliberate and controlled motion unsharpness. The principal purpose of tomography is to improve image contrast; however, this improvement occurs at the expense of increased patient dose.

Magnification radiography requires an increase in OID to produce a magnified image. The degree of magnification is given by the magnification factor (MF).

$$MF = \frac{Image\ size}{Object\ size} = \frac{SID}{SOD}$$

Magnification radiography works best with a small x-ray tube focal spot. It usually can be performed without radiographic grids, yet it still results in a somewhat higher patient dose.

EXERCISES

1. During conventional tomography, the image receptor:
   a. Is focused by the angle of movement
   b. Is focused to the automatic plane of interest
   c. Moves opposite the x-ray tube in a seesaw motion
   d. Moves with the x-ray tube similarly to the x-ray tube tower assembly in fluoroscopy
   e. Remains fixed

2. During conventional tomography, structures that lie outside the object plane are blurred because of which of the following?
   a. Absorption blur
   b. Geometric blur
   c. Image receptor blur
   d. Motion blur
   e. Subject blur

3. With linear tomography, which of the following is true?
   a. The source and the image receptor are the same distance from the focal plane.
   b. The source and the image receptor cover different tomographic angles.
   c. The source and the image receptor move at the same speed.
   d. The source and the image receptor move in opposite directions.
   e The source and the image receptor move the same distance.

4. Which of the following combinations determines the thickness of the cut in a tomograph?
   a. Collimation and filtration
   b. SID and length of tube travel
   c. OID and speed of tube travel
   d. SID and speed of tube travel
   e. SOD and length of tube travel

5. Conventional tomography uses which of the following principles?
   a. Tridimensional image
   b. Optical illusion
   c. Motion blur
   d. Random movement
   e. Stereoscopy

6. During conventional tomography, the fulcrum is in the:
   a. Film plane
   b. Focal plane
   c. Image receptor plane
   d. Object plane
   e. Tomographic layer

7. When the tomographic angle is 0 degrees, the tomographic layer is:
   a. Indefinable
   b. Infinity
   c. Thin
   d. Very thick
   e. Zero

8. To obtain a tomographic layer of approximately 1 mm, the tomographic angle should be approximately:
   a. 10 degrees
   b. 20 degrees
   c. 40 degrees
   d. 50 degrees
   e. 60 degrees

9. Which of the following is the major disadvantage of conventional tomography?
   a. Cost
   b. Enhanced contrast
   c. Image blur
   d. Lost spatial resolution
   e. Patient dose

147

10. The major advantage of conventional tomography is better:
    a. Contrast resolution
    b. Cost
    c. Image blur
    d. Patient dose
    e. Spatial resolution

11. Conventional tomography has been called which of the following?
    a. Cisternography
    b. Heel effect
    c. Laminography
    d. Myelography
    e. The line-focus principle

12. Which of the following tomographic angles would be considered for use in zonography?
    a. 5 degrees
    b. 15 degrees
    c. 25 degrees
    d. 35 degrees
    e. 60 degrees

13. The tomographic angle is the angle of x-ray tube movement during which of the following?
    a. Anode preparation
    b. Cathode boost
    c. Fulcrum adjustment
    d. Fulcrum motion
    e. X-ray exposure

14. Adequate magnification radiography requires that which of the following must have a large value?
    a. Focal spot
    b. OID
    c. SID
    d. SOD
    e. SSD

15. Magnification radiography normally is used to image what type of structure?
    a. High-contrast
    b. Large
    c. Low-contrast
    d. Moving
    e. Small

16. The magnification factor is equal to which of the following?
    a. SID + OID
    b. SID ÷ SOD
    c. SOD + OID
    d. SOD ÷ SID
    e. SSD × SID

17. For magnification cerebral angiography, which of the following focal-spot sizes would be best?
    a. 0.3 mm
    b. 0.6 mm
    c. 1.0 mm
    d. 2.0 mm
    e. 10 mm

18. The major disadvantage of magnification radiography is increased:
    a. Artifacts
    b. Blur
    c. Cost
    d. Noise
    e. Patient dose

Worksheet 14-1
History of Computers
Anatomy of a Computer

The hardware of a computer is the nuts, bolts, and chips of the system.

Hardware essentially exists in three stages: input devices, the elements involved in processing and storage, and output devices.

Everything visible and material about a computer is hardware.

The input and output devices, called I/O devices, are the most visible of the computer parts. Some serve only as input or output devices, but most perform a dual function.

Primary memory is provided by the least visible of all the hardware: small memory modules made up of very large-scale integrated circuits on very small silicon chips. The CPU also is located on such a chip.

EXERCISES

1. Which of the following best represents an analog device?
   a. A gasoline pump register
   b. A DVD player
   c. A traditional photograph
   d. A point-of-sale register
   e. A raffle ticket

2. Which of the following is a difference between random access memory (RAM) and read-only memory (ROM)?
   a. One cannot write to ROM.
   b. RAM is faster than ROM.
   c. RAM is on the hard drive and ROM is on a CD.
   d. RAM is solid state and ROM is tape.
   e. ROM is not found in primary memory.

3. Many milestones stand out in the development of the modern computer, but perhaps the *most* important is the:
   a. CPU
   b. Discovery of x-rays
   c. ENIAC
   d. Flip-flop
   e. Transistor

4. The arithmetic unit in a computer:
   a. Can be primary or secondary memory
   b. Contains the control unit
   c. Is an analog device
   d. Is an I/O device
   e. Is synchronized by an internal clock

5. Primary storage usually is found:
   a. On a DVD
   b. In the CPU
   c. On diskettes
   d. On a CD
   e. On the hard disk drive

6. Which of the following has the largest memory capacity?
   a. A floppy disk
   b. A DVD
   c. A CD
   d. A hard disc drive
   e. The CPU

7. A dumb terminal is one that:
   a. Can be programmed
   b. Does not do any processing
   c. Logically fits with the rest of the system
   d. Performs logic functions
   e. Can store data

8. In which of the following is RAM located?
   a. A floppy disk
   b. A magnetic tape
   c. A modem
   d. An optical disc
   e. The motherboard

9. The term *stored program* means which of the following?
   a. Digital instead of analog must be used.
   b. Instructions can be placed in memory.
   c. Memory can be expanded.
   d. Only binary data can be manipulated.
   e. The binary number system must be used.

149

10. The control unit:
    a. Can contain primary or secondary memory
    b. Contains the arithmetic unit
    c. Contains the LUT
    d. Is an I/O device
    e. Is synchronized by an internal clock

11. Which of the following is normally associated with the first generation of computers?
    a. An abacus
    b. Diodes
    c. Peg wheels
    d. Transistors
    e. Vacuum tubes

12. Most primary memory devices consist of which of the following?
    a. A disk
    b. A magnetic ferrite core
    c. A semiconductor
    d. A tape
    e. Transistors

13. Which of the following is an I/O device?
    a. CPU
    b. LUT
    c. Memory module
    d. Microphone
    e. Blu-Ray Disc

14. Which of the following is a type of fast access memory that the computer uses primarily during processing?
    a. Hard disk drive
    b. RAM
    c. CD
    d. DVD
    e. A solid state drive

15. A flatbed scanner is:
    a. A hardware device
    b. A software system
    c. A visual counter
    d. Part of the CPU
    e. Part of the cathode-ray tube (CRT)

16. Secondary memory is available as a:
    a. CPU
    b. Keypad
    c. DVD
    d. Network card
    e. Video display terminal (VDT)

17. Which of the following would be found in the CPU?
    a. Network card
    b. A DVD
    c. An arithmetic unit
    d. LUT
    e. Secondary storage

18. Which of the following would *least* likely be a part of a radiologic imaging VDT?
    a. Alphabetic keypad
    b. LCD
    c. Image receptor
    d. Network card
    e. Special function keypad

19. Which of the following is an arithmetic function?
    a. And/or
    b. Multiplication
    c. If/then
    d. Session
    e. Transfer file

Worksheet 14-2
Computer Software
Processing Methods

The written instructions that guide a computer through its various operations are called **computer programs.** These constitute the software of a computer. System software exists as instructions written in a very low-level computer language and based on the binary number system.

Individual application computer programs are written in various computer languages. High-level computer languages such as C++, BASIC, and Java are written in English-oriented symbols that can be assembled, compiled, or interpreted into a machine-oriented language.

Machine language is the lowest-level language used in computer programs. It consists of a series of binary digits (bits) assembled according to a code to represent instructions for the CPU or numeric and alphabetic characters.

The binary code is based on the binary number system, which contains only two digits—zero and one. Eight bits make a byte, and two bytes make a word. It is the bits, bytes, and words that move through a computer operation from input to output.

EXERCISES

1. Software includes which of the following?
   a. LUT
   b. The CPU
   c. The operating system
   d. The operating terminal
   e. The ROM

2. When a computer is turned on, the first interaction occurs through the:
   a. Applications program
   b. Bootstrap
   c. File manager and scheduler
   d. I/O manager
   e. Memory manager

3. The binary code for the decimal number 18 is:
   a. 10101
   b. 10001
   c. 1001
   d. 1010
   e. 10010

4. The sum of $2^3 + 2^2 + 2^0$ is:
   a. 8
   b. 13
   c. 84
   d. 842
   e. 96

5. The number 47 falls between:
   a. 2^4 and 2^5
   b. 2^5 and 2^6
   c. 2^6 and 2^7
   d. 2^7 and 2^8
   e. 2^8 and 2^9

6. Which of the following is a high-level computer language?
   a. Dbase
   b. Display writer
   c. FORTRAN
   d. LUT
   e. MS Windows

7. Which of the following is an applications program?
   a. C++
   b. Java
   c. Binary code
   d. Windows 7
   e. Microsoft Excel

8. Alphabetic characters usually are encoded by how many bits?
   a. 2
   b. 4
   c. 8
   d. 16
   e. 32

9. The operating system:
   a. Competes with the CPU
   b. Is found in the modem
   c. Is usually in decimal form
   d. Is an application program
   e. Organizes data flow through the computer

10. Which of the following terms does *not* fit with the others?
    a. Assembler
    b. Compiler
    c. Computer language
    d. Interpreter
    e. Operating system

11. Which of the following is a high-level language?
    a. Assembly
    b. Bootstrap
    c. C++
    d. Machine-oriented
    e. Windows 7

12. Which of the following is the oldest of currently used computer languages?
    a. ADA
    b. BASIC
    c. COBOL
    d. FORTRAN
    e. PASCAL

13. An algorithm is:
    a. A computer language
    b. An equation in a computer language
    c. An I/O device
    d. An operating system
    e. Rarely used in diagnostic imaging

14. The computer language that is particularly suited to programming in a design environment is which of the following?
    a. Java
    b. Visual Basic
    c. COBOL
    d. FORTRAN
    e. C++

15. Which type of computer processing is used in radiologic imaging?
    a. Batch processing
    b. Off-line processing
    c. On-line processing
    d. Real-time processing
    e. Time share processing

16. Which of the following equalities is *correct?*
    a. $2^8 = 512$
    b. $2^{10} = 1024$
    c. $3^4 = 27$
    d. $10^4 = 1000$
    e. $12^3 = 1654$

17. Which of the following is the programming language that is easiest to learn?
    a. COBOL
    b. BASIC
    c. FORTRAN
    d. PASCAL

18. The type of program that a user might write to classify radiologic images would be:
    a. A bootstrap program
    b. An applications program
    c. An assembler program
    d. An iterative program
    e. An operating system

19. The zero or one in the binary system is called a:
    a. Bit
    b. Byte
    c. Chomp
    d. CPU
    e. Word

20. To encode is to change from:
    a. Alphabetic characters to decimal characters
    b. Bits to bytes
    c. Bytes to bits
    d. Numbers to words
    e. Ordinary characters to binary digits

21. Which of the following number systems uses the greatest number of digits?
    a. Binary
    b. Decimal
    c. Duodecimal
    d. Exponential
    e. Hexadecimal

22. Which of the following computer measures is the largest?
    a. Bit
    b. Byte
    c. Chomp
    d. Smack
    e. Word

152

ACROSS

Use the following clues to solve the crossword puzzle on the next page.

1. Units that make up two bytes (plural)
2. Designed a system to record census data in 1890; started a company that eventually evolved into IBM
3. System of many transistors and other electronic elements fused onto a chip
4. One of two individuals who designed and built the first electronic digital computer
5. I/O device consisting of a keyboard and a cathode ray tube display
6. Tiny piece of semiconductor material, usually silicon
7. Computer programs that tell the computer what to do and how to store data
8. One of two mathematicians who built mechanical calculators using pegged wheels to automatically perform the four arithmetic functions
9. Type of data processing in which a computer performs operations on defined data without human input or intervention
10. One of the individuals involved in developing UNIVAC, the first commercially successful, general purpose, stored-program electronic digital computer
11. Primary control center unit that carries out instructions
12. Term indicating that a computer is powered by electrical devices rather than by a mechanical device

DOWN

1. Leader of a team of scientists at Bell Laboratories who in 1948 developed the transistor
2. Type of memory used for storing computational instructions or data that might change from time to time; sometimes called *read-write memory*
3. In microcomputers sometimes the CPU is referred to as the _____
4. Device that identifies the route of entry and directs data from an input device to destinations; transfers computed results to the output device selected
5. Operation in which information is transferred into primary memory
6. Type of memory module that consists of groups of silicon chips etched with extremely small storage circuits
7. Operation in which results of a computation are transferred from primary memory to storage or to the user
8. Secondary memory device that stores digital data on a mirrored surface by modulating the reflective properties of that surface
9. In 1842, designed an analytic engine to perform general calculations automatically
10. Visible components of a computer
11. Secondary memory device that stores data in a series of concentric magnetic tracks

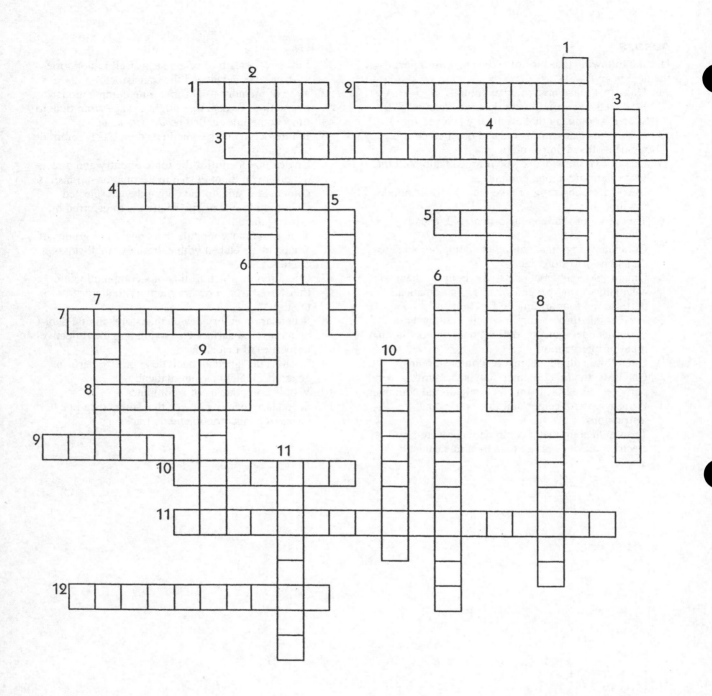

Worksheet 15-1
Computed Radiography Image Receptor

Computed radiography (CR) first appeared in 1984, but it took a decade for CR to become clinically acceptable. CR was the first example of digital radiography. Wet chemistry processing of a latent image is replaced with laser stimulation of metastable electrons that serve as the latent image.

The image receptor in CR is a photostimulable phosphor (PSP) made of barium fluorohalide such as barium fluorobromide (BaFlBr). It appears physically similar to much as a radiographic intensifying screen. With a PSP, however, no light is emitted in response to x-ray exposure. Rather, electrons are energized into a metastable state by the interaction of x-rays.

When an intense laser light is incident on the PSP, light is emitted as the metastable electrons return to their ground state. The intensity of this laser-stimulated light is proportional to the x-ray intensity at the image receptor.

EXERCISES

1. What is the principal difference between screen-film radiography and CR?
   a. Analog vs. digital
   b. Involves light
   c. Requires processing
   d. The cassette
   e. Uses an imaging plate

2. The laser light used in CR:
   a. Is in the ultraviolet light region
   b. Is more energetic than the emitted light
   c. Is pulsed across the PSP
   d. Has longer wavelength than the emitted light
   e. Produces light of intense fluorescence

3. Which of the following steps can be eliminated during switching from screen-film radiography to CR?
   a. Position patient
   b. Perform examination
   c. Process image
   d. Reload cassette
   e. Repeat examination

4. An electron that is described as being metastable:
   a. Is outside of the atom
   b. Is present in positive and negative form
   c. Is the transformation of an x-ray
   d. Has been captured by the nucleus
   e. Has higher energy than it should have

5. Doping of a PSP with europium results in:
   a. Better contrast resolution
   b. Better spatial resolution
   c. Higher x-ray absorption
   d. Lower patient dose
   e. More stimulable light emission

6. The activator in a PSP is there to:
   a. Define laser wavelength
   b. Enhance electron metastability
   c. Increase x-ray absorption
   d. Select the proper wavelength
   e. Shape the wavelength of stimulable emission

7. Which of the following is most intense?
   a. Laser light
   b. Normal visual light
   c. Optical lens support
   d. Stimulable emission
   e. X-ray beam

8. Which of the following is monochromatic?
   a. Infrared light
   b. Laser light
   c. Stimulated emission
   d. Visible light
   e. X-ray beam

9. PSP image receptors are effective because:
   a. Metastable states are produced.
   b. Optical density is proportional to dose.
   c. Spatial resolution is improved.
   d. Their response follows the H & D curve.
   e. They are composed of detector elements (DELs).

10. About how much time can pass between exposing a CR cassette and reading a CR cassette before image quality declines?
    a. 1 hour
    b. 10 minutes
    c. 8 hours
    d. 3 weeks
    e. 6 days

11. As a descriptor of a PSP, the term *turbid* refers to an appearance that is:
    a. Black
    b. Clear
    c. Colored
    d. Cloudy
    e. Gray

12. Europium is an activator in the PSP. An activator is responsible for:
    a. Contrast resolution
    b. Emitted light intensity
    c. Reduced patient dose
    d. Spatial resolution
    e. X-ray absorption

13. PSP image receptors:
    a. Are relatively insensitive to x-rays
    b. Become radiation fatigued with age
    c. Can be fogged by background radiation
    d. Have better spatial resolution than screen-film radiography
    e. Require higher patient dose

14. To remove the image of background radiation or a previous image, one should:
    a. Clear the image receptor with a cleaning solution.
    b. Expose the image receptor to intense light.
    c. Expose the image receptor to intense x-ray exposure.
    d. Store the image receptor for 3 days.
    e. Transfer the image receptor signal to digital storage.

15. Which of the following is the proper sequence for producing a computed radiographic image?
    a. Erase/read/expose
    b. Expose/erase/read
    c. Expose/read/erase
    d. Read/erase/expose
    e. Read/expose/erase

16. Thermoluminescent dosimeters (TLD) emit light when:
    a. Exposed to heat
    b. Exposed to light
    c. Exposed to x-rays
    d. Exposed to cold
    e. Exposed to gamma-rays

17. PSP emit light when:
    a. Exposed to heat
    b. Exposed to light
    c. Exposed to x-rays
    d. Exposed to cold
    e. Exposed to gamma-rays

18. Fog will appear on CR cassettes with exposure to:
    a. Light
    b. Background radiation
    c. Laser light
    d. Humidity
    e. Cold

19. CR cassettes eliminate the need for:
    a. A film processor
    b. Proper patient positioning
    c. Techniques that minimize dose
    d. A dark room
    e. Computers

Worksheet 15-2
Computed Radiography Reader

 The computed radiography (CR) reader (processor) appears much like a film daylight loader system. However, appearance is the only similarity between the two. Inside the CR reader are mechanical drive mechanisms, optical shaping lenses and mirrors, and photosensitive detectors.

The mechanical drive mechanism supports a "slow" scan of the imaging plate by moving the plate slowly through the reader. The optical assembly supports a "fast" scan mode by deflecting the laser beam back and forth across the imaging plate as it is slow scanned.

Interaction of the laser beam with the imaging plate results in photostimulable emission, which is measured by a photodiode and quantified. The intensity of photostimulable emission is proportional to the intensity of the x-ray exposure to that portion of the imaging plate. The diameter of the laser beam and scan motion determine the size of each pixel.

EXERCISES

1. The photostimulable emission in CR:
   a. Has longer wavelength than the laser-stimulating light
   b. Has shorter wavelength than the laser-stimulating light
   c. Is discrete, as is the laser-stimulating light
   d. Is in the far infrared region of the spectrum
   e. Is monochromatic, as is the laser-stimulating light

2. The slow scan portion of the CR reader:
   a. Has a speed that is determined by the emission rate
   b. Is under mechanical control
   c. Is under optical control
   d. Relies on a photometric response
   e. Requires mirrors and prisms

3. Spatial resolution in CR is principally determined by:
   a. Fast scan rate
   b. Field of view
   c. Laser beam diameter
   d. Phosphor size
   e. Slow scan rate

4. The source of the stimulating light is:
   a. Emitted light
   b. The laser
   c. The optical path
   d. The photometer
   e. X-radiation

5. What is the approximate diameter of the laser beam?
   a. <1 nm
   b. 10 nm
   c. 100 nm
   d. 1000 nm
   e. >1000 nm

6. How does the CR reader maintain the laser beam as a circle?
   a. Beam-shaping optics
   b. Fast scan regulation
   c. Intensity control
   d. Light-collecting optics
   e. Slow scan regulation

7. Which of the following is *not* a photodetector?
   a. ADC
   b. CCD
   c. CMOS
   d. PD
   e. PMT

8. The x-ray capture element of a CR imaging plate is the:
   a. BaFlBr
   b. Cassette
   c. CCD
   d. Laser beam
   e. Light-collecting optics

9. The characteristic curve of a CR imaging plate is described as:
   a. Detective quantum efficiency
   b. Image buffer
   c. Image receptor response function
   d. Modulation transfer function
   e. Sampling quantization

157

10. A screen-film image receptor is responsive over
    how many orders of magnitude?
    a. One
    b. Two
    c. Three
    d. Four
    e. Five

11. An advantage of CR over screen-film radiography,
    regardless of the type of examination, is the
    relatively constant:
    a. Image contrast
    b. Image processing
    c. Optical density
    d. Patient positioning
    e. Radiographic technique

12. Patient radiation dose reduction in CR is limited by:
    a. Fast scan mode
    b. Image contrast
    c. Patient size
    d. Slow scan mode
    e. System noise

13. Which of the following statements applies when CR
    is compared with screen-film radiography?
    a. kVp is less important.
    b. Image processing is faster.
    c. mAs is less important.
    d. Optical density is better.
    e. Patient positioning is easier.

14. Which of the following is an advantage of CR over
    screen-film radiography?
    a. Easier viewing
    b. Fewer repeats
    c. Patient positioning
    d. Patient scheduling
    e. Technique selection

15. A CR image receptor is responsive to an x-ray
    beam over how many orders of magnitude?
    a. One
    b. Two
    c. Three
    d. Four
    e. Five

16. Which of the following is a source of image noise
    that is apparent in CR and not in screen-film
    radiography?
    a. Latent image fading
    b. Electronic noise
    c. Noise due to properties of the phosphor
    d. Image receptor noise
    e. Scatter

17. CR imaging allows for the display of about:
    a. 30 shades of grey
    b. 100 shades of grey
    c. 3000 shades of grey
    d. 10,000 shades of grey
    e. 1,000,000,000 shades of grey

18. Screen-film radiography allows for the display of
    about
    a. 30 shades of grey
    b. 100 shades of grey
    c. 3000 shades of grey
    d. 10,000 shades of grey
    e. 1,000,000,000 shades of grey

Worksheet 16-1
Direct Radiography

Direct radiography produces digital radio-graphic images with a flat-panel, solid-state image receptor. Three designs are in use: photostimulable phosphor charge-coupled device (CCD), amorphous silicon (a-Si), and amorphous selenium (a-Se).

EXERCISES

1. Which of the following is the principal disadvantage of using an area beam versus a scanned projection radiography?
   a. Increased patient dose
   b. Lack of postexamination processing
   c. Reduced spatial resolution
   d. Scatter radiation
   e. Short exposure time

2. In scanned projection digital radiography, which of the following moves to produce an image?
   a. The x-ray tube
   b. A charge-coupled device (CCD)
   c. A laser
   d. The patient
   e. The image receptor

3. Digital imaging systems _____ than screen-film radiography:
   a. Have better spatial resolution
   b. Are slower
   c. Produce an initial image in analog form
   d. Require computer processing
   e. Use film as the image receptor

4. A scanned projection radiograph (SPR):
   a. Has better spatial resolution
   b. Has worse contrast than digital fluoroscopy
   c. Is like a tomograph
   d. Is virtually scatter-free
   e. Removes superposition of structures

5. Which of the following is a part of SPR?
   a. Analog-to-digital converter
   b. Area beam
   c. Data acquisition system
   d. Detector array
   e. Video monitor

6. Which of the following maintains the largest line spread function?
   a. Computed radiography
   b. Direct radiography
   c. SPR
   d. Digital mammography
   e. Screen-film radiography

7. The principal advantage of using an area beam versus an SPR is which of the following?
   a. Improved contrast resolution
   b. Low patient dose
   c. Postexamination processing
   d. Scatter radiation rejection
   e. Short exposure time

8. Which of the following is an advantage of an area beam over an SPR in digital radiography?
   a. Improved contrast
   b. Less scatter
   c. Less technique required
   d. Low noise
   e. Reduced motion blur

9. Which of the following is used as an image receptor in direct radiography?
   a. An image intensifier
   b. $CaWO_4$
   c. $CdWO_4$
   d. a-Se
   e. Rare earth phosphors

10. The principal disadvantage of digital radiography versus screen-film radiography is which of the following?
    a. Edge enhancement
    b. Longer exposure time
    c. More motion artifact
    d. Poorer contrast resolution
    e. Poorer spatial resolution

11. A digital image constructed on a 512 × 512 matrix will have how many pixels?
    a. 512
    b. 1024
    c. 512^2
    d. 1024^2
    e. 1636

159

12. All of the following are materials used in direct radiography, except:
   a. a-Se
   b. CsI
   c. GdOS
   d. CCD
   e. LaOBr

13. Which of the following is unique to direct radiography?
   a. A detector array
   b. Area x-ray beam
   c. Fast image access
   d. No cassette is required
   e. Reregistration

14. The image receptor in computed radiography could be:
   a. a-Se
   b. a-Si
   c. BaFlCl
   d. $CaWO_4$
   e. $CdWO_4$

15. Which of the following is used as a radiation detector in direct radiography?
   a. BGO
   b. $CdWO_4$
   c. Ceramic
   d. a-Se
   e. Xe

16. The principal limitation of the SPR mode of digital radiography is which of the following?
   a. Cost
   b. Examination time
   c. Image noise
   d. Patient dose
   e. Spatial resolution

17. An x-ray system used for direct radiography definitely has which of the following?
   a. A linear H & D curve
   b. A method of printing film
   c. A rapid film changer
   d. Access to the Internet
   e. At least two video monitors

18. Spatial resolution in digital imaging systems is primarily limited by:
   a. The speed of the examination
   b. The amount of collimation
   c. The tube's heat capacity
   d. Scatter
   e. The size and number of detectors

19. The principal advantage of a fan-shaped x-ray beam over an area x-ray beam is which of the following?
   a. Examination time
   b. Hybrid images
   c. Less heat generated
   d. Reduced patient dose
   e. Scatter radiation rejection

20. Which of the following has the highest spatial resolution?
   a. Computed radiography
   b. Direct radiography
   c. SPR
   d. Digital mammography
   e. Screen-film radiography

21. Which is most important for soft tissue contrast?
   a. Contrast resolution
   b. Spatial resolution
   c. High lp/mm
   d. Noise
   e. Scatter

Worksheet 17-1
Spatial Resolution

The ability of an imaging system to render on the image a faithful reproduction of a small, high-contrast object is termed **spatial resolution.** The smaller the object that can be imaged, the better the spatial resolution.

It is easy to image smaller and smaller objects and to state spatial resolution in terms of object size—1 cm, 1 mm, or 1 μm. In medical imaging, spatial resolution is expressed in terms of spatial frequency or frequency in space. Spatial frequency is a measure of how quickly an object changes in space.

Tissues can be identified by their spatial frequency. Calcified lung nodules or breast microcalcifications are high spatial frequency objects. Abdominal tissue, fat, and soft tissue masses are low spatial frequency objects. It is difficult for any imaging system to image both high-frequency objects and low-frequency objects.

As a generalization, digital imaging systems have better contrast resolution but poorer spatial resolution than screen-film imaging systems.

EXERCISES

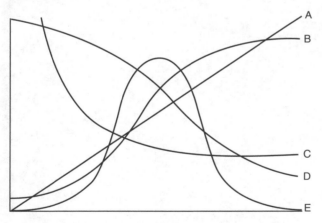

1. Which of the curves above represents a modulation transfer function?
   a. A
   b. B
   c. C
   d. D
   e. E

2. Which of the curves above represents a contrast-detail curve?
   a. A
   b. B
   c. C
   d. D
   e. E

3. Which of the curves above represents a characteristic screen-film response?
   a. A
   b. B
   c. C
   d. D
   e. E

4. Which of the curves above represents the digital image receptor radiation response?
   a. A
   b. B
   c. C
   d. D
   e. E

5. Which of the curves above represents a line spread function?
   a. A
   b. B
   c. C
   d. D
   e. E

6. Spatial frequency consists of units of:
   a. Line length
   b. Line pair
   c. Line pair/millimeter
   d. Millimeter
   e. Millimeter/line pair

7. As an object gets smaller, which of the following gets bigger?
   a. ll
   b. lp
   c. lp/mm
   d. mm
   e. mm/lp

8. A breast microcalcification is spherical and 300 μm in diameter. What is the spatial frequency of this tissue object?
   a. 0.5 lp/mm
   b. 0.6 lp/mm
   c. 1.0 lp/mm
   d. 1.7 lp/mm
   e. 2.7 lp/mm

9. Screen-film radiography can image to 8 lp/mm. This represents an object of approximately what size?
   a. 25 μm
   b. 63 μm
   c. 128 μm
   d. 250 μm
   e. 500 μm

10. A calcified lung nodule measures 1 cm. What spatial frequency does this represent?
    a. 0.05 lp/mm
    b. 0.1 lp/mm
    c. 0.5 lp/mm
    d. 1.0 lp/mm
    e. 5.0 lp/mm

11. The best a multislice computed tomography imaging system can image is 1.5 lp/mm. This represents an object of what size?
    a. 125 μm
    b. 333 μm
    c. 400 μm
    d. 550 μm
    e. 675 μm

12. The modulation transfer function for a digital imaging system has a cutoff spatial frequency of 5 lp/mm. What is the pixel size?
    a. 10 μm
    b. 25 μm
    c. 50 μm
    d. 100 μm
    e. 200 μm

13. Which of the curves above represents best spatial resolution?
    a. A
    b. B
    c. C
    d. D

14. Which of the curves above is most likely from a regular screen-film imaging system?
    a. A
    b. B
    c. C
    d. D

15. Which of the curves above represents digital radiography?
    a. A
    b. B
    c. C
    d. D

Worksheet 17-2
Contrast Resolution
Contrast Detail

Although it is clear that digital radiography has poorer spatial resolution than screen-film imaging, it is also becoming clearer that the superior contrast resolution of digital imaging is important for image quality and interpretation. Contrast resolution results in the ability to distinguish many shades of gray on an image.

The number of gray levels that an imaging system can produce is called **dynamic range.** The human visual system can see perhaps 30 shades of gray, and that is what we are stuck with when we use screen-film radiography. Today's digital imaging systems are capable of rendering up to 65,536 shades of gray (16 bits), all visible with postprocessing of the image.

One method for evaluating the relative spatial and contrast resolutions of imaging systems is the contrast-detail curve. Use of such a curve shows that spatial resolution is determined by the modulation transfer function (MTF) of the imaging system; contrast resolution is limited by the noise of the system.

EXERCISES

1. Which of the following reduces contrast resolution?
   a. Detective quantum efficiency
   b. kVp
   c. mAs
   d. Modulation transfer function
   e. Noise

2. If the dynamic range of a magnetic resonance imaging system is 12 bits, how many shades of gray are present?
   a. 1024
   b. 2048
   c. 4096
   d. 8192
   e. 16,384

3. Patient radiation dose should be lower when digital imaging is used than when screen-film imaging is used, principally because of:
   a. Detective quantum efficiency
   b. kVp
   c. mAs
   d. Modulation transfer function
   e. Noise

4. Contrast resolution in computed tomography is superior compared with other x-ray systems because of:
   a. Collimation
   b. Detective quantum efficiency
   c. The range of tissue values
   d. Modulation transfer function
   e. Spiral motion

5. "Technique creep" is an attempt to reduce patient radiation dose by instituting:
   a. Increased detective quantum efficiency (DQE)
   b. Increased kVp and reduced mAs
   c. Increased mAs and reduced kVp
   d. Increased mAs and reduced noise
   e. No repeats

6. The digital radiographic imaging repeat rate due to poor radiographic technique should not exceed:
   a. 0%
   b. 1%
   c. 5%
   d. 10%
   e. 25%

7. Detective quantum efficiency (DQE) is a measure of:
   a. Contrast resolution
   b. Digital data file size
   c. Image noise
   d. Spatial resolution
   e. X-ray absorption

8. The principal advantage of digital radiography over screen-film radiography is:
   a. Contrast resolution
   b. Easier patient positioning
   c. Fewer repeats
   d. Less noise
   e. Reduced radiographic technique

9. The x-ray beam incident on the image receptor compared with the one incident on the patient?
   a. Has higher energy
   b. Has higher mAs
   c. Has the same energy
   d. Has lower energy
   e. Has poorer image receptor absorption

10. What happens at the K-edge of the phosphor of a receptor?
    a. Higher noise
    b. Higher x-ray absorption
    c. Lower detective quantum efficiency
    d. Lower modulation transfer function
    e. Lower x-ray absorption

11. The dynamic range of screen-film radiography is:
    a. 4096
    b. 30
    c. 1000
    d. 3000
    e. 16,384

12. The dynamic range of a typical digital imaging system is:
    a. 4096
    b. 30
    c. 1000
    d. 3000
    e. 16,384

13. Why do digital imaging systems have a higher modulation transfer function at low spatial frequencies than does screen-film imaging?
    a. Better contrast resolution
    b. Fewer repeats
    c. Higher detective quantum efficiency (DQE)
    d. Less kVp dependence
    e. Lower patient dose

14. The postprocessing method used to allow humans to see all shades of gray in an image is referred to as:
    a. DQE
    b. Window and level
    c. Spatial resolution
    d. Contrast detail
    e. Technique optimization

15. Spatial resolution in screen-film radiography is determined principally by:
    a. The type of film
    b. Grid size
    c. Collimation
    d. Focal-spot size
    e. Pixel size

16. Spatial resolution in digital imaging systems is determined principally by:
    a. The type of film
    b. Grid size
    c. Collimation
    d. Focal-spot size
    e. Pixel size

17. A 2006 study comparing digital mammography to screen-film mammography indicated that digital mammography is:
    a. Inferior to screen film in all cases
    b. Superior to screen film in all cases
    c. Superior for younger, denser breasts
    d. Superior for older, less dense breasts
    e. Equivalent to screen film

Worksheet 18-1
Viewing the Digital Radiographic Image

The adoption of digital imaging brings with it a new set of required physics skills. In addition to the physics of ionizing radiation, we must have an understanding of the physics of visible light and how it affects image interpretation.

Photometry is the science of visible light, including its emission, reflection, and measurement. The basic unit of photometry is the lumen, which quantifies the intensity of light from a source. A digital image on a digital display device is called **soft copy,** and a screen-film image on a viewbox is referred to as **hard copy**.

A major advantage of digital imaging is that it allows one to preprocess and postprocess the image, to accentuate image detail. Further, the digital image can be viewed by different people in different locations through the picture archiving and communication system (PACS), which is not available with screen-film imaging.

EXERCISES

1. Photometry is the science of the:
   a. Anatomy of human vision
   b. Measurement of photographic images
   c. Quantity of light
   d. Reflection and refraction of light
   e. Measurement of the response of the human eye to light

2. The postprocessing manipulation called *image inversion* refers to:
   a. Changing from landscape to portrait format
   b. Exchange of images
   c. Reorienting right and left
   d. Reorienting top and bottom
   e. Turning white-black to black-white

3. Photopic vision is associated with:
   a. Color vision
   b. Cone vision
   c. Dim light
   d. Black and white vision
   e. Rod vision

4. How does one preprocess a digital image to correct for pixel, row, or column defects?
   a. Dark reference correction
   b. Extrapolation algorithms
   c. Interpolation algorithms
   d. Offset correction
   e. Pixel reregistration

5. Which of the following describes the luminous intensity from a light source such as a lightbulb?
   a. Cosine law
   b. Illuminance
   c. Luminance
   d. Luminance intensity
   e. Luminous flux

6. What is the approximate illuminance of an indoor tennis court?
   a. 5 ft-c
   b. 20 ft-c
   c. 30 ft-c
   d. 100 ft-c
   e. 200 ft-c

7. The luminance of a digital display device is measured in:
   a. Candelas
   b. Candelas per meter squared
   c. Foot-candles
   d. Lumens
   e. Luces

8. What is the matrix array of a 5 megapixel digital display device?
   a. 500×1000 pixels
   b. 1000×1000 pixels
   c. 1200×1800 pixels
   d. 1500×2000 pixels
   e. 2000×2500 pixels

9. Which of the following is characteristic of a CRT but not of an AMLCD?
   a. Active matrix address
   b. Flat face
   c. Light modulating
   d. Square pixel
   e. Veiling glare

10. What unit is used to describe illuminance, the intensity of light incident on a surface?
    a. Candela
    b. Candela per meter squared
    c. Foot-candle
    d. Lumen
    e. Nit

165

11. The luminance of a mammography viewbox must be uniform and at least 3000 nit. What is a nit?
    a. Candela per foot squared
    b. Candela per meter squared
    c. Lumen per foot squared
    d. Lumen per meter squared
    e. Lumen per steradian

12. With digital radiography, the cosine law applies to:
    a. Grayscale imaging
    b. Image inversion
    c. Inverse square law
    d. Off-axis viewing
    e. Reduced spatial resolution

13. Compared with photopic vision, scotopic vision:
    a. Has better spatial resolution
    b. Involves cones
    c. Is bright light vision
    d. Is more color vision
    e. Occurs at shorter wavelengths

14. An active matrix liquid crystal display is better than a cathode ray tube display because:
    a. Of its light-emitting property
    b. Of its phosphor face
    c. It has a curved face
    d. It is a light-modulating device
    e. It uses a scanning electron beam

15. Liquid crystals are:
    a. Linear organic molecules
    b. Phosphor grains
    c. Photo-detecting devices
    d. Thin film transistors
    e. Solid grains embedded in glass

16. The aperture ratio refers to the:
    a. Ability to control individual pixels
    b. Percent of light transmission
    c. Size of a pixel
    d. Size of the liquid crystals
    e. Viewing of an image off-axis

17. Ergonomics is the study of:
    a. Hospital information systems
    b. Human factors applied to system design
    c. Light levels in work areas
    d. Light illumination of workstations
    e. Picture archiving and communications systems

18. All of the following are examples of image preprocessing, except:
    a. Window and level
    b. Offset correction
    c. Flatfielding
    d. Gain correction
    e. Signal interpolation

19. Which of the following postprocessing methods helps improve visualization and spatial resolution?
    a. Annotation
    b. Magnification
    c. Image flip
    d. Image inversion
    e. Edge enhancement

20. PACS' primary use is to:
    a. Postprocess an image
    b. Preprocess an image
    c. Store digital images
    d. Invert an image
    e. Increase the size of the file room

166

Worksheet 19-1
Image Artifacts

 Perhaps the most important quality control program is that associated with the automatic processor. Daily monitoring of the automatic processor is essential, and this attention should be properly recorded.

An artifact is any irregular optical density on a radiograph that is not caused by the proper shadowing of the object by the primary x-ray beam. Processing, exposure, and handling and storage are the three types of artifacts a radiologic technologist is likely to encounter.

EXERCISES

1. Patient motion during exposure will result in which of the following?
   a. A handling artifact
   b. A processing artifact
   c. A storage artifact
   d. An exposure artifact
   e. An imaging system artifact

2. A guide shoe is a component of which of the following?
   a. A cassette
   b. A darkroom countertop
   c. A film bin
   d. An automatic processor
   e. An image receptor

3. The yellow appearance of a radiograph after a long time:
   a. Indicates that the developer was overreplenished
   b. Indicates that the developer was underreplenished
   c. Is a processing artifact
   d. Is a storage artifact
   e. Results from extended processing

4. Wet pressure sensitization would be classified as which of the following?
   a. A handling artifact
   b. A processing artifact
   c. A storage artifact
   d. An exposure artifact
   e. An imaging system artifact

5. Pi lines are so called because they:
   a. Are visible on the latent image
   b. Look like a section of pie
   c. Look like a whole sliced pie
   d. Occur at regular intervals
   e. Occur on the finished radiograph

6. Static artifacts appear *most often* during what conditions of temperature and humidity, respectively?
   a. High, high
   b. High, low
   c. This varies
   d. Low, high
   e. Low, low

7. If residual thiosulfate is *not* properly removed during washing, the radiograph will:
   a. Be overdeveloped
   b. Be underdeveloped
   c. Have to be repeated
   d. Turn blue
   e. Turn yellow

ACROSS

1. _____ fog looks like light or radiation fog and is usually a uniform, dull gray.
2. Warped cassettes cause _____ artifacts.
3. Dirt or chemical stain on a roller can cause _____ _____.
4. _____ fog and light fog look alike.
5. Chemistry not properly squeezed from the film creates a _____ effect.
6. When radiographers mix up cassettes, _____ _____ can occur.

DOWN

1. Dirty or _____ rollers can cause emulsion pickoff.
2. An artifact is any _____ on a radiograph that is not caused by superimposition of anatomy in the primary x-ray beam.

3. Cassettes that have not been checked for proper screen-film contact cause a _____ in the area of poor contact on the radiographic image.
4. _____-_____ sensitization is caused when irregular rollers cause pressure during development and produce small circular patterns.
5. Inadequate processing chemistry can result in a chemical fog called a _____ stain.
6. Crown, tree, and smudge are three distinct patterns of _____.
7. If a patient is placed under the tube when the tube is not centered to the table or Bucky tray, _____-_____ artifacts will occur.
8. Kinking or abrupt bending before processing can cause scratches that look like _____ marks.
9. A radiograph with patient motion appears blurred or _____.
10. Gelatin buildup can result in _____ deposits on the film.

Worksheet 20-1
Screen-Film Radiographic Quality Control

X-ray imaging systems are increasingly more sophisticated and complicated. Although the operation of such imaging systems often is made easier by continuing developments in design, the assurance that the equipment is functioning properly becomes more difficult to monitor. Such monitoring is called a **quality control program.**

A quality control program designed for an x-ray imaging system involves a number of observations and measurements of the various parts and subsystems of the system.

EXERCISES

1. Compared with a quality control program, a quality assurance program:
   a. Deals with equipment
   b. Deals with people
   c. Is normally performed weekly
   d. Is normally performed monthly
   e. Is normally performed annually

2. Which of the following is an essential element of a quality control program?
   a. Equipment performance evaluation
   b. Error correction
   c. Image interpretation
   d. Personnel performance evaluation
   e. Repair procedures

3. Radiographic kVp should be evaluated:
   a. Weekly
   b. Monthly
   c. Semiannually
   d. Annually
   e. Not required

4. The variable-aperture, light-localizing collimator must confine the x-ray beam to:
   a. ± 2% of the SID
   b. ± 5% of the SID
   c. Inside the light field
   d. Outside the light field
   e. Within the light field

5. The actual radiographic kVp should be within what value of the indicated kVp?
   a. ± 1%
   b. ± 2%
   c. ± 4%
   d. ± 6%
   e. ± 10%

6. Which of the following devices may be used to assess the accuracy of the exposure timer?
   a. Densitometer
   b. Penetrameter
   c. Ramp filter
   d. Sensitometer
   e. Solid-state detector

7. If the automatic exposure timer fails, a backup timer should terminate the exposure at:
   a. 3 s or 300 mAs
   b. 6 s or 600 mAs
   c. 9 s or 900 mAs
   d. 12 s or 1200 mAs
   e. 15 s or 1500 mAs

8. Output radiation intensity should be reproducible to within:
   a. 1%
   b. 3%
   c. 5%
   d. 10%
   e. 20%

9. Conventional tomography images should lie within what distance of the indicated tomographic plane?
   a. ± 1 mm
   b. ± 5 mm
   c. ± 10 mm
   d. ± 15 mm
   e. A range of values (depending on tube motion)

10. Which of the following organizations accredits hospitals?
    a. ACMP
    b. ACPM
    c. ACR
    d. CRCPD
    e. The Joint Commission

11. The minimum filtration required for general purpose radiography is:
    a. 2.0 mm Al
    b. 2.1 mm Al
    c. 2.3 mm Al
    d. 2.5 mm Al
    e. 3.0 mm Al

12. Which of the following can be used to measure effective focal-spot size?
    a. Densitometer
    b. Ion chamber
    c. Sensitometer
    d. Slit camera
    e. Solid-state detector

13. The ability of an x-ray imaging system to produce constant radiation output at various combinations of mA and exposure time, resulting in the same mAs, is called:
    a. Accuracy
    b. Linearity
    c. Precision
    d. Reproducibility
    e. Uniformity

14. A photometer is an instrument that is used to measure:
    a. Artifacts
    b. Contrast resolution
    c. Illumination
    d. Optical density
    e. Spatial resolution

15. Output radiation intensity linearity should be within what percent for adjacent mA stations?
    a. 1%
    b. 3%
    c. 5%
    d. 10%
    e. 20%

16. The exposure timer at exposures more than 10 ms should be accurate to within:
    a. 1%
    b. 3%
    c. 5%
    d. 10%
    e. 20%

17. The exposure timer at exposures 10 ms or less should be accurate to within:
    a. 1%
    b. 3%
    c. 5%
    d. 10%
    e. 20%

18. What is the minimum half-value layer (HVL) for a high-frequency 70 kVp x-ray beam?
    a. 0.4 mm Al
    b. 1.5 mm Al
    c. 1.5 mm Cu
    d. 2.0 mm Al
    e. 2.0 mm Cu

19. What instrument is the standard of measure for effective focal-spot sizes?
    a. Pinhole camera
    b. Star pattern
    c. Slit camera
    d. Diode
    e. Ionization chamber

20. How often should the wash water and developer temperatures be measured for effective film-processor QC?
    a. Hourly
    b. Daily
    c. Weekly
    d. Monthly
    e. Yearly

Worksheet 21-1
Digital Radiographic Artifacts

An artifact is any feature on an image that does not truly represent tissue. Artifacts can interfere with diagnosis and obscure lesions or normal anatomy.

Digital imaging artifacts can be classified into three categories: image receptor artifacts, object artifacts, and processing artifacts. The radiologic technologist must be able to identify the source of an artifact.

Artifacts associated with pixel failure are easily identified but may be difficult to correct. Environmental radiation or previous exposure of computed radiography image receptors can produce ghost images. These are easily corrected. Preprocessing and postprocessing artifacts also are easily corrected, and the correction is automatic.

In general, digital artifacts are easier to correct than screen-film artifacts.

EXERCISES

1. Which of the following is *not* a digital imaging artifact?
   a. Alignment
   b. Collimation
   c. Density difference
   d. Image compression
   e. Partition

2. When does the radiologic technologist have to be concerned with processing artifacts?
   a. When compression is employed
   b. When image histograms are used
   c. When images are printed
   d. When partition is involved
   e. When software is corrupted

3. Ghost images can appear when:
   a. Radiation fatigue is present.
   b. Dust remains on the image receptor.
   c. A CR image receptor has not been erased in 24 hours.
   d. A DR image receptor is not completely read out.
   e. A proper QC program is not instituted.

4. Which of the following should be presented to the radiologist for interpretation?
   a. For-compression image
   b. For-extrapolation image
   c. For-interpolation image
   d. For-presentation image
   e. For-processing image

5. Flatfielding is a preprocessing feature used to apply:
   a. Contrast resolution correction
   b. Geometric distortion correction
   c. Equalize response program
   d. Noise reduction algorithms
   e. Spatial resolution enhancement

6. What level of image compression is considered acceptable?
   a. 3:1
   b. 5:1
   c. 8:1
   d. 10:1
   e. 20:1

7. What does this artifact represent?

   a. Damaged imaging plate
   b. Debris on imaging plate
   c. Inadequate erasure
   d. Postprocessing artifact
   e. Preprocessing artifact

8. What does this artifact represent?

a. Inadequate erasure
b. Inappropriate reconstruction algorithm
c. Improper alignment
d. Improper collimation
e. Improper partition

9. What does this artifact represent?

a. Ghost image
b. Improper collimation
c. Improper partition
d. Inadequate erasure
e. Preprocessing artifact

Worksheet 22-1
AAPM TG-18

 Quality control programs supporting screen-film radiography are directed toward wet chemistry processing and viewbox illumination, among other activities. Times are changing, and rapidly. Similar quality control activities associated with digital imaging are associated with image receptor response and digital display devices used for image interpretation.

Digital display devices may have a number of deficiencies that can interfere with image interpretation. Several organizations have developed electronic test patterns to assess the image quality of a digital display device.

The American Association of Physicists in Medicine (AAPM) has taken the lead in developing electronic test patterns for quality control procedures for digital display devices. These test patterns are designed to be used regularly to evaluate characteristics of digital monitors such as geometric distortion, reflection, resolution, noise, and other features. Users should now use these test patterns in an ordered program of quality control.

EXERCISES

1. Which of the following organizations never developed electronic test patterns for digital display quality control?
   a. ANSI
   b. AAPM
   c. NEMA
   d. SMPTE
   e. VESA

2. GSDF stands for:
   a. Grand source of detected features
   b. Grayscale display function
   c. Great seal of dynamic function
   d. Gross scale of dynamic factors
   e. Ground source determined factor

3. Luminance response of a digital display device is properly accomplished with a/an:
   a. Charge-coupled device
   b. Densitometer
   c. Illuminator
   d. Photometer
   e. Sensitometer

4. This is the AAPM TG-18 QC test pattern. What is it used to evaluate?

   a. Artifacts
   b. Contrast resolution
   c. Geometric distortion
   d. Noise
   e. Spatial resolution

5. This is the AAPM TG-18 AD test pattern. What is it used to evaluate?

a. Artifacts
b. Contrast resolution
c. Diffuse reflection
d. Geometric distortion
e. Noise

6. Geometric distortion causes:
a. Poor overall image visibility
b. Displayed image to differ in size from original
c. Mirror images of surrounding objects
d. Difficulty seeing dark objects
e. Difficulty seeing small objects

7. Too much noise in an image causes:
a. Poor overall image visibility
b. Displayed image to differ in size from original
c. Mirror images of surrounding objects
d. Difficulty seeing dark objects
e. Difficulty seeing small objects

8. This is the AAPM TG-18 CT test pattern that contains 16 shades of gray. What is it used to evaluate?

a. Contrast resolution
b. Diffuse reflection
c. Geometric distortion
d. Luminance response
e. Noise

9. Poor luminance response often indicates:
a. Poor overall image visibility
b. Displayed image to differ in size from original
c. Mirror images of surrounding objects
d. Difficulty seeing dark objects
e. Difficulty seeing small objects

10. Poor display spatial resolution results in:
a. Poor overall image visibility
b. Displayed image to differ in size from original
c. Mirror images of surrounding objects
d. Difficulty seeing dark objects
e. Difficulty seeing small objects

11. This is the AAPM TG-18 LN test pattern that contains three images. What is it used to evaluate?

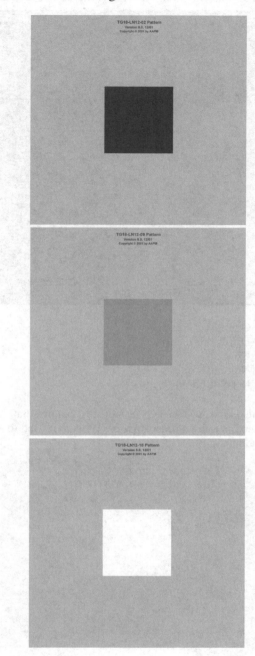

a. Artifacts
b. Contrast resolution
c. Diffuse reflection
d. Luminance uniformity
e. Luminance response

12. This is the AAPM TG-18 UN test pattern that contains three nine-section images. What is it used to evaluate?

a. Contrast resolution
b. Diffuse reflection
c. Geometric distortion
d. Luminance uniformity
e. Luminance response

175

13. This is the AAPM TG-18 CX test pattern. What is it used to evaluate?

    a. Artifacts
    b. Contrast resolution
    c. Geometric distortion
    d. Nonuniformity
    e. Spatial resolution

14. Specular reflection can result in:
    a. Poor overall image visibility
    b. Displayed image to differ in size from original
    c. Mirror images of surrounding objects
    d. Difficulty seeing dark objects
    e. Difficulty seeing small objects

15. Images from a digital modality store pixel information as an array of pixels with each pixel containing a:
    a. Digital driving level
    b. Luminance level
    c. Presentation value
    d. Brightness value
    e. Contrast value

16. This is the AAPM TG-18 PX test pattern with a rather uniform intensity. What is it used to evaluate?

    a. Contrast resolution
    b. Diffuse reflection
    c. Noise
    d. Nonuniformity
    e. Resolution uniformity

17. This is the AAPM TG-18 AFC test pattern that contains low-contrast squares. What is it used to evaluate?

    a. Artifacts
    b. Contrast resolution
    c. Luminance
    d. Noise
    e. Nonuniformity

Worksheet 23-1
Basis for Mammography
X-Ray Imaging System
Magnification Mammography

Mammography is an examination of the breast with the use of low-energy x-rays. General purpose x-ray imaging systems cannot be used successfully for mammography; a dedicated mammography x-ray imaging system is required.

Breast compression reduces motion blur, absorption blur, and patient dose and improves spatial and contrast resolution.

The mammographic imaging system must be able to accurately produce x-rays in the range of 23 to 30 kVp. The system should have a molybdenum/rhodium-targeted x-ray tube. Such a tube emits radiation with K-characteristic x-rays at 19 and 23 keV, respectively. Because of the low filtration of mammography, the radiation exposure of the patient can be considerably higher than in general radiography.

EXERCISES

1. Low kVp is required for mammography because of which of the following?
   a. High mAs
   b. Patient positioning and compression
   c. Composition of breast tissue
   d. Type of image receptor used
   e. Varying thickness of breast tissue

2. When molybdenum is used for the x-ray tube target:
   a. kVp can be higher.
   b. mAs can be lower.
   c. No added filtration is required.
   d. No bremsstrahlung x-rays are produced.
   e. Useful characteristic x-rays are used.

3. If the cathode of the x-ray tube is positioned toward the chest wall during a cranial-caudal view:
   a. Absorption blur will be reduced.
   b. Exposure time will be reduced.
   c. Geometric blur will be greater toward the chest wall.
   d. The central ray will miss the breast.
   e. Optical density on the nipple side will be greater.

4. In mammography, low kVp is selected to do which of the following?
   a. Improve spatial resolution.
   b. Increase Compton absorption.
   c. Increase photoelectric absorption.
   d. Reduce patient dose.
   e. Reduce skin reaction.

5. When a mammogram taken at 23 kVp is compared with one taken at 28 kVp:
   a. For the same exit dose, the 28 kVp examination will require a higher entrance dose.
   b. If the mAs is constant, exposure time will be less at 23 kVp.
   c. If the mAs is constant, the number of x-rays reaching the image receptor will be the same.
   d. Radiographic contrast will be enhanced at 28 kVp.
   e. The ratio of entrance dose to exit dose will be higher at 23 kVp.

6. The principal reason why molybdenum-targeted x-ray tubes are used in mammography is that molybdenum produces which of the following?
   a. A high atomic number
   b. A high melting point
   c. A higher heat capacity
   d. Useful bremsstrahlung x-rays
   e. Useful characteristic x-rays

7. Successful mammography cannot be done at 90 kVp because:
   a. Compton interactions are too few.
   b. Differential absorption is too low.
   c. Exposure time is too long.
   d. Patient dose is too high.
   e. X-ray tube heat is too great.

8. During mammography:
   a. More filtration is required.
   b. Radiographic contrast is low.
   c. The half-value layer is relatively low.
   d. Radiation quality is relatively high.
   e. X-ray transmission predominates.

9. Regarding the incidence of breast cancer in women, which of the following is *true?*
   a. Each year, about 10,000 new cases appear in the United States.
   b. It is on the decline.
   c. More than 80% of breast cancer results in death.
   d. The most critical decade is that of 30 to 40 years.
   e. The odds of developing breast cancer are 1 in 8.

10. In screen-film mammography, which of the following is *most* often responsible for image contrast?
    a. mAs
    b. kVp
    c. Tissue atomic number
    d. Tissue mass
    e. Tissue mass number

11. X-ray tube potential below 20 kVp is *not* used because:
    a. Characteristic x-rays are not produced.
    b. Compton interaction predominates.
    c. Generators are not available for such low voltage.
    d. There are no x-rays below 20 keV.
    e. X-ray penetration is not sufficient.

12. Why is SID reduced in mammography compared with conventional radiography?
    a. To decrease exposure time
    b. To decrease geometric unsharpness
    c. To improve differential absorption
    d. To improve spatial resolution
    e. To reduce patient dose

13. If an x-ray tube is positioned so that the anode is toward the chest wall during a cranial-caudal view:
    a. Image-forming x-rays will have more uniform intensity at the image receptor.
    b. Patient dose will be lower.
    c. Spatial resolution will be higher toward the nipple.
    d. Exposure time will be about one half.
    e. Radiation exposure will be greater at the nipple than at the chest wall.

14. The principal reason why mammography is widely used is that:
    a. It is easy.
    b. It is inexpensive.
    c. It is reimbursable.
    d. The incidence of breast cancer is high.
    e. The radiation dose is low.

15. Which of the following target/filter combinations is *most* appropriate for screening mammography?
    a. Mo/Al
    b. Mo/Mo
    c. Rh/Mo
    d. W/Al
    e. W/Mo

16. Compression during mammography is necessary to do which of the following?
    a. Comfort the patient
    b. Increase OID
    c. Increase SID
    d. Reduce geometric blur
    e. Use the small focal spot

17. Mammography grids are designed to do which of the following?
    a. Improve optical density
    b. Improve contrast
    c. Improve spatial resolution
    d. Reduce geometric blur
    e. Reduce patient dose

Worksheet 24-1
Quality Control Team
Quality Control Program

The purposes of a mammography quality control (QC) program are to produce the best possible diagnostic image through good equipment performance and to ensure that the patient receives the best available care with the least radiation exposure. QC falls under the larger umbrella of quality assurance (QA), which is an administrative program that ensures that all tasks of the QC team are carried out at the highest level. Continuous quality improvement is an extension of any QC/QA program and includes administrative protocols for the continuous improvement of mammographic quality.

The mammography QC team includes a radiologist, a medical physicist, and a mammographer. Radiologists oversee the QA program and track diagnostic results. Medical physicists examine and monitor the performance of imaging equipment, and they chart and record data to ensure compliance with the latest recommendations and standards. Mammographers perform many tests and evaluations that involve equipment, processing, and mammographic images.

EXERCISES

1. Which of the following describes the difference between QC and QA?
   a. QC deals with the performance of imaging apparatus.
   b. QC defines the quality of the QA team.
   c. QC is focused on patient scheduling, examination, and reporting.
   d. QA is concerned principally with image processing.
   e. QA is the responsibility of the mammographer.

2. Who is principally responsible for the QC/QA program?
   a. Administrator
   b. Mammographer
   c. Medical physicist
   d. QC technologist
   e. Radiologist

3. CQI stands for which of the following?
   a. Cautious quality improvement
   b. Competent quality imaging
   c. Continuous quality improvement
   d. Controlled quality insistence
   e. None of the above

4. The assessment of glandular dose in mammography is principally the responsibility of which of the following staff members?
   a. Administrator
   b. Mammographer
   c. Medical physicist
   d. QC technologist
   e. Radiologist

5. The responsibilities of the medical physicist must be carried out at *least:*
   a. Daily
   b. Weekly
   c. Monthly
   d. Quarterly
   e. Annually

6. Which member of the mammography QC/QA team is principally responsible for daily QC/QA?
   a. Administrator
   b. Mammographer
   c. Medical physicist
   d. The patient
   e. Radiologist

7. The duties of the QC mammographer include tasks that should be performed:
   a. Daily
   b. Daily and weekly
   c. Daily, weekly, and quarterly
   d. Daily, weekly, quarterly, and annually
   e. Daily, quarterly, and annually

8. Which of the following is a QC responsibility of the medical physicist?
   a. Collimation assessment
   b. Daily processor QC
   c. Fixer retention analysis
   d. Repeat analysis
   e. Screen-film contact assay

9. Which of the following tasks must the QC mammographer perform daily?
   a. Compression evaluation
   b. Darkroom cleanliness assessment
   c. Fixer retention assay
   d. Phantom image analysis
   e. Screen-film contact evaluation

10. Which of the following tasks must the QC mammographer perform daily?
    a. Compression evaluation
    b. Fixer retention assay
    c. Phantom image analysis
    d. Processor QC
    e. Screen-film contact evaluation

11. Which of the following tasks should the QC mammographer perform weekly?
    a. Compression evaluation
    b. Darkroom cleanliness assessment
    c. Fixer retention assay
    d. Phantom image analysis
    e. Screen-film contact evaluation

12. Which of the following tasks should the QC mammographer perform monthly?
    a. Darkroom cleanliness assessment
    b. Fixer retention assay
    c. Formal conference with the radiologist
    d. Screen-film contact evaluation
    e. Visual checklist

13. Which of the following tasks should the QC mammographer perform quarterly?
    a. Darkroom cleanliness assessment
    b. Darkroom fog analysis
    c. Fixer retention assay
    d. Formal conference with the radiologist
    e. Production of phantom images

14. Which of the following tasks should the QC mammographer perform semiannually?
    a. Darkroom cleanliness assessment
    b. Darkroom fog analysis
    c. Fixer retention assay
    d. Formal conference with the radiologist
    e. Production of phantom images

15. What is the principal reason to routinely require darkroom cleanliness?
    a. Ensure constant spatial resolution
    b. Improve image contrast
    c. Reduce chemical fog
    d. Reduce image artifacts
    e. Reduce light fog

16. Materials used for the construction of a mammography darkroom should be chosen with regard to which of the following properties?
    a. Ensuring abrasive surfaces
    b. Maximizing light absorption
    c. Minimizing dust collection
    d. Providing ease of chemical absorption
    e. Reducing light reflection

17. The film used to conduct a processor program should:
    a. Be that special film provided by the manufacturer
    b. Be the first sheets of each new box
    c. Be unprocessed discarded film
    d. Be used randomly throughout the clinical supply
    e. Come from a dedicated supply

18. Which of the following is *not* critical to the proper start of a processor QC program?
    a. Calibrated ion chamber
    b. Clean processor tanks and racks
    c. Dedicated box of film
    d. Proper chemistry, as specified by the manufacturer
    e. Proper temperature and replenishment rates

19. When performing processor QC, the sensitometric strip of film should be processed:
    a. In alternation with the guide rail
    b. While the least exposed end is fed first
    c. While the most exposed end is fed first
    d. With the long edge against the guide rail
    e. With the short edge against the guide rail

20. The mammography American College of Radiology (ACR) phantom consists of all of the following, except:
    a. Tissue equivalent material
    b. Specks
    c. Mass
    d. Fibers
    e. Rods

21. The densitometer is used in mammography QC to do which of the following?
    a. Ensure constant spatial resolution
    b. Evaluate exposure reproducibility
    c. Improve contrast resolution
    d. Measure average gradient
    e. Measure optical density

22. In the start-up phase of processor QC, a sensitometric strip should be evaluated:
    a. Each day for 5 consecutive days
    b. Each day for 1 month
    c. Twice daily for 3 consecutive days
    d. Twice daily for 5 consecutive days
    e. Twice daily for 1 month

23. The step on the sensitivity strip called the *speed index* is also the:
    a. Base step
    b. Contrast step
    c. Gamma point
    d. Middensity step
    e. Resolution step

24. The middensity step on the sensitometric strip is the one with optical density closest to:
    a. 1.2 but not less than 1.2
    b. 1.2 but not more than 1.2
    c. 1.2 but not less than 1.3
    d. 1.3 but not more than 1.3
    e. 1.4

25. The contrast index of a sensitivity strip is also known as the:
    a. Average gradient
    b. Base plus fog index
    c. Contrast difference
    d. Density difference
    e. Resolution index

26. Steps on the sensitometric strip assigned for density difference are those associated with the following optical densities:
    a. 0.5 and 2.2
    b. 0.5 and 2.5
    c. 1.0 and 2.2
    d. 1.2 and 2.2
    e. 1.2 and 2.5

27. The value for base plus fog on the sensitometric strip is determined from:
    a. An unexposed area of the strip
    b. The response with no film in the densitometer
    c. The step closest to OD equal to 1.2
    d. The step with the highest OD
    e. The step with the lowest OD

28. During evaluation of screens for cleanliness, if dust or dirt artifacts are observed:
    a. The density difference reading should be repeated.
    b. The middensity reading should be repeated.
    c. Phantom images should be repeated.
    d. The screen must be cleaned immediately.
    e. The screen should be cleaned as soon as possible.

29. What is the principal reason to measure middensity?
    a. Ensure clinical contrast
    b. Ensure constant spatial resolution
    c. Evaluate the constancy of image receptor speed
    d. Verify processor chemical replenishment rates
    e. Verify processor chemical temperature

30. What is the principal reason to evaluate density difference on a sensitivity strip?
    a. Detect light chemical fog
    b. Ensure constancy of image contrast
    c. Ensure proper processor chemistry
    d. Provide best spatial resolution
    e. Reduce base plus fog

31. During routine processor QC, middensity may vary by how much before corrective action is necessary?
    a. 0.05 OD
    b. 0.1 OD
    c. 0.15 OD
    d. 0.2 OD
    e. 0.3 OD

32. During a routine processor QC, density difference may vary by how much before corrective action is necessary (clinical images)?
    a. 0.05 OD
    b. 0.1 OD
    c. 0.15 OD
    d. 0.2 OD
    e. 0.3 OD

33. During processor QC, what is the reason for measuring the optical density of an unexposed portion of the sensitometric film?
    a. Ensure constant contrast
    b. Evaluate the level of fog in the processing chain
    c. Improve contrast resolution
    d. Maintain spatial resolution
    e. Monitor the chemical temperature and replenishment rate

34. The middensity assay of the sensitometric strip should be repeated if the value falls outside of the identified range by how much?
    a. 0.05 OD
    b. 0.1 OD
    c. 0.15 OD
    d. 0.2 OD
    e. 0.3 OD

35. The density difference assay of the sensitometric strip should be repeated if the value falls outside of the identified range by how much?
    a. 0.05 OD
    b. 0.1 OD
    c. 0.15 OD
    d. 0.2 OD
    e. 0.3 OD

36. The established base plus fog optical density value is allowed to vary by:
   a. +0.03
   b. ±0.3
   c. ±0.05
   d. ±0.15
   e. ±0.1

37. Screen cleanliness is a QC task that must be evaluated:
   a. Daily
   b. Weekly
   c. Monthly
   d. Quarterly
   e. Semiannually

38. When film is loaded for mammography:
   a. The base should be in contact with the screen.
   b. The emulsion should be in contact with the cover.
   c. The film should be on the x-ray tube side of the radiographic intensifying screen.
   d. The radiographic intensifying screen should be on the x-ray tube side of the film.
   e. The spatial resolution is the same as for routine radiography.

39. Mammographic screen-film systems offer what advantage over direct exposure examinations?
   a. Higher spatial resolution
   b. Lower cost
   c. Lower patient dose
   d. Patient comfort
   e. Less region blurring

40. A two view examination with a grid for a 4.5-cm compressed breast, 50-50 glandular/fat tissue, should result in a technique with an average glandular dose of:
   a. <2 mGy
   b. 4 mGy
   c. <6 mGy
   d. <6 mrad
   e. <2 mrad

41. Which of the following is *true* about the mammographic screen-film image receptor?
   a. A single screen is between the source and the film.
   b. Fixed grids are used.
   c. The receptor is nonscreen.
   d. The speed is approximately 200.
   e. Two screens with double-emulsion film are used.

42. When the radiographic intensifying screen is changed from screen "X" to screen "Y," which has twice the x-ray-to-light conversion efficiency with use of the same film:
   a. Exposure time is doubled.
   b. Geometric blur is accentuated.
   c. Image noise is increased.
   d. Motion blur is reduced.
   e. Patient dose is increased.

Worksheet 25-1
Illumination
Human Vision

The fluoroscopic examination has improved continually since its first demonstration in 1896 by Thomas A. Edison. Fluoroscopy used to require dark adaptation for scotopic vision (rod vision). Now, all fluoroscopic images are viewed under photopic vision (cone vision) with the use of a cathode ray tube or a flat panel display device for image viewing.

Image brightness is ensured through an automatic feedback loop called *automatic brightness control (ABC)*.

EXERCISES

1. In a modern fluoroscope, the fluoroscopic x-ray tube:
   a. Can be under or over the table
   b. Is always over the table
   c. Is always the same as the radiographic tube
   d. Is always under the table
   e. Must have very high capacity

2. The fluoroscope was invented by:
   a. Alexander Bell
   b. Hollis Potter
   c. Jan Marconi
   d. Thomas Edison
   e. Wilhelm Roentgen

3. Compared with a radiographic examination, the primary purpose of a fluoroscopic examination is to visualize:
   a. Cross-sectional images
   b. Dynamic images
   c. Longitudinal images
   d. Static images
   e. Transverse images

4. Fluoroscopy normally requires a tube current of:
   a. 0.1 to 1.0 mA
   b. 1 to 5 mA
   c. 5 to 10 mA
   d. 10 to 100 mA
   e. 10 to 1000 mA

5. Compared with radiography, the x-ray technique required for fluoroscopy calls for which of the following?
   a. Higher kVp
   b. Higher mA
   c. Lower kVp
   d. Lower mA
   e. Shorter exposure

6. ABS is designed to compensate for changes in which of the following?
   a. Examination time
   b. Patient composition
   c. Patient dose
   d. Patient positioning
   e. Technique selection

7. Where are rods located in the eye?
   a. Iris
   b. Retina
   c. Fovea centralis
   d. Pupil
   e. Cornea

8. Which of the following units of measurement is used to express fluoroscopic image brightness?
   a. cd/m^2
   b. Coulomb
   c. Coulomb/kilogram
   d. Lambert
   e. Roentgen

9. Which of the following structures is *most* sensitive to color?
   a. Cones
   b. Fovea centralis
   c. Rods
   d. Cornea
   e. Iris

10. What is the function of the iris?
    a. Control the light level
    b. Distinguish colors
    c. Focus the light onto the retina
    d. Protect the eye
    e. Sense visible-light photons

11. The cones are:
    a. Essentially color blind
    b. Located in the iris
    c. Located on the periphery of the retina
    d. Used for photopic vision
    e. Very sensitive to light

12. The fovea centralis is:
    a. Essential to focusing
    b. Next to the lens
    c. Part of the retina
    d. The blind spot
    e. The disclike structure

13. Visual acuity is the ability to do which of the following?
    a. Control the amount of light entering the eye
    b. Detect differences in brightness
    c. Distinguish colors
    d. Perceive fine detail
    e. Vary depth of field

14. The rods are used principally for which of the following?
    a. Bright vision
    b. Color perception
    c. Dim vision
    d. Focusing
    e. Visual acuity

15. In general, during fluoroscopy as compared with radiography:
    a. A smaller focal spot is used.
    b. Patient dose is lower.
    c. Spatial resolution is better.
    d. The mA is lower.
    e. The SID is longer.

16. Which of the following describes the fluoroscopic system designed to maintain constant image intensity?
    a. Automatic brightness stabilization (ABS)
    b. Automatic channel selector (ACS)
    c. Automatic programmed radiography (APR)
    d. Charge-coupled device (CCD)
    e. Positive-beam limitation (PBL)

17. Which of the following structures is responsible for the vision of dim objects?
    a. Cornea
    b. Fovea centralis
    c. Iris
    d. Pupil
    e. Rod

18. Which of the following ocular structures immediately precedes the vitreous humor along the path of incident light?
    a. Cone
    b. Cornea
    c. Fovea centralis
    d. Iris
    e. Lens

19. Which of the following properties is associated with rods but *not* with cones?
    a. Color detection
    b. Contrast perception
    c. Ray focusing
    d. Scotopic vision
    e. Visual acuity

20. What is the function of the iris?
    a. To see dark objects
    b. To see bright objects
    c. Magnification
    d. Controls brightness
    e. Focuses the eye

Worksheet 25-2
Image Intensification

 The image-intensifier tube was introduced to radiology in the 1950s for the principal purpose of reducing patient dose. The image-intensifier tube improves image quality and diagnostic accuracy.

The dose reduction produced by the image intensifier, called **brightness gain,** is the product of the geometric gain, or **minification,** and the **flux gain.**

Direct digital and solid-state flat-panel image receptors are beginning to completely replace the image-intensifier tube.

EXERCISES

1. Photoelectric emission:
   a. Is the emission of electrons from a heated wire
   b. Is the emission of electrons from an illuminated surface
   c. Is the emission of photons
   d. Occurs at the input phosphor of an image-intensifier tube
   e. Occurs at the output phosphor of an image-intensifier tube

2. At what stage of image-intensified fluoroscopy is the number of image-forming photons lowest?
   a. Entering the input phosphor
   b. Entering the photocathode
   c. Leaving the input phosphor
   d. Leaving the output phosphor
   e. Leaving the photocathode

3. Image-intensifier brightness gain increases with increasing:
   a. Flux gain
   b. kVp
   c. mA
   d. Output phosphor size
   e. Radiation exposure

4. When an image intensifier receives x-rays at the input phosphor, what is emitted at the output phosphor?
   a. Electrons
   b. Infrared light
   c. Ultraviolet light
   d. Visible light
   e. X-rays

5. Which of the following is the input phosphor of image intensifiers?
   a. Cadmium tungstate
   b. Calcium tungstate
   c. Cesium iodide
   d. Sodium iodide
   e. Zinc cadmium sulfide

6. Which of the following is the output phosphor of image intensifiers?
   a. Cadmium tungstate
   b. Calcium tungstate
   c. Cesium iodide
   d. Sodium iodide
   e. Zinc cadmium sulfide

7. The photocathode converts:
   a. Electrons into visible light
   b. Visible light into electrons
   c. Visible light into x-rays
   d. X-rays into electrons
   e. X-rays into visible light

8. Which of the following is the component of the image intensifier responsible for focusing the electron beam?
   a. Electrostatic lens
   b. Glass envelope
   c. Input phosphor
   d. Output phosphor
   e. Photocathode

9. The ability of an image intensifier to enhance image illumination is called:
   a. Automatic brightness
   b. Brightness gain
   c. Flux gain
   d. Illumination gain
   e. Minification gain

10. The minification gain of an image intensifier increases with increasing:
    a. Input phosphor size
    b. kVp
    c. mA
    d. Output phosphor size
    e. Tube voltage

11. Which of the following is a representative brightness gain for an image intensifier?
    a. 200
    b. 2000
    c. 20,000
    d. 200,000
    e. 2,000,000

12. If an image intensifier is described as a $^{25}/_{12}$ tube, $^{25}/_{12}$ refers to which of the following?
    a. Area of the input phosphor in square inches
    b. Diameter of the input phosphor in centimeters
    c. Diameter of the output phosphor in centimeters
    d. Radius of the input phosphor in inches
    e. Radius of the output phosphor in centimeters

13. When a multifocus image intensifier is operated in the magnification mode:
    a. A larger area of input phosphor is used.
    b. Contrast resolution is reduced.
    c. Patient dose is lower.
    d. Spatial resolution is reduced.
    e. The electron focal point is closer to the input phosphor.

14. An image that displays vignetting:
    a. Is dim around the periphery
    b. Is dim in the center
    c. Has higher contrast resolution
    d. Has higher spatial resolution
    e. Shows the barrel stay artifact

15. With a multifocus image intensifier in the magnification mode:
    a. Contrast resolution is reduced.
    b. Noise is increased.
    c. Patient dose is reduced.
    d. Spatial resolution is improved.
    e. Field of view is increased.

16. In a 10/7/5 image intensifier:
    a. Contrast resolution is best in the 10 mode.
    b. Spatial resolution is best in the 10 mode.
    c. The field of view is largest in the 10 mode.
    d. There are three different input phosphors.
    e. There are three different output phosphors.

17. An image intensifier has a 5-cm output phosphor and a 45-cm input phosphor. The brightness gain is 10,000. The flux gain is approximately:
    a. 10
    b. 80
    c. 120
    d. 1000
    e. 5000

18. Place the following in proper sequence for image-intensified fluoroscopy:
    1. Electric signal to light
    2. Electrons to light
    3. Light to electric signal
    4. Light to electrons
    5. X-ray to light
    a. 1, 2, 3, 4, 5
    b. 2, 3, 4, 5, 1
    c. 3, 5, 2, 1, 4
    d. 5, 3, 1, 4, 2
    e. 5, 4, 2, 3, 1

19. Which of the following applies to the output phosphor?
    a. Electrons emitted
    b. Light absorbed
    c. Light emitted
    d. X-rays absorbed
    e. X-rays emitted

Worksheet 25-3
Image Monitoring

The fluoroscopic image produced at the output phosphor of an image-intensifier tube is the size of a postage stamp and cannot be viewed directly. This image is manipulated for viewing, or **monitoring,** with a closed-circuit television system. The output image of the image-intensifying tube is detected by a television camera tube, usually a **vidicon,** or a CCD and then is displayed on a television or a flat-panel monitor.

Such images can be monitored with an optically coupled cine camera that usually is restricted to use during specialized examinations, such as cardiac catheterization, but has mainly been replaced by digital imaging. If static images are required during the examination, they are made with an optically coupled spot-film camera. Both spot-film and cine cameras use single-emulsion photographic film that has dimensional sizes of 16 to 105 mm.

EXERCISES

1. Vertical television resolution is limited principally by which of the following?
   a. Bandpass
   b. Field rate
   c. Frame rate
   d. Lines per frame
   e. Modulation

2. The electron beam in a television camera tube is produced by which of the following means?
   a. Electroemission
   b. Photoconduction
   c. Photoemission
   d. Thermionic emission
   e. Thermoluminescence

3. What is the camera tube most used in television fluoroscopy?
   a. Cesium iodide
   b. Electrons from light
   c. Minification
   d. Synchronized
   e. Vidicon

4. What is the photoemissive component of image-intensified fluoroscopy?
   a. Cesium iodide
   b. Electrons from light
   c. Minification
   d. Synchronized
   e. Vidicon

5. Which of the following is photoconductive?
   a. Electron gun
   b. Electrostatic grid
   c. Signal plate
   d. Target
   e. Window

6. What is the principal disadvantage of coupling the television camera to the image intensifier with the use of fiber optics?
   a. Cassette-loaded spot film cannot be used.
   b. Fragility is increased.
   c. Image noise is increased.
   d. Photospot camera cannot be used.
   e. Spatial resolution is reduced.

7. Which of the following refers to the image-intensifier input phosphor?
   a. Cesium iodide
   b. Electrons from light
   c. Minification
   d. Synchronized
   e. Vidicon

8. Which is a critical component in optically coupling an image intensifier with a photospot camera?
   a. Electrostatic lens
   b. Face plate
   c. Objective lens
   d. Signal plate
   e. Subjective lens

9. What is the *most* important component of a television monitor?
   a. Cathode ray tube
   b. Charge-coupled device
   c. Coupling device
   d. Electromagnetic coils
   e. Television camera tube

10. In an optical coupling arrangement, which is nearest the television camera?
   a. Beam splitter
   b. Camera lens
   c. Deflection coil
   d. Mirror
   e. Objective lens

11. What is the component of the television monitor in which the video signal is transformed into an image?
   a. Electron beam
   b. Electron gun
   c. Electrostatic grid
   d. Phosphor screen
   e. Target assembly

12. What is the electron beam of the television camera tube?
   a. A fan beam
   b. An area beam
   c. Blanked
   d. Collimated
   e. Modulated

13. One television frame is equivalent to which of the following?
   a. 17 ms
   b. 262½ lines
   c. 1024 lines
   d. One television field
   e. Two television fields

14. Fluoroscopic television operates at a frame rate of:
   a. 30 f/s
   b. 60 f/s
   c. 262½ f/s
   d. 525 f/s
   e. 1024 f/s

15. Horizontal television resolution is limited principally by which of the following?
   a. Bandpass
   b. Field rate
   c. Frame rate
   d. Lines per frame
   e. Modulation

16. What is normally the weakest imaging link in television fluoroscopy?
   a. Image-intensifier tube
   b. Optical coupling device
   c. Spot-film device
   d. Television camera
   e. Television monitor

17. Common frame rates during cinefluorography are 15, 30, and 60 f/s because:
   a. Flicker is not observed at these rates.
   b. It is linked to patient dose.
   c. Of the frame rate requirement of the television camera tube
   d. Of the frequency of the power supply
   e. The film format requires it.

18. When the electron beam of the CRT is blanked, it is:
   a. Demodulated
   b. In a vertical retrace
   c. In an active trace
   d. Modulated
   e. Turned on

19. What is the television camera tube component of image-intensified fluoroscopy?
   a. Cesium iodide
   b. Electrons from light
   c. Minification
   d. Synchronized
   e. Vidicon

Worksheet 26-1
Digital Fluoroscopy

Digital fluoroscopy has been developed as a replacement for some earlier angiographic procedures such as subtraction angiography. With digital fluoroscopy, such subtraction images are relatively easily and quickly produced, and postprocessing and manipulation of the image are possible.

In digital fluoroscopy, a high signal-to-noise ratio, high-resolution video system is coupled with a computer. The video signal is digitized, manipulated in the computer by one of several techniques, and finally displayed on the video monitor. Alternatively, solid-state flat-panel image receptors produce direct digital images.

EXERCISES

1. The principal reason for image integration is to:
   a. Improve contrast resolution
   b. Improve spatial resolution
   c. Reduce examination time
   d. Reduce image noise
   e. Reduce patient dose

2. The maximum frame acquisition rate in digital fluoroscopy is about:
   a. 1 frame per second
   b. 4 frames per second
   c. 10 frames per second
   d. 30 frames per second
   e. 60 frames per second

3. The signal-to-noise ratio of a conventional TV camera tube is about:
   a. 100:1
   b. 200:1
   c. 1000:1
   d. 2000:1
   e. 5000:1

4. Compared with conventional fluoroscopy, digital fluoroscopy is conducted:
   a. At much higher x-ray tube current
   b. At much lower x-ray tube current
   c. With a different type of image intensifier
   d. With a different type of video monitor
   e. With higher-capacity x-ray tubes

5. Digital imaging systems can display images on a 1024 × 1024 matrix. How many pixels are present in such a matrix?
   a. 1000
   b. 1024
   c. 2048
   d. 1,048,576
   e. It depends on the gray scale.

6. A conventional radiograph is which of the following?
   a. A digital image
   b. A geometric image
   c. A linear image
   d. An analog image
   e. An exponential image

7. Which of the following components found in digital fluoroscopy is *not* found in conventional fluoroscopy?
   a. A video monitor
   b. An automatic brightness stabilizer (ABS)
   c. An analog-to-digital converter (ADC)
   d. An image intensifier
   e. A source-to-image receptor distance (SID) indicator

8. During digital fluoroscopy, the image receptor is which of the following?
   a. Film
   b. The cassette
   c. The image-intensifier tube
   d. The TV camera tube
   e. The video monitor

9. A principal advantage of digital fluoroscopy over conventional fluoroscopy for subtraction studies is:
   a. Contrast enhancement
   b. Examination speed
   c. Less contrast material
   d. Low patient dose
   e. Noise enhancement

10. The approximate pixel size for a 12-inch image-intensifier tube and a 256 reconstruction matrix is:
    a. 0.4 mm
    b. 0.8 mm
    c. 1.0 mm
    d. 2.5 mm
    e. 4 mm

11. During digital fluoroscopy:
    a. Both cine and spot film modes can be used.
    b. Neither cine nor spot film modes can be used.
    c. The x-ray beam is continuous and at high mA.
    d. The x-ray beam is continuous and at low mA.
    e. The x-ray beam is pulsed.

12. Digital fluoroscopy is conducted:
    a. At relatively low mA
    b. In the progressive TV mode
    c. With direct-exposure film
    d. With low patient dose
    e. With low signal-to-noise ratio

13. How many video monitors are required for digital fluoroscopy?
    a. None
    b. One
    c. Two
    d. Three
    e. Four

14. The time-interval difference mode is best used for which of the following?
    a. Dynamic studies
    b. Extremities
    c. High-dose examinations
    d. Large fields
    e. Long exposure times

15. Reregistration of an image is used to do which of the following?
    a. Correct any error in patient identification
    b. Correct for motion
    c. Increase edge enhancement
    d. Reduce noise
    e. Reduce patient dose

16. The combination of temporal subtraction and energy subtraction techniques is called:
    a. Enhanced subtraction
    b. Hybrid subtraction
    c. No subtraction
    d. Radiographic subtraction
    e. Resonance subtraction

17. The minimum acceptable TV signal-to-noise ratio for digital fluoroscopy is:
    a. 100:1
    b. 200:1
    c. 1000:1
    d. 2000:1
    e. 5000:1

18. Interrogation time:
    a. Is the time spent questioning the patient
    b. Is the time needed to switch off the x-ray tube
    c. Is the time needed to switch on the x-ray tube
    d. Is the total exposure time
    e. Refers to the total examination time

19. A digital imaging system with a dynamic range of 2^{10} will be able to reproduce how many shades of gray?
    a. 32
    b. 256
    c. 512
    d. 1024
    e. 4096

20. An advantage of temporal subtraction over energy subtraction angiography is:
    a. Motion artifacts
    b. Higher patient dose
    c. Increased spatial resolution
    d. Higher contrast at lower dose
    e. More types of subtraction are possible

21. An advantage of digital imaging over conventional imaging is which of the following?
    a. Increased latitude
    b. Increased resolution
    c. Postprocessing
    d. Reduced noise
    e. Reduced speed

22. A pixel is a:
    a. Matrix of numbers
    b. Range of numbers
    c. Three-dimensional digital image cell
    d. Two-dimensional digital image cell
    e. Unit of fluoroscopy dose

23. Between the TV camera and the computer of a digital fluoroscopic system is a/an:
    a. Analog-to-digital converter
    b. Digital-to-analog converter
    c. Image-intensifier tube
    d. Image storage device
    e. Second video monitor

24. The mask image is usually the:
    a. First image
    b. Image at the peak of contrast
    c. Image just preceding contrast
    d. Last contrast image
    e. Last image

25. Energy subtraction is based on which of the following?
    a. Changing mAs
    b. Contrast enhancement
    c. K-edge absorption
    d. Noise reduction
    e. Time differences

190

26. As one integrates video frames in digital fluoroscopy:
    a. Image noise is lower.
    b. Patient dose increases.
    c. Spatial resolution is improved.
    d. The signal-to-noise ratio increases.
    e. Video noise is louder.

27. Which of the following components is uniquely essential to digital fluoroscopy?
    a. ADC
    b. CRT
    c. High-frequency generator
    d. TV camera pickup tube
    e. TV monitor

28. A misregistration artifact:
    a. Cannot be corrected or compensated
    b. Is not really an artifact
    c. Occurs when a patient moves
    d. Requires more hardware than is usually available
    e. Usually follows a change in kVp

29. Remasking:
    a. Can correct for patient motion
    b. Reduces spatial resolution
    c. Requires a change in kVp
    d. Requires a repeat examination
    e. Will increase patient dose

30. A matrix of what size can be held by 10 bytes of memory?
    a. 256 × 256
    b. 512 × 512
    c. 1024 × 1024
    d. 2084 × 2084
    e. 4096 × 4096

31. A 7-bit pixel can display how many shades of gray?
    a. 7
    b. 49
    c. 64
    d. 128
    e. 256

32. The idea behind digital subtraction angiography is:
    a. To decrease patient dose
    b. To see bone better
    c. To image vessels
    d. To increase SNR
    e. To decrease noise

33. How many numbers can be stored in 7 bits?
    a. 64
    b. 128
    c. 256
    d. 512
    e. 1024

34. How many bits are required to display 512 shades of gray?
    a. 5
    b. 6
    c. 7
    d. 8
    e. 9

35. How many shades of gray are possible in a pixel of size 2^{10}?
    a. 64
    b. 128
    c. 256
    d. 512
    e. 1024

36. In a venous entry during digital subtraction angiography, a bolus of about how many milliliters is typically used?
    a. 10 ml
    b. 20 ml
    c. 40 ml
    d. 60 ml
    e. 100 ml

37. The standard contrast material used in digital subtraction angiography is:
    a. Cesium
    b. Barium
    c. Gadolinium
    d. Sodium
    e. Iodine

38. If the same amount of imaging time occurs, compared to the dose in conventional fluoroscopy, the dose in digital fluoroscopy is:
    a. Higher
    b. Lower
    c. About the same
    d. It depends
    e. None of the above

39. Which of the following is not an advantage of CCD devices with regard to medical imaging?
    a. High SNR
    b. Low patient dose
    c. High spatial resolution
    d. Low cost
    e. Linear response

40. What is a typical bolus size in milliliters for an arterial injection in digital subtraction angiography?
    a. 20 ml
    b. 40 ml
    c. 60 ml
    d. 80 ml
    e. 100 ml

Worksheet 26-1 **Digital Fluoroscopy**

41. In a typical digital subtraction angiography cardiac study, how many images are taken?
    a. 10
    b. 5
    c. 60
    d. 120
    e. 3

42. Reregistration of the mask involves:
    a. Acquiring more images
    b. Increasing patient dose
    c. Shifting image pixels
    d. Injecting more contrast
    e. Significant computation time

43. The k-edge for iodine is what energy?
    a. 16 keV
    b. 74 kVp
    c. 53 keV
    d. 33 keV
    e. 90 keV

44. During 5 minutes of digital fluoroscopy, a typical dose is:
    a. 200 mGy
    b. 5 mGy
    c. 200 rad
    d. 500 mGy
    e. 500 rad

45. Which of the following is not an advantage of flat panel image receptors over CCDs coupled to image intensifiers in digital fluoroscopy?
    a. Distortion-free images
    b. Higher spatial resolution
    c. Constant image quality
    d. Improved contrast resolution
    e. High DQE

Worksheet 27-1
Types of Procedures
Basic Principles
IR Suite

IR stands for *interventional radiography*. Radiographers who have passed the American Registry of Radiologic Technologists (ARRT) examination for cardiovascular and interventional radiography have the letters (CV) in their credentials.

Angiography refers to methods of imaging contrast-filled vessels. Vascular imaging and therapeutic intervention through vessels require a special suite equipped with advanced radiographic and fluoroscopic imaging systems. Special guidewires and catheters are used in interventional radiology to access the vascular network without surgery. Different catheter tips are designed to access specific arteries.

Charge-coupled devices (CCDs) are rapidly replacing the television camera tube as the image recorder. CCDs are photosensitive silicon chips that can be used anywhere that light will be converted to a digital video image. The advantages of CCDs for IR are many and include high spatial resolution, lack of spatial distortion, a linear response, lower patient dose, and the lack of warm-up and maintenance requirements.

EXERCISES

1. The term *angiography* refers to which of the following?
   a. Contrast examinations of arteries
   b. Contrast examinations of veins
   c. Contrast examinations of vessels
   d. Examination of brain vessels
   e. Examination of leg vessels

2. Transbrachial select coronary angiography refers to examination of which of the following?
   a. Angiointerventional radiography
   b. Angioplasty
   c. Coronary arteries through an artery of the arm
   d. Coronary arteries through an artery of the leg
   e. The brachial artery

3. What is the principal reason to use guidewires in cardiovascular angiography and interventional radiology?
   a. Better visualization under fluoroscopy
   b. Ease of entry at the puncture site
   c. Safe introduction of the catheter into the vessel
   d. Visualization of arteries
   e. Visualization of veins

4. What is the approximate length of a conventional guidewire?
   a. 50 cm
   b. 100 cm
   c. 145 cm
   d. 200 cm
   e. 300 cm

5. To prevent clotting of blood within the catheter, what is the normal procedure?
   a. Saline flush
   b. Water flush
   c. Aspirin administration
   d. Heparinized saline flush
   e. Catheter occlusion

6. For vascular studies, choice of radiopaque contrast medium is based on which of the following?
   a. Air
   b. Barium
   c. Calcium
   d. Iodine
   e. Gadolinium

7. After angiography:
   a. A physical examination is necessary to assess the patient's medical history for allergies and other conditions.
   b. Manual compression on the femoral site is not necessary once the catheter is removed.
   c. The patient usually can be released immediately.
   d. The patient is instructed to remain immobile for several hours.
   e. The patient is visited by the radiologist to establish rapport.

193

8. What does *osmolality* refer to when applied to contrast media?
   a. Atomic number of the media
   b. Concentration of ions in the media
   c. Mass density of the media
   d. Risk of the media
   e. Viscosity of the media

9. What is a principal complication of transfemoral angiography?
   a. Blood loss
   b. Hemorrhage of the puncture site
   c. Oxygen deprivation
   d. Patient anxiety
   e. Vessel collapse

10. Which of the following is an imaging procedure that would be conducted in an IR suite?
    a. Angioplasty
    b. Arthrectomy
    c. Embolization
    d. Myelography
    e. Thrombolysis

11. Which of the following is an interventional procedure that would be conducted in an IR suite?
    a. Arteriography
    b. Arthrography
    c. Cardiac catheterization
    d. Myelography
    e. Stent placement

12. In an IR suite, a door between the operating console and the examination room:
    a. Is a protective barrier
    b. Is not required
    c. Must be double-hinged
    d. Must be double-wide
    e. Should accommodate a stretcher

13. Which of the following is a minimum requirement for an IR x-ray tube?
    a. 0.3-mm small focal spot
    b. 5-cm diameter anode
    c. 80-kW power rating
    d. 300,000-kHU anode heat capacity
    e. Molybdenum-targeted anode

14. For the spatial resolution requirements of the magnification of small vessels, the focal spot must be:
    a. No smaller than 0.3 mm
    b. No larger than 0.3 mm
    c. No smaller than 0.5 mm
    d. No larger than 0.5 mm
    e. None of the above

15. What is a characteristic of an IR x-ray tube?
    a. Large target angle
    b. Small-diameter anode disk
    c. Small target angle
    d. 50-kW power rating
    e. 300,000-kHU anode heat capacity

16. If an aortogram is performed with a 0.3-mm focal spot and an SID of 100 cm and the artery is 15-cm from the image receptor, what is the magnification factor?
    a. 0.85
    b. 1.08
    c. 1.10
    d. 1.18
    e. 1.25

17. If a carotid arteriogram is performed with a 0.3-mm focal spot at 100 cm SID and the artery is 10 cm from the image receptor, what is the focal-spot blur?
    a. 0.033
    b. 0.33
    c. 0.27
    d. 2.7
    e. 3.3

Worksheet 28-1
Principles of Operation of CT

 Computed tomography (CT) represents one of the most important developments in medical imaging of the 20th century. The development of slip-ring technology and high-frequency generators promoted the introduction of helical computed tomography. This was followed by multislice computed tomography for faster imaging of a larger tissue volume.

The CT imaging system has three principal sections: the gantry, the operating console, and the computer. The gantry assembly includes a high-voltage generator, an x-ray tube, a detector array, and the patient couch.

EXERCISES

1. A CT imaging system produces which type of image?
   a. Axial
   b. Biaxial
   c. Fulcrum plane
   d. Longitudinal
   e. Transverse

2. In its simplest configuration, the CT imaging system consists of an x-ray source and which of the following?
   a. A detector
   b. A selenium plate
   c. A video display terminal
   d. An image intensifier
   e. An x-ray beam collimator

3. Which of the following is characteristic of first-generation CT imaging systems?
   a. A pencil x-ray beam
   b. A selenium or film image receptor
   c. Multiple sources and multiple detectors
   d. Rotate-only geometry
   e. Slip rings

4. CT imaging systems incorporate:
   a. Charged electrostatic plates
   b. High-frequency radiographic grids
   c. Light-localizing, variable-aperture collimators
   d. Automatic brightness control
   e. A gantry

5. Sensitivity profile in CT is determined principally by the:
   a. Bow-tie filter
   b. Predetector collimator
   c. Prepatient collimator
   d. Reconstruction algorithm
   e. Ramp function

6. Spatial resolution for CT imaging systems is approximately:
   a. 1 cm
   b. 10 cm
   c. 100 mm
   d. 1 mm
   e. 10 mm

7. Second-generation CT imaging systems:
   a. Have a multiple detector array
   b. Have rotate-rotate geometry
   c. Require imaging speeds from 1 to 5 minutes
   d. Require special patient preparation
   e. Use increments of 1 degree per view

8. Third-generation CT imaging systems have which of the following?
   a. Multiple-detector, area-beam geometry
   b. Rotate-rotate geometry
   c. Rotate-translate geometry
   d. Single-detector, fan-beam geometry
   e. Translate-translate geometry

9. Fourth-generation CT imaging systems:
   a. Are faster than third-generation CT imaging systems
   b. Have rotate-rotate geometry
   c. Incorporate area-beam geometry
   d. May use selenium or film as the image receptor
   e. Require prepatient collimation

10. Which of the following subsystems would normally be associated with the gantry assembly?
    a. Image postprocessing
    b. The algorithms
    c. The detector array
    d. The physician's viewing console
    e. The software

11. Which of the following has been used as a detector in a CT imaging system?
    a. Bismuth germanate
    b. $CaWO_4$
    c. High-pressure air
    d. Selenium
    e. Silver halide

12. A comparison of scintillation and gas-filled detectors shows that:
    a. Both have approximately the same total detection efficiency.
    b. Both rely heavily on Compton interaction.
    c. Only scintillation detectors require prepatient collimation.
    d. The gas-filled detectors have higher intrinsic efficiency.
    e. The scintillation detectors have higher geometric efficiency.

13. Noise on a CT image can be reduced by:
    a. Increasing kVp
    b. Increasing mAs
    c. Increasing matrix size
    d. Reducing image time
    e. Reducing pixel size

14. In a CT imaging system, prepatient collimation:
    a. Controls pixel size
    b. Controls scatter radiation that reaches the detector
    c. Determines image noise
    d. Determines patient dose
    e. Determines slice thickness

15. The translate-rotate mode:
    a. Collects data only during the rotate portion
    b. Describes both first- and second-generation CT imaging systems
    c. Requires higher heat capacity x-ray tubes
    d. Requires only solid-state detectors
    e. Results in imaging times as short as 1 s

16. Each translation of a source detector assembly produces which of the following?
    a. A matrix
    b. A pixel
    c. A projection
    d. A voxel
    e. An image

17. Slice thickness can also be expressed as which of the following?
    a. Dose profile
    b. Low-contrast profile
    c. Resolution profile
    d. Sensitivity profile
    e. Spatial profile

18. The thickness of section in CT depends primarily on:
    a. kVp
    b. mAs
    c. Matrix size
    d. Predetector collimation
    e. Prepatient collimation

19. CT mA is modulated to:
    a. Improve image contrast
    b. Minimize beam hardening
    c. Reduce patient dose
    d. Reduce scatter radiation
    e. Reduce x-ray tube loading

Worksheet 28-2
Image Characteristics
Image Quality
Quality Assurance

 Every medical image has two principal characteristics: spatial resolution and contrast resolution.

Spatial resolution refers to the ability of an imaging system to image small, high-contrast objects such as calcifications in soft tissue. Spatial resolution is best measured by **spatial frequency** and **modulation transfer function (MTF).**

Contrast resolution refers to the ability of the imaging system to reproduce objects such as cysts and tumors that do not vary much from surrounding tissue in their x-ray absorption properties.

EXERCISES

1. A 120 × 120 matrix will consist of how many pixels?
   a. 120
   b. 240
   c. 625
   d. 14,400
   e. 65,536

2. What is the pixel size of an image reconstructed from a 24-cm diameter region of interest (ROI) in a 320 × 320 matrix?
   a. 0.25 mm
   b. 0.5 mm
   c. 0.75 mm
   d. 1.3 mm
   e. 1.5 mm

3. A CT image is made with a 5-mm slice thickness and a 0.5-mm pixel size. What is the size of the voxel?
   a. 0.75 mm^3
   b. 1.00 mm^3
   c. 1.25 mm^3
   d. 1.5 mm^3
   e. 25 mm^3

4. Which of the following Hounsfield unit (HU) values *most* closely represents the value for blood?
   a. −80 HU
   b. −40 HU
   c. −2 HU
   d. 20 HU
   e. 100 HU

5. A CT imaging system has a limiting resolution of 7 lp/cm. An object of what size can be resolved?
   a. 0.35 mm
   b. 0.5 mm
   c. 0.7 mm
   d. 1.4 mm
   e. 3.5 mm

6. Which of the following is characteristic of a CT image but *not* of a conventional radiograph?
   a. Anatomic structures are superimposed.
   b. Better contrast resolution is obtained.
   c. Better spatial resolution is obtained.
   d. More scatter radiation reaches the image receptor.
   e. Overlying and underlying tissues are blurred.

7. An image matrix contains which of the following?
   a. Algorithms
   b. Equations of information
   c. Picture elements
   d. Silver halide information units
   e. Slice sensitivity 1.00

8. A Hounsfield unit:
   a. Has a value from −100 to +100
   b. Has a value from −500 to +500
   c. Is the numeral value of a pixel
   d. Is the numeral value of anode heat generated
   e. Is the volume of a voxel expressed in mm^3

9. The precise pixel value in HU depends on which of the following?
   a. 32 shades of gray
   b. Light field, x-ray beam coincidence
   c. Pixel size
   d. The x-ray attenuation coefficient
   e. X-ray beam size

10. Spatial resolution refers to which of the following?
    a. The ability to classify large low-contrast objects
    b. The ability to identify small high-contrast objects
    c. The ability to identify tissues of varying composition
    d. The binary number system
    e. The constancy of the imaging system over time

11. When a CT image is described, contrast resolution:
    a. Is limited by the MTF of the system
    b. Is limited by the noise of the system
    c. Is not as good as in conventional radiography
    d. Is the same as spatial resolution
    e. Means that contrast material was injected

12. Partial volume artifacts are more likely with:
    a. Higher kVp
    b. Higher mA
    c. Larger pixel size
    d. Thicker slices
    e. Thinner slices

Exercises 13 through 15 refer to the figure below.

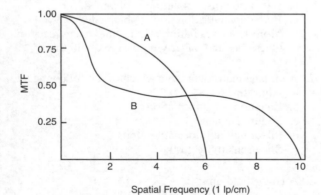

13. The MTF curves describe two imaging systems. Which of the following statements is *true?*
    a. System A detects smaller objects than system B.
    b. System A has better spatial resolution than system B.
    c. System A has more image noise than system B.
    d. System B has better contrast for coarse details than system A.
    e. System B has better spatial resolution than system A.

14. A device has the MTF characteristics represented by B. Which of the following statements is *true* for that device?
    a. At 2 lp/cm, only one half of an object can be imaged.
    b. At 10 lp/cm, the response is excellent.
    c. It can image a 0.5-mm object.
    d. Its imaging ability increases with increasing spatial frequency.
    e. Longer imaging time than in A will be required.

15. The MTF characteristics of system A suggest that it:
    a. Can image down to approximately 0.8 mm
    b. Can image down to approximately 6 cm
    c. Images large objects better than small objects
    d. Images small objects better than large objects
    e. Is a better system than B

Worksheet 28-3
Computed Tomography

 Helical computed tomography (CT) reduces motion blur, imaging time, and partial volume artifact. It is made possible by slip-ring technology that allows the gantry to rotate continuously without interruption. Interpolation allows collected data to be reconstructed at any position along the z-axis, which is the long axis of the body. The volume of the tissue image is determined by examination time, couch travel, pitch, and collimation.

The spiral CT pitch is the relationship between patient couch movement and x-ray beam collimation. Increasing the pitch ratio to above 1.0 increases the volume of tissue that can be imaged and reduces patient dose.

Multislice helical CT uses several parallel detector arrays, each of which contains thousands of individual detectors, to produce four or more helical slices at the same time. The signal from each radiation detector is connected to a computer-controlled electronic amplifier and switching device called a *data acquisition system (DAS)*.

The DAS selects detector combinations for signal summation and sends the signals to a computer for reconstruction of the image. Multislice helical CT can image larger tissue volume faster than single-slice helical CT.

EXERCISES

1. Which of the following terms is equivalent to *helical?*
   a. Elliptical
   b. Spiral
   c. Interpolation
   d. Paraboloid
   e. Trispiral

2. Which of the following molecules takes on a helical structure?
   a. Carbohydrate
   b. Deoxyribonucleic acid
   c. Free radical
   d. Lipid
   e. Protein

3. Which of the following is specifically characteristic of helical CT?
   a. Continuous bidirectional rotation of the x-ray tube
   b. Continuous x-ray tube rotation in one direction
   c. Rotating detector array
   d. Stationary patient couch
   e. Steplike motion of the patient couch

4. During spiral CT examination of a supine patient, the z-axis:
   a. Is the anterior-posterior axis
   b. Is the lateral axis, left to right
   c. Is the lateral axis, right to left
   d. Is the long axis of the body
   e. Varies with the examination

5. The ability to reconstruct an image at any z-axis position is due to:
   a. Extrapolation
   b. Filtered back projection
   c. Fourier transformation
   d. Interpolation
   e. Linear estimation

6. A principal advantage of reconstruction in any z-axis position is:
   a. Image acquisition during a single breath-hold
   b. Improved contrast resolution
   c. Improved spatial resolution
   d. Larger volume of tissue imaged
   e. Reduction of partial volume

7. The simplest form of three-dimensional imaging is:
   a. Isometric
   b. Maximum-intensity projection
   c. Shaded surface display
   d. Shaded volume display
   e. Slip-ring technology

8. Today all CT scanners are what generation?
   a. First generation
   b. Second generation
   c. Third generation
   d. Fourth generation
   e. Fifth generation

9. During a 360-degree x-ray rotation, the patient couch moves 15 mm during each revolution. Slice thickness is 10 mm. What is the slice pitch?
   a. 0.66
   b. 1.25
   c. 1.5
   d. 1.66
   e. 2.0

10. Which of the following is one advantage of helical CT over conventional CT?
    a. Better patient dose use
    b. Improved contrast resolution
    c. Improved spatial resolution
    d. Lack of motion artifact
    e. Large matrix reconstruction

11. Which of the following is another advantage of helical CT over conventional CT?
    a. Better patient dose use
    b. Improved contrast resolution
    c. Improved spatial resolution
    d. Large matrix reconstruction
    e. Reduced scanning time

12. If a 20-s helical CT examination is acquired at a pitch of 1.5 with collimation of 10 mm, what was the length of the scan if gantry rotation time was 1 s?
    a. 3 cm
    b. 30 cm
    c. 300 cm
    d. 3 mm
    e. 30 mm

13. Thirty centimeters of tissue along the z-axis is to be imaged with a 5-mm slice thickness at a pitch of 2.0. What imaging time is required if gantry rotation time is 1 s?
    a. 20 s
    b. 25 s
    c. 30 s
    d. 35 s
    e. 40 s

14. How much z-axis tissue will be imaged during a 20-s procedure if the slice width is 5 mm at a pitch of 1 and the gantry rotation time is 2 s?
    a. 5 cm
    b. 10 cm
    c. 100 cm
    d. 5 mm
    e. 10 mm

15. Why is it recommended that beam pitch should *not* exceed 2.0?
    a. Increased noise
    b. Poor contrast resolution
    c. Poor patient dose use
    d. Poor spatial resolution
    e. Poor z-axis resolution

16. Which of the following is another term for slice thickness?
    a. Dose profile
    b. Interpolation profile
    c. Reconstruction index
    d. Section sensitivity profile
    e. Z-axis profile

17. With increasing slice pitch:
    a. Image noise is reduced.
    b. Patient dose is increased.
    c. Sagittal/coronal reconstruction is improved.
    d. The section sensitivity profile decreases in width.
    e. The section sensitivity profile increases in width.

18. When a shaded surface display reformation is implemented, the image will appear:
    a. As CT angiography
    b. As z-axis reformation
    c. Isometric
    d. Surface-rendered
    e. Volume-rendered

19. Which of the following technique developments made helical CT possible?
    a. Dose-efficiency detectors
    b. High-frequency generators
    c. Interpolation algorithms
    d. Slip rings
    e. Volume imaging

20. CT angiography relies on a reconstruction process that is called:
    a. Longitudinal reformation
    b. Maximum intensity projection
    c. Shaded surface display
    d. Surface-rendered
    e. Volume-rendered

21. Which of the following characteristics is specific to a helical CT x-ray tube?
    a. High anode heat capacity
    b. High rotation speed
    c. Large effective focal spots
    d. Large target angle
    e. Small effective focal spots

22. Approximately what is the minimum power requirement for the high-voltage generator and x-ray tube for helical CT?
    a. 10 kW
    b. 20 kW
    c. 30 kW
    d. 40 kW
    e. 50 kW

23. The single *most* important advantage of helical CT is which of the following?
    a. Imaging of a large volume of anatomy at a low patient dose
    b. Imaging of a large volume of anatomy in one breath-hold
    c. Improved contrast resolution
    d. Improved spatial resolution
    e. Improved z-axis resolution

24. What range of beam pitch is recommended for multislice spiral CT?
    a. 0.5 to 1
    b. 0.5 to 2
    c. 0.5 to 4
    d. 1
    e. 1 to 2

25. DAS stands for which of the following?
    a. Data acquisition system
    b. Digital acquired space
    c. Digital activation signal
    d. Digital analog server
    e. Digital analog system

26. The largest number of individual detectors in a multislice CT imager is approximately:
    a. Two
    b. Four
    c. Ten
    d. Hundreds
    e. Thousands

27. Which of the following statements about multislice CT is *true?*
    a. Higher-resolution multislice helical CT results in low patient radiation dose.
    b. Larger detector size results in better spatial resolution.
    c. Narrower slice scanning results in better contrast resolution at the same mA.
    d. The simplest approach to multislice scanning is the use of eight detector arrays, each of equal width.
    e. Wider multislices allow imaging of a greater tissue volume.

28. A principal advantage of multislice helical CT compared with step-and-shoot CT is all of the following, except:
    a. Better spatial resolution
    b. Faster imaging
    c. Larger tissue volume
    d. Lower patient dose
    e. None of the above

29. Noise on a CT image increases with an increase in:
    a. kVp
    b. mA
    c. Matrix size
    d. Pixel size
    e. Slice thickness

30. During CT imaging, beam hardening artifacts:
    a. Are due to the polyenergetic beam
    b. Can be corrected by preprocessing
    c. Produce CT numbers higher in the periphery
    d. Result in brighter pixels in the center of the patient
    e. Result in higher attenuation in the center of the patient

31. Spatial resolution in CT imaging depends principally on:
    a. Focal-spot size
    b. kVp
    c. Pixel size
    d. Postpatient collimation
    e. Slice thickness

32. What was originally the primary disadvantage of third-generation CT scanners?
    a. Long imaging time
    b. Low spatial resolution
    c. Motion artifact
    d. Ring artifact
    e. High heat load

33. What type of material is least likely to produce artifact in a CT image?
    a. High Z-material
    b. Low Z-material
    c. Lead-based material
    d. Aluminum
    e. Copper

34. Which of the following is an advantage of iterative reconstruction methods?
    a. Higher patient dose
    b. Higher spatial resolution
    c. Faster scan time
    d. Higher contrast resolution
    e. Shorter reconstruction time

35. The quantity that describes the ability to distinguish between two different tissues is called:
    a. Contrast resolution
    b. Spatial resolution
    c. Point spread function
    d. Filtered backprojection
    e. Signal-to-noise ratio

36. The standard deviation of a uniform image can help determine:
    a. Spatial resolution
    b. Image noise
    c. Contrast resolution
    d. Patient dose
    e. Scan time

37. What is the primary advantage of a dual source multislice helical CT?
    a. Lower patient dose
    b. Higher spatial resolution
    c. Less noise
    d. Higher signal-to-noise ratio
    e. Faster scan time

38. What is the Hounsfield unit for water?
    a. 0
    b. 30
    c. −100
    d. 1000
    e. −20

39. A weekly test should be performed to ensure that the Hounsfield unit for water is within what range of its standard value?
    a. ±1
    b. ±5
    c. ±10
    d. ±20
    e. ±100

40. How often should patient dose measurements be taken on a multislice helical CT?
    a. Daily
    b. Weekly
    c. Monthly
    d. Semiannually
    e. Annually

Worksheet 29-1
Human Radiation Response
Composition of the Body

An understanding of how radiation affects biologic tissue is essential to the radiologic technologist's task of producing high-quality x-ray images with a minimum of radiation exposure. The composition of the human body has its basis in atoms, and it is at the atomic level that radiation interacts.

The atomic composition of the body determines the character and degree of the radiation interaction, and molecular and tissue composition define the nature of the radiation response.

The following list summarizes the atomic composition of the body and shows that more than 85% of the body is hydrogen and oxygen.

- 0.1% phosphorus
- 0.1% sulfur
- 0.2% calcium
- 0.8% trace elements
- 2.4% nitrogen
- 10.7% carbon
- 25.7% oxygen
- 60.0% hydrogen

EXERCISES

1. The effects of fetal irradiation include all of the following, *except*:
   a. Childhood malignancy
   b. Congenital malformation
   c. Diminished growth and development
   d. Erythema
   e. Neonatal death

2. Which of the following human responses to ionizing radiation would be categorized as a stochastic effect?
   a. Central nervous system syndrome
   b. Gastrointestinal syndrome
   c. Leukemia
   d. Extremity damage
   e. Hematologic depression

3. Most radiobiologic research is conducted with animals. Approximately how many human population groups have shown radiation effects?
   a. None
   b. Fewer than 5
   c. 5 to 10
   d. 10 to 20
   e. More than 20

4. Human responses to radiation that do *not* have a threshold dose are called:
   a. Large effects
   b. Stochastic effects
   c. Latent response
   d. Law effects
   e. Deterministic effects

5. Which of the following is the first step in producing a radiation response?
   a. Ionization
   b. Latent effect
   c. Manifestation of a lesion
   d. Molecular alteration
   e. Removal and isolation of a lesion

6. Approximately what percentage of the body is water?
   a. 20
   b. 35
   c. 50
   d. 65
   e. 80

7. Which element is *most* abundant in the body?
   a. Calcium
   b. Carbon
   c. Hydrogen
   d. Nitrogen
   e. Oxygen

8. Which molecule is *most* abundant in the body?
   a. Carbohydrate
   b. Lipid
   c. Nucleic acid
   d. Protein
   e. Water

9. A radiation effect that increases in severity with an increase in dose is called a:
   a. Stochastic effect
   b. Deterministic effect
   c. Late effect
   d. Delayed effect
   e. DNA

10. There are two main categories that we use to describe radiation damage; what are these categories called?
    a. Mitosis effect/meiosis effect
    b. Late effect/early effect
    c. Stochastic effect/deterministic effect
    d. Close effect/far-away effect
    e. Low dose effect/high dose effect

11. The stochastic effects of radiation on humans include effects that have these characteristics:
    a. Linear; threshold dose
    b. Nonlinear; threshold dose
    c. Linear; nonthreshold dose
    d. Nonlinear; nonthreshold dose
    e. None of the above

12. Radiation damage
    a. Only can be observed immediately
    b. Only can be observed after years of waiting
    c. Cannot be repaired
    d. Can only be observed in humans
    e. Can be repaired at each stage in the damage sequence

13. An ionization event occurs:
    a. After telophase
    b. When an electron moves to an outer-orbital shell
    c. When an atom loses an electron potentially resulting in the breaking of a chemical bond
    d. While a ribosome is eating a lysosome
    e. At all phases of the cell cycle

14. *ALARA* stands for
    a. As Long As Rooms are Available
    b. As Low As Reasonably Achievable
    c. As Low As Responsibly Achievable
    d. As Long As Resting Allows
    e. None of the above

15. Which one of the following is not a deterministic effect of radiation?
    a. Lymphoma
    b. Skin erythema
    c. Lymphocyte depression
    d. Skin desquamation
    e. All of the above

16. A scientist who studies the effects of ionizing radiation on the body is called a/an:
    a. Medical physicist
    b. Radiologist
    c. X-ray technologist
    d. Radiation biologist
    e. Molecular biologist

Worksheet 29-2
Cell Theory

 To understand the effects of radiation on the human body, one must have a basic knowledge of the composition and function of cells. The cell is considered the biologic building block. Every organ and tissue structure in the body is composed of many cells. Radiation injury begins when the cell is injured, and therefore an understanding of cellular components and roles is important to understand how radiation damage occurs.

The single most important molecule and cellular component in the body is deoxyribonucleic acid (DNA). DNA contains all of the genes and is responsible for controlling the body's growth, development, and function.

It is assumed that the principal type of radiation damage is inflicted on the cell's control center—the DNA—and results in errors in metabolism that can produce a visible radiation effect.

EXERCISES

1. Anton van Leeuwenhoek:
   a. Accurately described a living cell in 1673 on the basis of microscopic observations
   b. Described atoms as having eyes and hooks
   c. Described the molecular structure of DNA in 1953
   d. First named the cell in 1665
   e. Showed conclusively that all plants and animals contain cells as their basic functional units

2. Schleiden and Schwann:
   a. Accurately described a living cell in 1673 on the basis of microscopic observations
   b. Described the molecular structure of DNA in 1953
   c. Developed the original periodic table
   d. First named the cell in 1665
   e. Showed conclusively that all plants and animals contain cells as their basic functional units

3. Watson and Crick:
   a. Accurately described a living cell in 1673 on the basis of microscopic observations
   b. Described the molecular structure of DNA in 1953
   c. Discovered x-ray crystallography
   d. First named the cell in 1665
   e. Showed conclusively that all plants and animals contain cells as their basic functional units

4. The production of large molecules from small ones is called:
   a. Anabolism
   b. Catabolism
   c. Hormesis
   d. Metabolism
   e. Mitosis

5. Which of the following are present in all tissues of the body and are the structural components of cell membranes?
   a. Carbohydrates
   b. Lipids
   c. Nucleic acids
   d. Proteins
   e. Sugars

6. The chief function of carbohydrates in the body is to:
   a. Assist in maintaining body temperature
   b. Exercise regulatory control over functions such as growth and metabolic rate
   c. Provide a defense mechanism against infection and disease
   d. Provide fuel for cell metabolism
   e. Provide structure and support

7. Which of the following is the concept of the relative constancy of the internal environment of the human body?
   a. Homeostasis
   b. Hormesis
   c. Meiosis
   d. Molecular composition
   e. Radiation hormesis

8. RNA:
   a. Contains all the hereditary information that represents a cell
   b. Is a principal component of a hormone
   c. Is located principally in the cytoplasm of the cell
   d. Is located principally in the nucleus of the cell
   e. Serves as the command or control molecule for all functions

205

9. Which of the following is an example of a macromolecule?
   a. A free radical
   b. A lipid
   c. An amino acid
   d. Salt
   e. Water

10. The breaking down of macromolecules into water and carbon dioxide is:
    a. Anabolism
    b. Catabolism
    c. Homeostasis
    d. Hormesis
    e. Metabolism

11. Which of the following molecules is a protein?
    a. A lipid
    b. A nucleic acid
    c. A salt
    d. An amino acid
    e. An enzyme

12. Lipids are:
    a. Energy storehouses
    b. Electrical conductors
    c. Inorganic compounds
    d. Micromolecules
    e. The sites of protein synthesis

13. Lipids store which of the following?
    a. Antibodies
    b. Enzymes
    c. Fat
    d. Salt
    e. Sugar

14. Organic molecules are defined as molecules that contain:
    a. Calcium
    b. Carbon
    c. Nitrogen
    d. Oxygen
    e. Sulfur

15. Which of the following is a principal component of protein?
    a. Amino acid
    b. Enzyme
    c. Lipid
    d. Peptide bond
    e. Sugar

16. The general formula $(C_6H_{10}O_5)_n$ represents which of the following?
    a. Amino acids
    b. Polysaccharides
    c. Genes
    d. Nucleic acids
    e. Proteins

17. Polysaccharides are which of the following?
    a. Carbohydrates
    b. Free radicals
    c. Lipids
    d. Nucleic acids
    e. Proteins

18. Which of the following base pairs is allowed for DNA?
    a. Adenine-cytosine
    b. Adenine-guanine
    c. Cytosine-thymine
    d. Guanine-cytosine
    e. Thymine-guanine

19. Homeostasis refers to what property of the body?
    a. Atomic composition
    b. Constancy of the internal environment
    c. Molecular composition
    d. Resistance to radiation
    e. Water content

20. Which of the following is the nitrogenous organic base found in RNA but *not* in DNA?
    a. Adenine
    b. Cytosine
    c. Guanine
    d. Thymine
    e. Uracil

21. The nucleic acids of the cell:
    a. Are found only in the nucleus
    b. Are macromolecules
    c. Consist of DNA and RNA
    d. Have a backbone of peptide bonds
    e. Store energy

Worksheet 29-3
Human Cells
Tissues and Organs

To understand the effects of radiation on the human body, one must have a basic knowledge of human anatomy and physiology. The body is an extremely organized system, but it is composed mostly of water. Radiation interactions at the atomic level are transferred through the various levels of organization and can result in visible radiation effects.

Understanding human cell division and the role of DNA helps in understanding how and why radiation effects occur. The phases of cell division include:

Prophase: nucleus swells and DNA becomes more prominent, beginning to take structural form

Metaphase: chromosomes line up in the central area of the cell

Anaphase: each chromosome splits at the centromere, creating sister chromatids

Telophase: chromosomes disappear into a mass of DNA and the cytoplasm divides into two parts

Different tissues and organs have different radiosensitivities, depending on the type of cells they are composed of. Radiation injuries tend to be more severe if a cell is injured when it is immature. Injury severity also depends on the type of cell damaged and which part of the cell life cycle it is in.

EXERCISES

1. "Crossing over":
   a. Is a process that occurs during meiosis, resulting in changes in genetic constitution and inheritable traits
   b. Is characterized by the disappearance of structural chromosomes into a mass of DNA
   c. Is the final phase of mitosis
   d. Is the period of cell growth between divisions
   e. Is the phase of the cell cycle during which the nucleus swells and the DNA becomes more prominent and begins to take structural form

2. Ribosomes:
   a. Are called the workhorses of the cell
   b. Are helpful in the control of intracellular contaminants
   c. Are sites of protein synthesis that are essential to normal function
   d. Are small, pealike sacs that are capable of digesting cellular fragments and even the cell itself
   e. Digest macromolecules to produce energy for the cell

3. Lysosomes:
   a. Are called the workhorses of the cell
   b. Are sites of protein synthesis that are essential to normal cellular function
   c. Contain enzymes capable of digesting cell fragments
   d. Deliver energy to target molecules
   e. Digest macromolecules to produce energy for the cell

4. During which of the following subphases of meiosis does each chromosome split at the centromere, so that two chromatids are connected by a fiber to the poles of the nucleus?
   a. Anaphase
   b. Metaphase
   c. Prophase
   d. Telophase
   e. None of the above

5. In the human cell:
   a. Both the cytoplasm and the nucleus are surrounded by membranes.
   b. Lysosomes contain nucleic acid.
   c. Macromolecules are digested in the ribosomes.
   d. Macromolecules are synthesized in the mitochondria.
   e. The DNA passes through the endoplasmic reticulum.

6. Which of the following is part of interphase?
   a. DNA synthesis phase
   b. G_0 phase
   c. Prophase
   d. Protein synthesis phase
   e. Telophase

7. At metaphase, the chromosomes:
   a. Are visible in the microscope
   b. Line up at the poles of the cell
   c. Ooze through the cellular membrane
   d. Remain dominant
   e. Split apart and replicate

8. At what phase in mitosis are the chromosomes *most* visible?
   a. Anaphase
   b. Interphase
   c. Metaphase
   d. Prophase
   e. Telophase

9. Messenger RNA (mRNA) moves from:
   a. Cytoplasm to mitochondria
   b. Cytoplasm to nucleus
   c. Nucleus to lysosome
   d. Nucleus to mitochondria
   e. Nucleus to ribosome

10. During which of the following subphases of meiosis do the chromosomes appear and line up along the equator of the nucleus?
    a. Anaphase
    b. Metaphase
    c. Prophase
    d. Telophase
    e. None of the above

11. Which of the following make(s) up the bulk of the cell and contain(s) all of the molecular components in great quantity?
    a. Cellular inclusions
    b. Cytoplasm
    c. Endoplasmic reticulum
    d. Membranes
    e. Nucleus

12. Which of the following searches the cytoplasm for the amino acid for which it is coded, attaches to that amino acid, and then carries it to the ribosome?
    a. A codon
    b. DNA
    c. mRNA
    d. The endoplasmic reticulum
    e. tRNA

13. Meiosis:
    a. Results in two cells with 46 chromosomes each
    b. Is the process of division and reduction that occurs in genetic cells
    c. Is the process of division that occurs in somatic cells
    d. Results in the formation of two genetically identical daughter cells that look precisely like the parent cell
    e. None of the above

14. The body is organized in such a way that:
    a. Differentiated cells are immature.
    b. Epithelial cells usually are found inside organs.
    c. Mature cells are called stem cells.
    d. Organs combine to form tissues.
    e. Tissues and organs form an organ system.

15. Which of the following tissues is most radiosensitive?
    a. Bone marrow
    b. Brain
    c. Thyroid
    d. Muscle
    e. Skin

16. The nucleolus in particular contains which of the following?
    a. Amino acids
    b. DNA
    c. Lipids
    d. Proteins
    e. RNA

Worksheet 30-1
Law of Bergonié and Tribondeau
Physical Factors That Affect
Radiosensitivity

Linear energy transfer (LET) expressed in keV/ μm is the rate at which energy is transferred from ionizing radiation to tissue. In general, high-LET radiation is more damaging than low-LET radiation.

Different types of ionizing radiation have different LET, and the efficiency for producing a given response is related to LET. Such efficiency is measured by the relative biologic effectiveness (RBE), which is determined experimentally.

$$RBE = \frac{\text{Dose of standard radiation necessary to produce a given effect}}{\text{Dose of test radiation necessary to produce the same effect}}$$

EXERCISES

1. Which of the following is a part of the law of Bergonié and Tribondeau?
   a. A fetus is less radiosensitive than an adult.
   b. Stem cells are radiosensitive.
   c. The more mature a cell is, the more radiosensitive it is.
   d. When metabolism is high, radiosensitivity is low.
   e. When the proliferation rate is high, so is radio-resistance.

2. The law of Bergonié and Tribondeau states that:
   a. Mature cells are more sensitive than stem cells.
   b. Metabolic activity results in radioprotection.
   c. Radiosensitivity increases with increasing hypoxia.
   d. Radiosensitivity increases with the proliferation rate.
   e. The older a cell is, the more radiosensitive it is.

3. The response of tissue to radiation is principally a function of which of the following?
   a. Dose
   b. Fractionation
   c. LET
   d. Oxygen enhancement ratio (OER)
   e. RBE

4. The RBE:
   a. Describes tissue radiosensitivity
   b. Increases as x-ray energy increases
   c. Is a descriptor of the type of radiation
   d. Is equal to 3 keV/μm for alpha particles
   e. Is equal to 3 keV/μm for diagnostic x-rays

5. The law of Bergonié and Tribondeau relates to which of the following?
   a. Radiocurability and tumor size
   b. Radioresistance and cell lethality
   c. Radioresistance and oxygenation
   d. Radiosensitivity and cellular differentiation
   e. Radiosensitivity and oxygenation

6. The RBE:
   a. Has a value of 1 to 100
   b. Is a ratio of effects needed to produce a given dose
   c. Is a ratio of effects produced at a given dose
   d. Is higher for high-LET radiation than for low-LET radiation
   e. Refers to type of effect

7. LET is measured in which of the following?
   a. Gray
   b. keV/rad
   c. keV/μm
   d. rad
   e. rad/μm

8. Which of the following has the highest LET?
   a. Alpha particles
   b. Cobalt-60 gamma rays
   c. Diagnostic x-rays
   d. Neutrons
   e. Protons

9. Diagnostic x-rays have an RBE of:
   a. 0.5
   b. 1
   c. 2
   d. 3
   e. 10

10. Dose fractionation is less effective than a single dose because:
    a. Dose fractionation has a low LET.
    b. Dose fractionation has a low OER.
    c. Fractionated doses are lower.
    d. Recovery occurs between doses.
    e. The RBE is less.

11. The LET, OER, and RBE are interrelated. Therefore, which of the following statements is *true?*
    a. Diagnostic x-rays are considered low LET and RBE and high OER.
    b. Diagnostic x-rays have a lower LET than cobalt-60 gamma rays.
    c. Diagnostic x-rays have an LET of 3.0 keV/μm and an OER of 3.
    d. High-LET radiation has low RBE.
    e. High-RBE radiation has high OER.

12. LET is useful for expressing radiation:
    a. Dose
    b. Production
    c. Quality
    d. Quantity
    e. Response

13. What is related to radiation protection as LET is related to radiobiology?
    a. Dose
    b. Quantity factor
    c. Radiation weighting factor (WR)
    d. Response
    e. Tissue weighting factor (WT)

14. Which of the following has the lowest LET?
    a. Alpha particles
    b. Cobalt-60 gamma rays
    c. Diagnostic x-rays
    d. Fast neutrons
    e. Protons

15. Dose protraction relates principally to which of the following?
    a. Dose
    b. Dose accumulation
    c. Dose integration
    d. Dose rate
    e. Dose response

16. Which of the following is considered a physical dose-modifying factor?
    a. Age
    b. Cell progression
    c. Dose protraction
    d. Oxygen
    e. Recovery

17. Which of the following factors has no influence on response to radiation exposure?
    a. Age
    b. Dose protraction
    c. Occupation
    d. Oxygen tension
    e. Sex

18. Dose fractionation is less effective than an equal single dose because of which of the following?
    a. Cellular recovery
    b. Oxygenation and proliferation
    c. RBE and LET
    d. Reduced LET
    e. Reduced OER

19. Why do we develop radiation dose-response relationships?
    a. To establish benefit-risk coefficients
    b. To establish estimates of diagnostic accuracy
    c. To predict the harmful effects of radiation at low doses
    d. To predict the therapeutic value of an occupational exposure
    e. To predict the value of a radiologic examination

Worksheet 30-1 **Law of Bergonié and Tribondeau**

Worksheet 30-2
Biologic Factors That Affect Radiosensitivity
Radiation Dose-Response Relationships

Tissue irradiated in the presence of oxygen (aerobic) responds to radiation more than does tissue irradiated under reduced levels of oxygen or in the absence of oxygen (hypoxic, anoxic, or anaerobic). The magnitude of this ratio in response is called the **oxygen enhancement ratio (OER).**

$$OER = \frac{\text{Radiation dose necessary to produce an effect under anaerobic conditions}}{\text{Radiation dose necessary to produce same effect under aerobic conditions}}$$

Most radiobiologic research is designed to establish the nature of radiation dose-response relationships. Such relationships generally can be classified as **linear** or **nonlinear** and **threshold** or **nonthreshold.** Knowledge of the precise nature of the radiation dose-response relationship allows one to predict human response after a given dose of radiation.

EXERCISES

1. Radiation-induced damage in tissue:
   a. Is caused by interaction at the tissue level
   b. Is greater in the presence of oxygen
   c. Is greater with protracted delivery
   d. Is irreversible
   e. Results in only latent effects

2. When one considers the biologic modifying factors to radiation response:
   a. Age is a factor.
   b. Nitrogen pressure is a factor.
   c. Pharmaceutical agents are capable only of protection.
   d. Pharmaceutical agents are capable only of sensitization.
   e. Sex is a factor.

3. Why is the linear, nonthreshold dose-response relationship used as a model for radiation protection guides?
   a. Because a linear response is directly proportional to the dose
   b. Because in a nonthreshold dose-response relationship, any dose is expected to produce a response
   c. Because of ALARA
   d. Because such guides are concerned exclusively with the deterministic effects of radiation exposure
   e. Because such guides are concerned exclusively with the stochastic effects of radiation exposure

4. The *least* sensitive time in life to radiation exposure is which of the following?
   a. Adulthood
   b. Childhood
   c. In utero
   d. Old age
   e. There is no least sensitive time.

5. Which of the following effects exhibits a threshold type of radiation dose-response relationship?
   a. Cataracts
   b. Leukemia
   c. Life span shortening
   d. Lung cancer
   e. Thyroid cancer

6. When a radiation dose-response relationship intercepts the response axis at a positive value:
   a. That response is acute.
   b. That response is not related to radiation.
   c. The radiation has a high LET.
   d. The relationship is linear.
   e. The relationship is nonlinear.

211

7. Which of the ensuing effects follows a nonlinear, threshold type of dose-response relationship?
   a. Breast cancer
   b. Skin effects
   c. Leukemia
   d. Life span shortening
   e. Prostate cancer

8. Dose limits (DLs) are based on which type of radiation dose-response relationship?
   a. Linear, nonthreshold
   b. Linear, quadratic
   c. Linear, threshold
   d. Nonlinear, nonthreshold
   e. Nonlinear, threshold

9. The stochastic effects of diagnostic x-rays probably follow which type of radiation dose-response relationship?
   a. Linear, nonthreshold
   b. Linear, quadratic
   c. Linear, threshold
   d. Nonlinear, nonthreshold
   e. Nonlinear, threshold

10. A wide error bar on a graphic data point indicates which of the following?
    a. A late effect
    b. Great confidence
    c. High LET
    d. Little confidence
    e. Low LET

11. The OER:
    a. Has a maximum value of about 10
    b. Is higher for protons than for photons
    c. Is highest for high-LET radiation
    d. Is highest for low-LET radiation
    e. Is independent of LET

12. Which of the following is considered a biologic dose-modifying factor?
    a. Dose per fraction
    b. Dose protraction
    c. Geometry
    d. LET
    e. The oxygen effect

13. Which of the following have the highest OER?
    a. Alpha particles
    b. Cobalt-60 gamma rays
    c. Diagnostic x-rays
    d. Neutrons
    e. Protons

14. Humans are *most* sensitive to radiation:
    a. At no special time
    b. During childhood
    c. During old age
    d. During preconception
    e. In utero

15. When an irradiated cell dies before the next mitosis, this is called:
    a. Clonal death
    b. Cytogenetic death
    c. Interphase death
    d. Metaphase death
    e. Mitotic death

16. A linear, nonthreshold dose-response relationship:
    a. Describes most deterministic effects
    b. Has a maximum response followed by a minimum response
    c. Is shaped like an "S"
    d. States that there is a range of very low doses that are totally safe
    e. Suggests that even the smallest dose may be risky

17. When a linear, nonthreshold dose-response relationship intersects the response axis at zero dose, this means that:
    a. It is not really linear.
    b. It is really threshold.
    c. Recovery and repair have occurred.
    d. There is a natural incidence of the response.
    e. There is no natural incidence of the response.

Worksheet 31-1
Molecular Radiobiology

 When irradiated in vitro (outside the body), molecules are relatively resistant to radiation damage. However, when irradiated in vivo (inside the body), even relatively minor molecular damage can produce visible and sometimes significant effects at the whole-body level.

Irradiation of macromolecules can result in main-chain scission, cross-linking, or point lesions. The macromolecule of principal importance in vivo is DNA.

Irradiation of water produces free radicals, hydrogen peroxide (H_2O_2), and the hydroperoxyl radical (HO_2), each of which is considered a harmful molecular by-product.

If radiation interacts with a macromolecule of importance, the subsequent effect is said to be **direct**. Alternatively, if radiation interacts with water, thereby creating one of the harmful by-products, which then diffuses through the cell to the macromolecule, the effect is said to be **indirect**.

EXERCISES

1. After a low radiation dose, most cellular radiation damage that results in a late total-body effect occurs because of which of the following?
   a. Cross-linking
   b. In vitro effects
   c. Main-chain scission
   d. Point lesions
   e. Reduced viscosity

2. The biologically reactive molecular by-products formed during radiolysis of water are thought to be which of the following?
   a. H_2O
   b. H^* and OH^*
   c. O_2 and H_2
   d. O and H
   e. SH compounds

3. Which of the following is the most radiosensitive molecule?
   a. DNA
   b. tRNA
   c. mRNA
   d. Ribosomes
   e. H_2O

4. Which of the following may occur in DNA molecules as a result of irradiation?
   a. Free radical formation
   b. Hydrogen bond breakage
   c. H_2O_2 formation
   d. A double-strand break
   e. Peroxy radical formation

5. When water is irradiated, products of the *initial* interaction are which of the following?
   a. H_2O_2
   b. H_2O and e^-
   c. HOH^+ and e^-
   d. OH^* and e^-
   e. OH^* and H^*

6. Which of the following is an example of anabolism?
   a. Hormesis
   b. Main-chain scission
   c. Protein synthesis
   d. Radiolysis of water
   e. Transfer RNA

7. Radiation-induced changes in DNA that result in genetic damage follow which type of dose-response relationship?
   a. Linear, nonthreshold
   b. Linear, quadratic
   c. Linear, threshold
   d. Nonlinear, nonthreshold
   e. Nonlinear, threshold

8. Which of the following is a free radical?
   a. e^-
   b. H_2O_2
   c. HO_2^*
   d. HOH^+
   e. HOH^-

9. When molecules are irradiated:
   a. Directly, it is with x-rays
   b. In solution in vitro, they are in free radicals
   c. In suspension, they are irradiated in solution
   d. In suspension, they are irradiated in vivo
   e. Inside the cell or body, they are irradiated in vitro

213

10. Radiation effects at the total-body level occur mainly because of which of the following?
    a. Alterations in viscosity
    b. Direct effect
    c. Increased radiosensitivity
    d. Indirect effect
    e. Irradiation in vitro

Ionization of water yields the following:

$$H_2O + Energy \rightarrow H_2O^+ + e^-$$

H_2O^+ is unstable and instantly produces two subunits as follows:

$$H_2O^+ \rightarrow H^+ + OH^*$$
$$(A) \quad (B) \quad (C)$$

and

$$H_2O^+ + e^- \rightarrow H_2O^-$$
$$(D) \quad (E) \quad (F)$$

followed by

$$H_2O^- \rightarrow H^* + OH^-$$
$$(G) \quad (H) \quad (I)$$

Match the ionization products given above (labeled A through I) with the description below:

11. Which of the above is the hydrogen ion?
    a. A
    b. B
    c. C
    d. H
    e. I

12. Which of the above is the hydroxyl free radical?
    a. B
    b. C
    c. G
    d. H
    e. I

13. Which of the above is positively ionized water?
    a. A
    b. B
    c. C
    d. D
    e. F

14. Which of the above is the hydroxyl ion?
    a. B
    b. C
    c. G
    d. H
    e. I

15. Which of the above is the hydrogen free radical?
    a. E
    b. F
    c. G
    d. H
    e. I

Worksheet 32-1
Cellular Radiobiology

 Radiation effects at the total-body level occur because of radiation damage to cells. Cellular damage, in turn, occurs because of molecular responses to radiation.

It is thought that certain critical molecules constitute sensitive targets within the cell, each of which must be inactivated to produce the ultimate response—cell lethality. This is the **target theory.**

The radiation dose-response relationship for cell lethality is **nonlinear** and **nonthreshold.** Cell survival follows the single-target, single-hit model or the multitarget, single-hit model of radiation-induced lethality. These models are the consequence of target theory and incorporate parameters useful for measuring the efficiency of various conditions of irradiation and the sensitivity of different types of cells.

D_{37} = Radiation dose after which 37% of cells will survive, whereas, conversely, 63% will die

D_O = Mean lethal dose; similar to D_{37} but applicable only to the straight-line portion of the multitarget, single-hit model

n = Extrapolation number

D_Q = Threshold dose or shoulder dose

EXERCISES

1. Which of the following phases of the cell cycle is considered *most* resistant?
   a. Early S phase
   b. G_1 phase
   c. G_2 phase
   d. Late S phase
   e. M phase

2. When cell-survival curves are used, the measure of cell radiosensitivity is which of the following?
   a. D_O
   b. D_Q
   c. n
   d. O_{37}
   e. RBE

3. When irradiated with high-LET radiation, human cells follow which of the following models?
   a. The linear, quadratic model
   b. The multitarget, multihit model
   c. The multitarget, single-hit model
   d. The single-target, multihit model
   e. The single-target, single-hit model

4. The probability of human cell death can be computed:
   a. If only D_O is known
   b. If only D_Q is known
   c. If only n is known
   d. Using the normal distribution
   e. Using the Poisson distribution

5. If a dose equal to D_{37} were *uniformly* distributed, what percentage of cells would survive?
   a. 0%
   b. 37%
   c. 50%
   d. 63%
   e. 100%

6. Which of the following is the mean lethal dose?
   a. D_O
   b. D_Q
   c. D_{37}
   d. D_n
   e. n

7. The multitarget, single-hit model:
   a. Contains D_O, which is the threshold dose
   b. Contains n, which is the mean lethal dose
   c. Is characterized by D_{37}
   d. Is not a part of target theory
   e. Presumes a threshold

8. The difference in generation time among different types of cells is due mainly to the length of which of the following?
   a. The G_1 phase
   b. The G_2 phase
   c. The G_O phase
   d. The M phase
   e. The S phase

9. Which of the following factors does *not* affect the radiation response of mammalian cells?
   a. Dose rate
   b. LET
   c. Presence of oxygen
   d. Sex of the cell
   e. Stage of the cell in its cycle

215

10. According to the multitarget model of cell lethality:
    a. Cells have more than one critical target, each of which has to be inactivated for cell death.
    b. Cells have one critical target and several secondary targets.
    c. Only cell death can be measured with accuracy.
    d. The cell can accumulate a radiation dose.
    e. The critical target is considered to be the RNA.

11. In the following graph that shows two survival curves, which of the following is true?

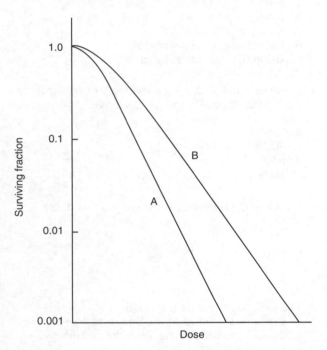

a. Both curves have the same D_{37}.
b. Both curves have the same D_Q.
c. Both curves have the same mean lethal dose.
d. Curve A could represent oxygenated cells if curve B represented anoxic cells.
e. Curve A could represent protracted exposure if curve B represented single exposure.

12. According to target theory:
    a. A hit can occur only by direct effect.
    b. A hit can occur only by indirect effect.
    c. Radiation favors the target molecule.
    d. Radiation interacts randomly.
    e. Radiation interacts uniformly.

13. When irradiated with x-rays, human cells follow which of the following models?
    a. The linear, quadratic model
    b. The multitarget, multihit model
    c. The multitarget, single-hit model
    d. The single-target, multihit model
    e. The single-target, single-hit model

14. To explain radiation effects on living cells, target theory states that:
    a. A target can receive a hit by direct or indirect effect.
    b. Once hit, targets can be replaced.
    c. Only one target exists within the cell.
    d. Only one target must be hit to cause cell death.
    e. There is only one type of target.

15. If a dose equal to D_{37} were randomly distributed, what percentage of cells would die?
    a. 0%
    b. 37%
    c. 50%
    d. 63%
    e. 100%

Worksheet 33-1
Acute Radiation Lethality
Local Tissue Damage

The degree of radiation effect is related to the radiation dose and is predicted by a dose-response relationship. These conclusions are drawn from experimentation with animals and from observations of humans irradiated both accidentally and intentionally.

Effects of radiation exposure at the whole-body level that occur within weeks of exposure are referred to as acute, or early, effects of radiation exposure. These effects include radiation lethality and radiation effects on local tissues. They are generally due to the death of many cells within the tissue.

EXERCISES

1. The $LD_{50/60}$ for humans is closest to which of the following?
   a. 1.6 Gy_t
   b. 2.5 Gy_t
   c. 3.5 Gy_t
   d. 4.5 Gy_t
   e. 6.0 Gy_t

2. A whole-body dose equivalent of 30 Gy_t would probably cause death in 4 to 10 days by which of the following mechanisms?
   a. Central nervous system death
   b. Gastrointestinal death
   c. Hemopoietic death
   d. Latent effects
   e. Prodromal syndrome

3. With regard to the radiation exposure of mammalian gonads:
   a. A linear, nonthreshold dose-response relationship prevails for sterility.
   b. Effects are apparently independent of LET.
   c. Spermatocyte depression has been measured at as low as 0.1 Gy_t.
   d. Sterility is induced at doses as low as 0.5 Gy_t.
   e. The spermatocyte represents the most sensitive stage in the male.

4. The minimum testicular dose for transient infertility is approximately:
   a. 0.05 Gy_t
   b. 0.1 Gy_t
   c. 0.5 Gy_t
   d. 2.0 Gy_t
   e. 5.0 Gy_t

5. The $LD_{50/30}$ refers to a:
   a. Lethal dose delivered within 30 to 50 days
   b. Lethal dose of total-body radiation for 30% of the people so exposed in 50 days
   c. Lethal dose of total-body radiation for 30% to 50% of the people so exposed
   d. Lethal dose of total-body radiation for 50% of the people so exposed in 30 days
   e. Lovely dance for half the people younger than 30 years

6. The $LD_{50/60}$ represents the dose:
   a. Equivalent to 37% cell survival (D_{37})
   b. Required to kill 50% of the cells in 60 days
   c. Required to kill 60% of the cells in 50 days
   d. Resulting in 60% human death within 2 months
   e. That will kill half the people in 60 days

7. Human radiation lethality follows which dose-response relationship?
   a. Linear, quadratic
   b. Linear, nonthreshold
   c. Linear, threshold
   d. Nonlinear, nonthreshold
   e. Nonlinear, threshold

8. Which dose range, applied to both ovaries, is needed to induce permanent sterility?
   a. 0.1 to 1.0 Gy_t
   b. 1.0 to 2.0 Gy_t
   c. 2.0 to 5.0 Gy_t
   d. 5.0 to 12.0 Gy_t
   e. More than 12.0 Gy_t

217

9. Which syndrome has a mean survival time that is independent of dose?
   a. Central nervous system
   b. Gastrointestinal
   c. Hematologic
   d. Latent
   e. Prodromal

10. The dose of x-rays necessary to produce erythema in half of those exposed is approximately:
    a. 0.5 Gy_t
    b. 1.0 Gy_t
    c. 3.0 Gy_t
    d. 5.0 Gy_t
    e. 10.0 Gy_t

11. The acute radiation syndrome consists of all of the following, *except:*
    a. Central nervous syndrome
    b. Gastrointestinal syndrome
    c. Hematologic syndrome
    d. Latent injury syndrome
    e. Latent period

12. Which of the following is *not* an early response to radiation exposure?
    a. Breast cancer
    b. Chromosome aberrations
    c. Epilation
    d. Intestinal distress that occurs 1 week after exposure
    e. Skin erythema that occurs 2 weeks after exposure

13. Which of the following is a delayed local tissue effect?
    a. Cataracts
    b. Epilation
    c. Moist desquamation
    d. Skin erythema
    e. Transient sterility

14. Five days after a whole-body dose of 10 Gy_t is received, physiologic alterations in the small intestine include all of the following, *except:*
    a. Crypt cell death
    b. Diarrhea
    c. Epilation
    d. Leakage of proteins from the intestinal lumen
    e. Loss of electrolytes and water

15. The acute radiation syndrome:
    a. Begins at a threshold dose of 0.5 Gy_t
    b. By gastrointestinal death indicates a mean survival time of about 4 to 10 days
    c. Can occur after high doses administered over a short time or over several months
    d. Includes the gastrointestinal syndrome, which occurs after doses of approximately 50 to 100 Gy_t
    e. Includes the most sensitive of the syndromes—the gastrointestinal syndrome

16. The mean survival time after a lethal radiation dose is constant:
    a. Between 2.0 and 10.0 Gy_t
    b. For gastrointestinal death
    c. For hematologic death
    d. With increasing the dose to more than 50 Gy_t
    e. With increasing the dose to more than 100 Gy_t

Worksheet 33-2
Hematologic Effects
Cytogenetic Effects

All of the acute radiation effects observed at the whole-body level have been studied thoroughly in experimental animals. Most have been observed in human populations, including atomic bomb survivors, radiation accident victims, and patients with radiation-induced cancer.

Blood is a body tissue that has received considerable attention as a biologic in vivo radiation dosimeter. Because blood is radiosensitive and is easy to sample, it often is used to predict the likely outcome of an unknown radiation exposure.

Cell counts and cytogenetic analysis of lymphocytes are conducted on all radiation accident victims to determine the aggressiveness of supportive therapy and to help guide treatment.

EXERCISES

1. Which of the following cell types is most severely depressed by radiation?
   a. Erythrocytes
   b. Granulocytes
   c. Lymphocytes
   d. Megakaryocytes
   e. Neurons

2. The normal human karyotype consists of:
   a. 23 chromosomes
   b. 23 chromosome pairs
   c. 42 autosomes
   d. 46 autosomes
   e. Two sex chromosome pairs

3. Of the following chromosome aberrations, which requires a karyotype for analysis?
   a. Chromatid deletion
   b. Dicentric chromosome
   c. Isochromatid fragments
   d. Reciprocal translocation
   e. Ring chromosome

4. Which of the following blood observations is *most* appropriate during monitoring for radiation response?
   a. Erythrocyte count
   b. Granulocyte count
   c. Hematocrit
   d. Lymphocyte count
   e. Thrombocyte count

5. A whole-body radiation dose of 0.25 Gy_t is *most* likely to produce which of the following?
   a. Cytogenetic damage
   b. Depletion of oogonia
   c. Epilation
   d. Erythrocyte depression
   e. Skin erythema

6. Which of the following is *not* a mature blood cell?
   a. Cystocyte
   b. Erythrocyte
   c. Granulocyte
   d. Lymphocyte
   e. Thrombocyte

7. Radiation effects on the hematologic system:
   a. Are first observed as a lymphocyte depression
   b. Are measurable at whole-body doses as low as 5 rad
   c. Are permanent
   d. Cannot result in a late response
   e. Suggest that radiation workers should undergo routine blood analysis

8. Which of the following blood observations is *most* appropriate for routine monitoring of radiation workers?
   a. Erythrocyte count
   b. Lymphocyte count
   c. Shilling differential
   d. Thrombocyte count
   e. None of the above

9. Which of the following chromosome aberrations obeys a linear, nonthreshold dose-response relationship?
   a. Chromatid break
   b. Dicentric
   c. Reciprocal translocation
   d. Ring chromosome
   e. Tricentric

10. Which cells are involved in the human immune response?
    a. Erythrocytes
    b. Granulocytes
    c. Lymphocytes
    d. Spermatocytes
    e. Thrombocytes

11. Which cells are *most* sensitive to radiation exposure?
    a. Cystocytes
    b. Erythrocytes
    c. Granulocytes
    d. Lymphocytes
    e. Thrombocytes

12. What phase of the cell cycle has the *most* variable length?
    a. G_0
    b. G_1
    c. G_2
    d. M
    e. S

13. Which of the following is the precursor to a thrombocyte?
    a. Cystocyte
    b. Lymphocyte
    c. Megakaryoblast
    d. Myeloblast
    e. Reticulocyte

14. Which two cell lines are the *most* radiosensitive?
    a. Granulocytes, lymphocytes
    b. Granulocytes, oogonia
    c. Granulocytes, spermatogonia
    d. Spermatogonia, lymphocytes
    e. Spermatogonia, oogonia

15. Which of the following human cells are *most* often used for cytogenetic analysis?
    a. Lymphocytes
    b. Oogonia
    c. Skin cells
    d. Spermatogonia
    e. Thrombocytes

16. How long after radiation exposure do chromosome aberrations first appear in peripheral blood cells?
    a. Hours
    b. Months
    c. Years
    d. Decades
    e. Never

17. The principal response of the blood to radiation exposure is:
    a. A decrease in cell number
    b. Stimulation of cell proliferation
    c. Cellular transformation
    d. Fragmentation of chromosomes
    e. Rearrangement of chromosomes

18. After radiation exposure, the first blood cells to respond are the:
    a. Cystocytes
    b. Erythrocytes
    c. Granulocytes
    d. Lymphocytes
    e. Thrombocytes

19. A chromosomal karyotype is:
    a. A description of the radiation response
    b. A point mutation
    c. An analysis of chromosome fragments
    d. An orderly map of chromosomes
    e. Unrestrained growth of chromosomes

20. Evidence suggests that the most harmful male genetic mutations occur in which of the following?
    a. Leydig cells
    b. Sertoli cells
    c. Spermatocytes
    d. Spermatids
    e. Postspermatogonia cells

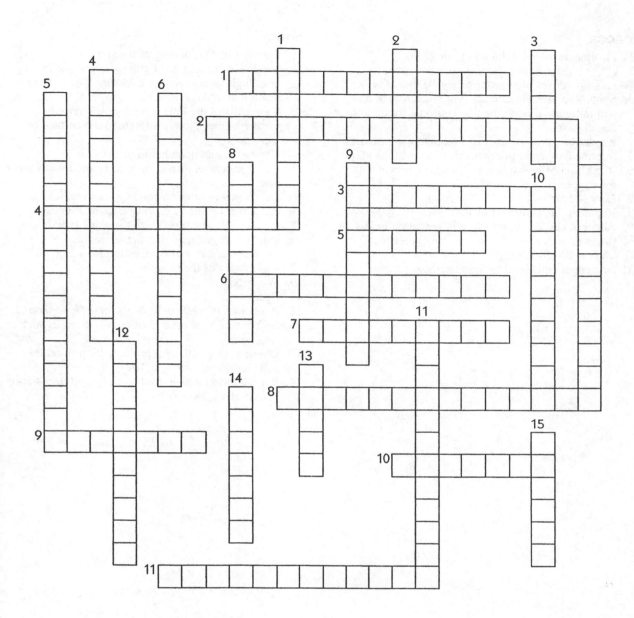

ACROSS

1. Platelets involved in blood clotting
2. _____ Radiation Syndrome is produced by radiation doses of approximately 10 to 50 Gy_t.
3. Syndrome of acute clinical symptoms that occur within hours of exposure and continue for up to a day or two
4. Reduction in the number of immune response cells
5. Intermediate layer of connective tissue in the skin
6. Red blood cells that are the transportation agents for oxygen
7. Loss of hair
8. Rapid rise in scavenger cells
9. Effect of cell death, resulting in reduction in size of tissue or organ
10. Stem cells of the ovaries
11. Scavenger cells used to fight bacteria

DOWN

1. Sunburn-like reddening of the skin
2. Syndrome represented by the sequence of events after high-level radiation exposure that leads to death within days or weeks
3. Stem cells in the lowest layer of the skin that mature as they slowly migrate to the surface of the epidermis
4. Ulceration and denudation of the skin
5. Rapid decrease, then slower decrease, in scavenger cells
6. Development of germ cells by both ovaries and testes that occurs at varying rates and times
7. _____ illness refers to the acute radiation lethality stage, including hematologic, gastrointestinal, and neuromuscular symptoms.
8. Outer layer of the skin
9. White cells
10. Platelets
11. Reduction in white cells of the peripheral blood
12. Soft x-rays once used to treat skin diseases such as ringworm
13. Ovarian stem cells encapsulated by primordial follicles during late fetal life
14. Period during which a subject exposed to radiation is free of visible effects

Worksheet 34-1
Local Tissue Effects
Life Span Shortening
Risk Estimates

Delayed or late responses to radiation exposure include genetic effects and those somatic effects that require months or even years to develop. Radiobiologists rely heavily on data extrapolated from observations of humans who have suffered high radiation doses or on large-scale epidemiologic studies.

These late effects generally follow low doses of radiation. Precise dose-response relationships are seldom possible to determine; therefore, radiation scientists resort to various estimates of risk.

Principal late effects of concern are the induction of malignant disease and genetic effects. Each of these is presumed to follow a linear, nonthreshold dose-response relationship. Late local tissue effects are for the most part threshold in nature.

EXERCISES

1. Which of the following is an example of a linear, nonthreshold dose-response relationship?
   a. Cataracts
   b. CNS syndrome
   c. Epilation
   d. Lethality
   e. Leukemia

2. Which of the following statements about radiation-induced cataracts after a computed tomography examination of the head is *most* appropriate?
   a. Cataracts are possible because there is no threshold.
   b. Lens shields should be used.
   c. The dose is certainly below the threshold for such an effect.
   d. The dose is probably in the neighborhood of the threshold for such an effect.
   e. The probability of cataracts is high.

3. The best estimate for radiation-induced life span shortening is:
   a. 1 hr/mGy$_t$ (= 10 hr/rad)
   b. 1 day/mGy$_t$ (= 10 days/rad)
   c. 2.4 hrs/mGy$_t$ (= 24 hr/rad)
   d. 2.4 days/mGy$_t$ (= 24 days/rad)
   e. 0.1 mo/mGy$_t$ (= 1 mo/rad)

4. Diagnostic x-rays have been shown to produce which of the following?
   a. Cataracts
   b. Chromosome aberrations
   c. Leukemia
   d. Organ atrophy
   e. Shortening of life

5. Supporting evidence for radiation carcinogenesis comes from:
   a. British radiologists
   b. Fluoroscopic monitoring of patients with tuberculosis
   c. ^{131}I therapy for hyperthyroidism
   d. Pelvimetry
   e. People living in areas with high background radiation (e.g., Denver)

6. If the incidence of cancer is 1:5000, what is the relative risk if an irradiated population shows an incidence of 4:10,000?
   a. 2:1
   b. 4:1
   c. 10:1
   d. 1000:1
   e. 4000:1

7. Which of the following groups has suffered a harmful radiation effect?
   a. Patients receiving diagnostic x-rays
   b. Nuclear power plant workers
   c. Radiologic technologists
   d. Radium watch dial painters
   e. The last generation of radiologists

8. Radiation-induced cataracts:
   a. Appear on the posterior pole of the lens
   b. Exhibit a threshold to x-rays of approximately 0.1 Gy$_t$ (10 rad)
   c. Follow a linear, nonthreshold type of dose-response relationship
   d. Follow a nonlinear, threshold type of dose-response relationship
   e. Have a latent period of approximately 1 year

9. Approximately how many Americans will die of malignant disease from natural causes?
   a. 5%
   b. 10%
   c. 20%
   d. 40%
   e. 50%

10. Significant gonadal radiation exposure occurs:
   a. In whole-body MRI
   b. Only when no collimator is used
   c. When radiation is scattered from other parts of the body
   d. When radiation is scattered internally
   e. When the gonads are in the primary beam

11. Epidemiology is the study of which of the following?
   a. Early radiation effects
   b. Late radiation effects
   c. Populations
   d. Radiation
   e. Statistics

12. Radiation-induced chromosome aberrations are which of the following?
   a. Early or late effects
   b. Observable following 0.1 Gy$_t$ (10 rad)
   c. Only early effects
   d. Only late effects
   e. Present only after whole-body irradiation

13. The average latent period for radiation-induced cataracts is:
   a. 5 years
   b. 15 years
   c. 30 years
   d. 50 years
   e. Life

14. The approximate acute x-ray dose required to produce a 100% incidence of cataracts is:
   a. 1 Gy$_t$
   b. 10 Gy$_t$
   c. 100 Gy$_t$
   d. 1000 Gy$_t$
   e. 10,000 Gy$_t$

15. When engaged in a busy fluoroscopy schedule, who should wear protective lens shields?
   a. Both radiologists and technologists
   b. Neither radiologists nor technologists
   c. Not enough information is given
   d. Only radiologists
   e. Only technologists

16. Which of the following has the greatest loss-of-life expectancy?
   a. Accidents
   b. Being male
   c. Cancer
   d. Occupation
   e. Radiation

17. Patients should use protective lens shields:
   a. Always
   b. Never
   c. When the lens is in the primary beam and such use does not interfere with the examination
   d. Whenever the lens is in the primary beam
   e. Not enough information is given.

18. Breast cancer is observed in 30 of 450 patients. If the normal incidence is 2:1000, what is the approximate relative risk in these patients?
   a. 10:1
   b. 30:1
   c. 50:1
   d. 100:1
   e. 300:1

Worksheet 34-2
Radiation-Induced Malignancy
Total Risk of Malignancy
Radiation and Pregnancy

It is undeniable that humans are most sensitive to the harmful effects of radiation while in utero. Furthermore, the fetus is most radiation-sensitive early in pregnancy. Radiation effects include prenatal and postnatal mortality, congenital abnormalities, and latent malignant disease.

Low-dose irradiation (e.g., 10 rad [0.1 Gy_t]) has never caused such effects in humans. Only epidemiologic studies such as the Oxford survey have suggested an increased risk of latent malignant disease after low-dose in utero irradiation.

No direct evidence of radiation-induced genetic effects has been found in humans.

Observations of flies and mice, however, have shown the following:

1. Radiation-induced genetic mutations follow a linear, nonthreshold dose-response relationship.
2. The passage of time leads to some recovery from the genetic effects of radiation.
3. Radiation does not induce specific genetic mutations but rather increases the incidence of already existing mutations.
4. Radiation-induced genetic mutations are usually recessive.
5. For humans, the doubling dose is approximately 50 rad (0.5 Gy_t).

EXERCISES

1. The relative risk of leukemia after low-dose radiation in utero is approximately:
   a. 0.5
   b. 1.5
   c. 3.5
   d. 5.0
   e. 10

2. The generally accepted absolute risk factor for radiation-induced breast cancer is:
   a. 0.006 cases/10^6/mGy_t/yr = (0.06 cases/10^6/rad/yr)
   b. 0.06 cases/10^6/mGy_t/yr = (0.6 cases/10^6/rad/yr)
   c. 0.6 cases/10^6/mGy_t/yr = (6 cases/10^6/rad/yr)
   d. 6 cases/10^6/mGy_t/yr = (60 cases/10^6/rad/yr)
   e. 60 cases/10^6/mGy_t/yr = (600 cases/10^6/rad/yr)

3. Radiation-induced leukemia:
   a. Can be reversed
   b. Does not occur after long-term, low-level radiation exposure
   c. Follows a linear, threshold dose-response relationship
   d. Has been demonstrated in both animals and humans
   e. Probably does not occur at doses of less than approximately 0.25 Gy_t (25 rad)

4. Which of the following dose-response relationships best describes radiation-induced lung cancer?
   a. Linear, nonthreshold
   b. Linear, quadratic
   c. Linear, threshold
   d. Nonlinear, nonthreshold
   e. Nonlinear, threshold

5. Which of the following numbers approximates the total cases of leukemia observed in the 100,000 atomic bomb survivors?
   a. 50
   b. 150
   c. 500
   d. 1500
   e. 5000

6. Which of the following statements about the development of radiation-induced liver cancer in Thorotrast-injected patients is *true?*
   a. The findings are negative.
   b. The findings are positive and statistically significant.
   c. The findings are positive but not statistically significant.
   d. The radiation source was iodine.
   e. The suspected principal radiation dose comes from beta emission.

7. After a dose of 0.1 Gy_t (10 rad) at 6 weeks of gestation, the increase in congenital abnormalities is approximately:
   a. 0.1%
   b. 1%
   c. 10%
   d. 25%
   e. 50%

8. The latent period of radiation-induced leukemia is considered to be:
   a. 1 year
   b. 1 to 3 years
   c. 4 to 7 years
   d. 8 to 12 years
   e. >12 years

9. Analysis of the survivors of the atomic bomb shows that the induction of leukemia:
   a. Does not exist
   b. Peaked 10 years after the bomb
   c. Principally implicates chronic lymphocytic leukemia
   d. Suggests a threshold of 3 Gy_t (300 rad)
   e. Supports a linear, nonthreshold dose-response relationship

10. Which of the following populations has shown an increased incidence of leukemia after radiation exposure?
    a. American radiologic technologists
    b. Atomic bomb survivors
    c. Chernobyl survivors
    d. Diagnostic imaging patients
    e. Radium watch-dial painters

11. Which of the following types of cancer has *not* been demonstrated in humans after irradiation?
    a. Breast
    b. Colon
    c. Liver
    d. Lung
    e. Skin

12. Which type of radiation-induced cancer exhibits a threshold dose-response relationship?
    a. Bone
    b. Breast
    c. Liver
    d. Lung
    e. Skin

13. The radiation dose-response relationship for genetic mutations is:
    a. Exponential
    b. Independent of dose
    c. Linear
    d. Nonlinear
    e. Threshold

14. The relative risk of leukemia after irradiation in utero:
    a. Is approximately 50
    b. Is approximately 100
    c. Is less than 1.0 at zero dose
    d. Would equal 1.0 if there were no risk
    e. Would equal 100 if there were no risk

15. Which of the following radiation responses in utero is *most* likely when exposure occurs during organogenesis?
    a. Childhood cancer
    b. Congenital abnormalities
    c. Leukemia
    d. Neonatal death
    e. Prenatal death

16. With regard to radiation-induced genetic mutations:
    a. The dose-response relationship is nonlinear.
    b. The dose-response relationship is threshold.
    c. The doubling dose is approximately 0.5 to 2.5 Gy_t (50 to 250 rad).
    d. The male is more sensitive than the female.
    e. The most frequent types are dominant.

17. The data and conclusions of the Oxford survey:
    a. Are based on exposure of mice
    b. Show a 100% incidence of effects after an exposure of 2 Gy_t (200 rad)
    c. Suggest a relative risk of approximately 8:1 during the first trimester of pregnancy
    d. Suggest a threshold for cataracts of approximately 2 Gy_t (200 rad)
    e. Suggest a shortening of the life span by 1 day/mGy_t (= 10 days/rad)

Worksheet 35-1
Cardinal Principles of Radiation Protection
Dose Limits

Time and experience have led to a body of rules, regulations, and recommendations known as the principles of radiation protection. Exposure levels considered to be safe have been established, and these have been supplemented by the concept of **ALARA** (*as low as reasonably achievable*). Procedures and techniques have been developed to maintain occupational exposure below recommended limits and to ensure that all exposures are ALARA.

The cumulative **dose limit (DL)** is the dose that, if received each year during a 40-year occupational span, would result in an acceptable risk of injury.

Three principles of radiation control are known as the cardinal principles:

1. Keep the time of radiation exposure as short as possible.
2. Increase the distance from the source.
3. Place shielding between the source and the person who is being shielded.

These cardinal principles of radiation protection must be applied. Nearly all of the protective procedures and devices used in diagnostic radiology incorporate some aspect of these principles.

EXERCISES

1. Half-value layer (HVL) is related to which of the following principles of radiation protection?
   a. Distance
   b. Exposure
   c. Monitoring
   d. Shielding
   e. Time

2. If all other factors remain constant, radiation dose is related to x-ray beam-on time:
   a. By the inverse square
   b. Directly
   c. Exponentially
   d. Geometrically
   e. Inversely

3. If all other factors remain constant, radiation dose is related to source-to-object distance (SOD):
   a. By the inverse square
   b. Directly
   c. Exponentially
   d. Inversely
   e. Proportionately

4. If all other factors remain constant, radiation dose is related to shielding:
   a. By the inverse square
   b. Directly
   c. Exponentially
   d. Inversely
   e. Proportionately

5. One tenth-value layer (TVL) is defined as:
   a. $\frac{1}{10}$ the initial dose
   b. $\frac{1}{10}$ the initial shielding
   c. 10 times the HVL
   d. The shielding necessary to reduce exposure to $\frac{1}{10}$
   e. The shielding that will produce 10 times the dose

6. One TVL is equal to approximately how many HVLs?
   a. 2.0
   b. 2.2
   c. 3.3
   d. 5.0
   e. 10.0

7. During radiography, the best position for the radiologic technologist is:
   a. Behind the operating console barrier
   b. Down the hall
   c. Holding the patient
   d. In the examination room and as far from the patient as practical
   e. In the examination room and next to the patient

8. The HVL for 70 kVp is greater:
   a. For long exposure time than for short exposure time
   b. Than that for 90 kVp
   c. Than the TVL for 70 kVp
   d. With high filtration than with low filtration
   e. With single-phase power than with three-phase power

9. The exposure rate from a point source is 1 mGy$_a$/hr (100 mR/hr) at 120 cm. If a radiologic technologist moves to within 30 cm of the source of radiation, how many HVLs would be needed to reduce the exposure rate to 1 mGy$_a$/hr (100 mR/hr)?
   a. 1
   b. 2
   c. 4
   d. 6
   e. 8

10. If a survey meter reads 0.25 mGy$_a$/hr (25 mR/hr), how long can a person stay at that location before receiving an exposure of 1 mGy$_a$/hr (100 mR/hr)?
    a. 1 hour
    b. 2 hours
    c. 4 hours
    d. 6 hours
    e. 8 hours

11. If the exposure rate 1 m from a source is 90 mGy$_a$/hr (9000 mR/hr), what is the exposure rate at 3 m from the source?
    a. 1 mGy$_a$/hr (100 mR/hr).
    b. 9 mGy$_a$/hr (900 mR/hr).
    c. 10 mGy$_a$/hr (1000 mR/hr).
    d. 30 mGy$_a$/hr (3000 mR/hr).
    e. 90 mGy$_a$/hr (9000 mR/hr).

12. The exposure rate alongside a fluoroscopic table (distance = 60 cm from the source) is 4 mGy$_a$/hr (400 mR/hr). Therefore, if the radiologic technologist:
    a. Completed a 3-minute barium enema, the exposure would be 0.2 mGy$_a$ (20 mR)
    b. Completed a procedure at a distance of 120 cm, the total exposure would be 0.4 mGy$_a$ (40 mR)
    c. Completed a procedure that required 10 minutes, the exposure would be 0.4 mGy$_a$ (40 mR)
    d. Moved 60 cm farther from the table, the exposure rate would be 2 mGy$_a$/hr (200 mR/hr)
    e. Moved 60 cm farther from the table, the exposure rate would be increased

13. The DL for a radiologic technologist is:
    a. 1 mSv (100 mrem) per year
    b. 5 mSv (500 mrem) per 9 months
    c. 5 mSv (500 mrem) per year
    d. 50 mSv (5000 mrem) per 9 months
    e. 50 mSv (5000 mrem) per year

14. You are a 17-year-old radiologic technologist student. How much occupational exposure are you allowed?
    a. 1 mSv (100 mrem) per 9 months
    b. 1 mSv (100 mrem) per year
    c. 5 mSv (500 mrem) per 9 months
    d. 5 mSv (500 mrem) per year
    e. 50 mSv (5000 mrem) per year

15. During fluoroscopy, the exposure rate at the technologist's position is 3.5 mGy$_a$/hr (350 mR/hr). How much x-ray beam-on time is allowed before the technologist reaches a weekly DL?
    a. 8 minutes
    b. 17 minutes
    c. 35 minutes
    d. 1 hour
    e. 2 hours

16. The cumulative DL is computed as follows:
    a. 5 to 18N
    b. 5(N − 18)
    c. 5N − 18
    d. 10 mSv × N
    e. 50 mSv × N

17. A protective apron is equivalent to 2 HVLs. How much more time can the radiologic technologist remain in the room during fluoroscopy with such an apron than without one?
    a. Half as much time
    b. Twice as much time
    c. Four times as much time
    d. Eight times as much time
    e. Not enough information is given

Worksheet 36-1
Design of X-Ray Apparatus
Design of Protective Barriers

Designers of equipment and x-ray facilities exercise considerable care and attention. Much of this attention results from the need for radiation protection.

X-ray imaging systems have filters, collimators, and shields to reduce radiation exposure to patients and personnel. Attention is given to proper design and calibration of kVp, mA, and exposure timers so that radiographic techniques can be accurately and consistently used. This accuracy reduces the number of reexaminations, which in turn reduces human exposure. This is why periodic radiation control surveys and performance evaluation of x-ray apparatus are recommended.

Nearly all diagnostic x-ray rooms have lead in the walls. Sometimes, floor and ceiling barriers also require lead shielding.

EXERCISES

1. Every diagnostic x-ray tube housing must be sufficiently shielded to limit the level of exposure 1 m from the housing to:
   a. 0.1 mGy$_a$/hr (10 mR/hr).
   b. 1 mGy$_a$/hr (100 mR/hr).
   c. 10 mGy$_a$/hr (1000 mR/hr).
   d. A factor that varies according to kVp
   e. A factor that varies according to use

2. During mammography, at tube potentials less than 30 kVp, the minimum acceptable total equivalent filtration is:
   a. 0.05 mm Al
   b. 0.1 mm Al
   c. 0.25 mm Al
   d. 0.5 mm Al
   e. 2.5 mm Al

3. The minimum permissible filtration for general purpose radiographic or fluoroscopic tubes is:
   a. 0.05 mm Al
   b. 0.1 mm Al
   c. 0.25 mm Al
   d. 0.5 mm Al
   e. 2.5 mm Al

4. The fluoroscopic tube should *not* be positioned closer than 38 cm to the tabletop because the:
   a. Bucky slot would interfere
   b. Geometric unsharpness would increase
   c. Heat load on the tube would increase
   d. Patient radiation dose would be excessive
   e. Resultant magnification would be objectionable

5. Which of the following is regulated in a controlled area?
   a. Patient flow
   b. Public access
   c. Radiation exposure
   d. Type of procedure
   e. X-ray operation

6. Radiographic work load (W) has units of:
   a. mAmin/wk
   b. mR/mAmin
   c. mR/mAs
   d. R/mAmin/wk
   e. R/wk

7. The radiographic workload in a busy radio fluoroscopy room is approximately:
   a. 10 mAmin/wk
   b. 50 mAmin/wk
   c. 100 mAmin/wk
   d. 500 mAmin/wk
   e. 5000 mAmin/wk

8. Which of the following locations in a hospital should have the highest occupancy factor (T)?
   a. Laboratory
   b. Elevator
   c. Corridor
   d. Restroom
   e. Waiting room

9. Which of the following usually is considered to be a secondary protective barrier?
   a. All walls
   b. Chest wall
   c. Control booth barrier
   d. Floor
   e. Lateral wall

10. Fluoroscopic x-ray units must:
    a. Be image-intensified
    b. Have at least 2.5 mm Al equivalent filtration
    c. Have spot-film capability
    d. Limit leakage radiation to 10 mGy$_a$/hr (1000 mR/hr) at 1 m from the tube
    e. Never exceed 100 mGy$_a$/min (10 R/min) at the tabletop

11. Which of the following contributes to the exposure of radiologic personnel?
    a. Off-focus radiation
    b. Primary radiation
    c. Remnant x-rays
    d. Scatter radiation
    e. Useful beam

12. The design limit for exposure of occupants in controlled areas is:
    a. 0.01 mSv/wk (1 mrem/wk)
    b. 0.1 mSv/wk (10 mrem/wk)
    c. 1 mSv/wk (100 mrem/wk)
    d. 5 mSv/wk (500 mrem/wk)
    e. 10 mSv/wk (1000 mrem/wk)

13. The use factor (U):
    a. Applies only to radiography, not fluoroscopy
    b. Describes the use of the room
    c. Describes the use of the x-ray tube
    d. Is always 1 for secondary barriers
    e. Takes on values from 0 to 10

14. All fluoroscopes have a 5-minute reset timer:
    a. Because no patient shall ever receive more than 5 minutes of x-ray beam-on time
    b. To allow image receptor change
    c. To permit a tube cooldown period
    d. To protect the patient
    e. To protect the x-ray tube

15. A test to ensure that radiation intensity is doubled when radiographic mA is doubled is called a test of:
    a. Alignment
    b. Coincidence
    c. Linearity
    d. Reproducibility
    e. Uniformity

16. When the fluoroscopic x-ray tube is mounted farther under the table, what is reduced?
    a. Beam alignment
    b. Filtration
    c. Image receptor speed
    d. Patient dose
    e. Scatter radiation

17. Which of the following would definitely be a secondary barrier?
    a. All walls of a dedicated chest room
    b. Any wall in a CT room
    c. The chest wall in an RF room
    d. The door
    e. The floor

18. What is the weekly workload if 20 patients are examined each day at an average of 78 kVp/60 mAs per view and 3.4 views per patient?
    a. 68 mAmin/wk
    b. 340 mAmin/wk
    c. 442 mAmin/wk
    d. 500 mAmin/wk
    e. >700 mAmin/wk

19. A dedicated chest examination room is used to image 40 patients per day, two views per patient, and the PA technique is 110 kVp/1.5 mAs; the LAT technique is 120 kVp/3 mAs. What is the workload?
    a. 5 mAmin/wk
    b. 15 mAmin/wk
    c. 30 mAmin/wk
    d. 65 mAmin/wk
    e. 100 mAmin/wk

Worksheet 36-2
Radiation Detection and Measurement

For many years, film was the only type of detector available to indicate the presence of x-radiation.

As a radiation detector, photographic emulsion has many advantages, but it also has many disadvantages. Its advantages continue to qualify it for personnel radiation monitoring—the film badge.

Other methods of radiation detection and measurement are now available, and some of them are more sensitive, more accurate, and more applicable for certain situations.

Gas-filled detectors are used for x-ray output calibration and radiation monitoring of areas for exposure levels. Thermoluminescent dosimetry (TLD) and optically stimulated luminescence (OSL) are used for personnel monitoring and patient dose estimation. Scintillation detectors are used principally in nuclear medicine imaging apparatuses such as the gamma camera.

Instruments that incorporate nearly all of these methods can be designed for many different uses. To apply the best possible instrumentation to a given situation, one must understand the basic operating principles of each method and the associated characteristics of sensitivity, accuracy, range, and type of radiation detected.

EXERCISES

1. Which of the following is a characteristic of the ionization chamber survey meter?
   a. Geiger-Müller counter
   b. Detection of individual ionizations
   c. Highly sensitive, 1 uGy$_a$/hr (0.01 mR/hr)
   d. Narrow range, 0 to 0.5 mGy$_a$/hr (0 to 50 mR/hr)
   e. Wide range, 0 to 10 mGy$_a$/hr (0 to 1000 mR/hr)

2. Gas-filled radiation detectors are used:
   a. As a proportional counter to measure the output of an x-ray machine
   b. As an integration type of ionization chamber
   c. Because they are more sensitive than scintillation detectors
   d. For occupational radiation monitoring
   e. In the Geiger region to map the radiation exposure levels in fluoroscopy

3. If each stage of a photomultiplier tube has a gain of approximately 4, a 10-stage photomultiplier tube will have a gain of approximately:
   a. 10^4
   b. 4^9
   c. 4^{10}
   d. 40
   e. 400

4. Which of the following is used in thermoluminescent dosimetry?
   a. Barium fluorochloride
   b. Cadmium tungstate
   c. Calcium tungstate
   d. Lithium fluoride
   e. Polyester

5. Which of the following detectors can be used to identify an unknown gamma emitter?
   a. Geiger-Müller counter
   b. Ionization chamber
   c. Lithium fluoride
   d. Multichannel crystal spectrometer
   e. Photographic emulsion

6. Which of the following normally operates in the rate mode?
   a. A proportional counter
   b. A thermoluminescence dosimeter
   c. An ion chamber
   d. Photographic emulsion
   e. Photoluminescence dosimeter

7. Operation in which region of a gas-filled chamber results in the lowest output?
   a. Continuous discharge
   b. Geiger-Müller region
   c. Ionization chamber
   d. Proportional
   e. Recombination

8. The resolving time of a radiation detector is the time required:
   a. For the meter to respond
   b. To detect sequential ionizations
   c. To identify different types of radiation
   d. To read the meter
   e. To reset the meter

9. The amount of light emitted by a scintillation phosphor is proportional to what feature of photon energy?
   a. Absorbed
   b. Attenuated
   c. Incident
   d. Scattered
   e. Transmitted

10. In thermoluminescence dosimetry, a plot of output intensity versus temperature is called a:
    a. Glow curve
    b. Glow worm
    c. Pulse height
    d. Pulse height analysis
    e. Pulse height spectrum

11. Which of the following statements correctly applies to the voltage response plot of the ideal gas-filled detector?
    a. Instrument sensitivity is highest in the Geiger-Müller region.
    b. The ionization region is most sensitive.
    c. The lowest voltage of operation corresponds to the Geiger-Müller region.
    d. Voltage is higher in the proportional region than in the Geiger-Müller region.
    e. The curve has three distinct regions.

12. Which of the following is a gas-filled detector?
    a. Film badge
    b. Geiger-Müller counter
    c. Recombination chamber
    d. Scintillation counter
    e. Thermoluminescent dosimeter

13. When an accurate measurement of radiation exposure is made in the air, which should be used?
    a. Film badge
    b. Geiger-Müller counter
    c. Ionization chamber
    d. Scintillation detector
    e. TLD

14. Which of the following is characteristic of a Geiger-Müller counter?
    a. For laboratory use only
    b. Measures counts per minute
    c. Measures integrated radioactivity
    d. Useful personal monitor
    e. Wide range {0.01 to 100 mGy_a/hr (1 to 10^4 mR/hr)}

15. Which of the following is characteristic of scintillation detectors that are used as survey instruments?
    a. Can detect individual photons
    b. Are independent of energy
    c. Need extremely high voltage
    d. Suffer from saturation effects
    e. Have very low detection efficiency

16. Sodium iodide is a good gamma ray detector because:
    a. It has a high Z.
    b. It has excellent energy resolution.
    c. It is gas-filled.
    d. Photoelectrons are easily collected.
    e. The resultant charge is stored.

17. Compared with Geiger-Müller counters, scintillation counters:
    a. Are more sensitive to gamma rays
    b. Are sensitive to beta particles
    c. Have a lower background counting rate
    d. Make better occupational radiation monitors
    e. Will count longer

18. The signal detector of a gas-filled radiation detector is the:
    a. Central electrode
    b. Chamber case
    c. Ionization region
    d. Planchet
    e. Scintillation crystal

Worksheet 37-1
Patient Radiation Dose
Reduction of Unnecessary Patient Dose

In diagnostic radiology, radiation control procedures are designed to maintain patient radiation dose ALARA while producing quality images. This requires measurement and estimation of patient dose.

Patient dose is expressed in three ways. The first, entrance skin dose (ESD), can be measured easily. One can directly measure the output intensity of an x-ray unit at the source-to-skin distance (SSD), or one can position dosimeters such as those used in thermoluminescence dosimetry (TLD) on the skin of the patient for direct measurement during examination.

The second method of expressing patient dose is to state the radiation dose to the bone marrow. This dose, of course, cannot be measured directly; it must be computed from phantom exposures and skin measurements. The marrow dose is used to estimate the population **mean marrow dose,** which is considered to be an indication of the leukemogenic radiation hazard.

A third method of expressing patient dose relates to organ dose and usually to gonad dose. Gonad dose can be directly measured in males, but it can only be estimated in females. This is an important patient dose quantity because from it is estimated the **genetically significant dose (GSD).** The GSD is the dose of radiation that, if received by the entire population, would result in the same dose to the gene pool that is actually received by those irradiated.

EXERCISES

1. To protect a patient from soft radiation, one should use which of the following?
   a. Cone
   b. High-speed screen
   c. Small focal spot
   d. Increased filtration
   e. Tighter collimation

2. The GSD from medical radiation exposure depends on all of the following, *except* the:
   a. Average gonad dose per examination
   b. Future childbearing expectancy of the population during any given year
   c. Number of people examined during any given year
   d. Occupational exposure
   e. Total population

3. Which of the following units is *most* appropriate when patient dose is expressed?
   a. Coulombs/kilogram
   b. Gray
   c. Rem
   d. Roentgen
   e. Sievert

4. Which of the following procedures helps to reduce patient dose during radiographic examination?
   a. Cones
   b. Digital detectors
   c. Filtration
   d. Grids
   e. Single-emulsion film

5. In the production of an acceptable radiograph, patient dose increases as _____ increases.
   a. Added filtration
   b. The grid ratio
   c. Image receptor speed
   d. kVp
   e. The SID

6. Which of the following is *most* important in determining patient dose during radiography?
   a. Grid ratio
   b. SID
   c. Single-phase or three-phase power
   d. Size of the field exposed
   e. Size of the focal spot

7. Which of the following procedures might result in an ESD that exceeds 100 mGy_a (10^4mR)?
   a. 5 minutes of fluoroscopy
   b. A 10-minute sonogram
   c. A mammogram
   d. An intravenous pyelogram
   e. Spiral CT

233

8. The GSD is:
   a. A radiation dose that will produce chromosome aberrations
   b. An index of radiation received by the gene pool
   c. Determined from A-bomb survivor data
   d. The radiation dose considered to be the threshold for genetic mutations
   e. Used to predict the level of genetic damage

9. The mean marrow dose is:
   a. Approximately 2 mGy_t (200 mrad/yr)
   b. Considered an important indicator of somatic radiation hazard
   c. Greater than the gonad dose for examinations of the abdomen and pelvis
   d. An index of radiation response
   e. That which results in leukemia

10. In the United States, the GSD from medical radiation exposure is approximately:
    a. 0.05 mGy_t/yr (5 mrad/yr)
    b. 0.2 mGy_t/yr (20 mrad/yr)
    c. 0.5 mGy_t/yr (50 mrad/yr)
    d. 2 mGy_t/yr (200 mrad/yr)
    e. 5 mGy_t/yr (500 mrad/yr)

11. If a 26-year-old female undergoes a KUB (radiography of the *k*idneys, *u*reters, and *b*ladder) examination, which will be highest?
    a. Bone marrow dose
    b. Gonad dose
    c. Kidney dose
    d. Mean marrow dose
    e. Skin dose

12. Which of the following examinations results in the highest ESD?
    a. Abdomen
    b. Cervical spine
    c. Lateral chest
    d. Lateral skull
    e. Lumbar spine

13. If the skin dose from a single CT image is compared with that from multiple images:
    a. The dose will be the same for both.
    b. The multiple-image dose will be proportionally higher in relation to the number of images.
    c. The multiple-image dose will be slightly higher.
    d. The multiple-image dose will be twice as high.
    e. The single-image dose will be slightly higher.

14. Which of the following devices is designed specifically for patient protection purposes?
    a. Dental pointer cone with an integral diaphragm
    b. Fixed diaphragm
    c. Positive beam-limiting (PBL) system
    d. Fluoroscopic shutters
    e. 2.5 mm Al added filtration

15. At 70 kVp, 10 mAs, the patient dose is 50 mrad. What is it at 86 kVp, 5 mAs?
    a. 0.25 mGy_t (25 mrad)
    b. 0.31 mGy_t (31 mrad)
    c. 0.38 mGy_t (38 mrad)
    d. 1.51 mGy_t (151 mrad)
    e. 1.72 mGy_t (172 mrad)

16. In radiography of the lumbar spine, which of the following techniques would provide the *least* patient ESD?
    a. 84 kVp, 100 mAs
    b. 90 kVp, 100 mAs
    c. 95 kVp, 50 mAs
    d. 95 kVp, 100 mAs
    e. 84 kVp, 200 mAs

Worksheet 37-2
X-Rays and Pregnancy

 Exposure to radiation during diagnostic radiology, whether as a patient or as a technologist, is extremely low. Nevertheless, because of the increased sensitivity of the fetus to radiation, the portion of a radiation safety program that deals with x-rays and pregnancy requires some extra effort.

Pregnant patients should be alerted by information posted in the waiting area. Pregnant technologists should be assigned a second personal radiation monitor with instructions that it be worn under the protective apron at waist level.

If, after a radiologic examination, a patient is found to be pregnant, the extent of the examination should be reviewed, the fetal dose should be estimated, and the time of gestation at which the dose was delivered should be determined. **Termination of pregnancy is rarely indicated.** However, should the fetal dose exceed 25 rad, such termination should be seriously considered.

The pregnant technologist should inform her supervisor as soon as she knows of her condition so that a second monitor can be provided. The dose limit to the fetus is 50 mrem/mo (0.5 mSv/mo).

EXERCISES

1. If an AP examination of the pelvis results in an ESD of 300 mR, the approximate fetal dose will be:
   a. 0.05 mGy$_t$ (5 mrad)
   b. 0.5 mGy$_t$ (50 mrad)
   c. 1 mGy$_t$ (100 mrad)
   d. 2 mGy$_t$ (200 mrad)
   e. 3 mGy$_t$ (300 mrad)

2. When a second radiation monitor is provided to a pregnant radiologic technologist:
   a. It should be worn at collar position.
   b. It should be worn outside the apron at waist level.
   c. It should be worn under the apron at waist level.
   d. She should alternate wearing the two.
   e. She should wear both under the apron at waist level.

3. What could a radiologic technologist do to reduce the radiation dose to the fetus of a pregnant patient?
   a. Decrease kVp and increase mAs
   b. Increase OID
   c. Increase SID and mAs
   d. Reduce exposure time
   e. Use specific area shields if appropriate

4. A patient is to undergo radiographic examination because of low back pain. As she is being positioned, she asks whether this will affect her current pregnancy. What should the radiologic technologist do?
   a. Ignore the patient
   b. Reassure her and proceed with the examination
   c. Refuse to do the examination
   d. Seek advice from the radiologist before proceeding
   e. Use a high-kVp technique and a gonad shield

5. Which of the following techniques results in the lowest exposure to the fetus?
   a. 60 kVp, 80 ms, 100 mA
   b. 85 kVp, 200 ms, 300 mA
   c. 90 kVp, 200 ms, 100 mA
   d. 100 kVp, 200 ms, 100 mA
   e. 120 kVp, 100 ms, 100 mA

6. After a skull series, a brain scan, a barium enema, and an intravenous pyelogram, it is discovered that the patient is pregnant. What is the *correct* course of action?
   a. Estimate the fetal dose
   b. Do nothing
   c. Perform a hysterosalpingogram
   d. Reassure the patient and send her home
   e. Terminate the pregnancy

7. Radiation dose to the fetus from radiographic procedures is usually:
   a. < 0.01 Gy$_t$ (1 rad)
   b. 0.02 to 0.04 Gy$_t$ (2 to 4 rad)
   c. 0.05 to 0.1 Gy$_t$ (5 to 10 rad)
   d. 0.1 to 0.2 Gy$_t$ (10 to 20 rad)
   e. > 0.2 Gy$_t$ (20 rad)

8. What effects of diagnostic radiation exposure are possible in a newborn?
   a. Chromosome aberrations
   b. Extrauterine growth retardation
   c. IUGR
   d. Microcephaly
   e. Neonatal death

235

9. A patient who is 2 months pregnant is to undergo intravenous pyelography. Which of the following is *correct?*
   a. No more than two radiographs should be made.
   b. Normal precautions are adequate because fetal damage is least likely during this period of gestation.
   c. Order a pregnancy test first.
   d. The examination should be delayed if possible.
   e. The possibility of spontaneous abortion is high.

10. The greatest nonlethal radiation hazard to an embryo or fetus occurs:
    a. During the first 2 weeks of gestation
    b. At 2 to 8 weeks of gestation
    c. At 8 to 15 weeks of gestation
    d. During the second trimester
    e. During the third trimester

11. The National Council on Radiation Protection and Measurements (NCRPM) recommends a therapeutic abortion if the fetal dose exceeds:
    a. 1 rad
    b. 5 rad
    c. 10 rad
    d. 25 rad
    e. No recommendation is made

12. In pelvic radiography, a dose to the shielded female gonads is primarily due to the:
    a. Characteristic x-rays released by high atomic number atoms in the pelvis
    b. Internally scattered x-rays
    c. Leakage radiation and air scatter
    d. Secondary electrons scattered out of the x-ray field
    e. X-rays scattered from nearby objects

13. When a radiologic technologist becomes pregnant, she should be:
    a. Counseled on proper radiation safety
    b. Fired
    c. Given a temporary leave of absence
    d. Given an additional lead apron
    e. Reassigned to nonfluoroscopy work

14. For a pregnant radiologic technologist, required radiation protection practice includes which of the following?
    a. Assignment to a low-exposure job
    b. No fluoroscopy
    c. Providing an additional apron
    d. Providing two radiation monitors
    e. Use of a gonad shield

15. Which of the following is needed to calculate the dose received by a fetus after a radiographic procedure?
    a. Fetal sex
    b. Gestation period
    c. Grid ratio
    d. Image receptor speed
    e. X-ray output

16. The fetal dose below which termination of pregnancy need *not* be considered is approximately:
    a. 0.02 Gy_t (2 rad)
    b. 0.0 Gy_t (5 rad)
    c. 0.1 Gy_t (10 rad)
    d. 0.2 Gy_t (20 rad)
    e. 0.5 Gy_t (50 rad)

Worksheet 38-1
Occupational Exposure
Reduction in Occupational Exposure

The dose limit (DL) applies only to occupationally exposed persons—not to patients. The DL is the dose of radiation below which the probability of harmful somatic or genetic effects is negligibly small, even when the DL is received each year of a working career.

Personnel monitoring is a program designed to measure the occupational exposure of workers. The quantity measured is the dose equivalent (DE), and the unit of DE is the rem (sievert).

Fluoroscopy is responsible for nearly all occupational radiation exposure among radiology personnel. Consequently, fluoroscopy requires maximum care with attention to good radiation safety practices. When a protective apron is worn, the monitor should be positioned above the apron in the collar region.

EXERCISES

1. What is the approximate annual occupational exposure received by a radiologic technologist?
   a. 0.5 mSv (50 mrem)
   b. 1 mSv (100 mrem)
   c. 3 mSv (300 mrem)
   d. 10 mSv (1000 mrem)
   e. 30 mSv (3000 mrem)

2. Which of the following should *not* be part of a personnel radiation monitoring program?
   a. Film badges
   b. Optically stimulated luminescence (OSL)
   c. Photoluminescence dosimetry (PLD)
   d. Routine blood examination
   e. Thermoluminescence dosimeter (TLD)

3. To reduce occupational exposure during mobile x-ray examination:
   a. The patient should be given a film badge.
   b. The patient should be given a protective apron.
   c. The radiographic tube head should have a photoluminescence dosimeter.
   d. The radiologic technologist should wear a personnel monitor.
   e. The radiologic technologist should wear a protective apron.

4. In evaluation of a personnel monitoring report:
   a. Beta radiation is considered to contribute to the whole-body dose.
   b. Extremity dose is most limiting.
   c. Lens dose is most limiting.
   d. The skin dose is considered the sum of the whole-body dose and the extremity dose.
   e. Whole-body dose is usually highest.

5. Which of the following is required on the personnel monitoring report?
   a. Activity in millicuries
   b. Birth date
   c. Cumulative annual skin exposure
   d. Occupational position
   e. Position of monitor

6. Recommendations proposed for mobile x-ray imaging systems state that the exposure cord length should be at least:
   a. 1 m
   b. 1.5 m
   c. 1.8 m
   d. 3 m
   e. 5 m

7. Personnel monitoring is required:
   a. For all radiology employees
   b. Only for radiologic technologists and radiologists
   c. When a pregnant patient is deliberately examined
   d. When it is likely that one will receive $\frac{1}{10}$ the DL
   e. When it is likely that one will receive the DL

8. A nurse is 3 feet to the patient's side during a portable chest x-ray exposure. What is likely to be her exposure?
   a. <0.01 mGy$_a$ (1 mR)
   b. 0.01 to 0.05 mGy$_a$ (1 to 5 mR)
   c. 0.05 to 0.1 mGy$_a$ (5 to 10 mR)
   d. 0.1 to 0.25 mGy$_a$ (10 to 25 mR)
   e. >0.25 mGy$_a$ (25 mR)

9. Which of the following personnel monitors can be worn the longest?
   a. Film badge
   b. Geiger-Müller tube
   c. Pocket ionization chamber
   d. Scintillation monitor
   e. TLD device

10. During fluoroscopy, the personnel radiation monitor should be worn:
    a. Anywhere; it really does not matter
    b. At waist level, outside the apron
    c. At waist level, under the apron
    d. On the chest
    e. On the collar, outside the apron

11. Personnel monitoring must be conducted at least:
    a. Every 2 weeks
    b. Monthly
    c. Every 2 months
    d. Quarterly
    e. Annually

12. A 0.5 mm Pb equivalent apron attenuates a 75 kVp x-ray beam by approximately:
    a. 10%
    b. 30%
    c. 70%
    d. 90%
    e. 99%

13. Which of the following people is the *most* appropriate choice to hold a patient during a radiologic examination?
    a. Nurse
    b. Orderly
    c. Radiologic technologist
    d. Radiology secretary
    e. Relative

14. Which of the following statements about the use of protective apparel is *true?*
    a. Aprons are required even when a technologist is behind a protective barrier.
    b. During pregnancy, two aprons should be worn.
    c. Gloves should be worn by all who hold patients during the x-ray examination.
    d. It is unnecessary during mobile radiography.
    e. It is unnecessary while in the room during CT.

15. Which of the following personnel radiation monitors is *most* sensitive?
    a. Film badge
    b. Geiger-Müller tube
    c. Pocket ionization chamber
    d. Scintillation detector
    e. TLD device

16. Which of the following is an advantage of film over TLD for personnel monitoring?
    a. Can be reused
    b. Can be used for longer periods
    c. Is cheaper
    d. Is less energy-dependent in the diagnostic range
    e. Is less sensitive to heat and humidity

17. Personnel monitoring of the extremities is necessary:
    a. During angiointerventional procedures
    b. During contrast injections
    c. During mobile radiography
    d. When the dose to the hands may exceed $\frac{1}{10}$ the DL
    e. When the dose to the hands may exceed 50 mSv/yr (5000 mrem/yr)

18. Filters are used in film badges to:
    a. Correct for film fog
    b. Correct for length of wear
    c. Estimate radiation energy
    d. Identify the wearer
    e. Increase the sensitivity

19. For radiologists, protective eyewear:
    a. Is unnecessary
    b. Must be used for C-arm fluoroscopy
    c. Must be used with fluoroscopy with no protective curtain
    d. Must have 0.5 mm Pb equivalent shielding
    e. Must have side shields for scatter

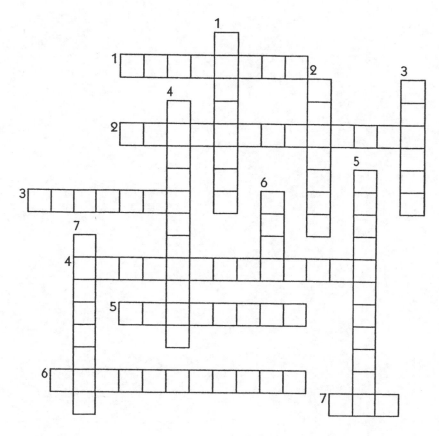

ACROSS

1. Proper unit for measuring occupational exposure
2. Proper unit for measuring radiation exposure
3. Monitoring periods and associated exposure records must not exceed a calendar_____.
4. Biologic effectiveness of radiation energy absorbed (2 words)
5. Term that refers to radiation intensity in air
6. The population gonad dose of importance is the _____ significant dose.
7. The unit of effective dose used for radiation protection purposes; usually applied to occupationally exposed persons

DOWN

1. Proper unit for measuring radiation dose
2. The _____ monitor is used to measure background exposure during transportation, handling, and storage.
3. One of the factors considered when GSD is computed
4. Diagnostic x-ray procedure that leads to one of the highest occupational exposures
5. Exposure to the skin (ESE) (2 words)
6. Measures radiation energy absorbed as a result of radiation exposure during patient examinations
7. The GSD is a _____-average gonad dose.

MATH TUTOR

Contributed by Quinn B. Carroll, MEd, RT

Name _____

Date _____

Working With Decimal Timers

EXERCISE 1: CALCULATING TOTAL mAs VALUES

One of the first things you will learn in any radiographic imaging course is the relationship between milliamperage (mA) and exposure time (s) in producing a total milliampere-seconds (mAs). The total mAs value is very important because it directly relates to how dark the radiograph will be. Exposure time cannot be considered alone, nor can mA, when it comes to controlling the *total* density of the resultant image.

A key point to remember is that mA is a *rate*. It tells us how many x-rays are emitted from the x-ray tube per second or, to phrase it another way, how "fast" they are coming out.

The speedometer in your car measures a rate as well. It does not tell you what the end result of your trip will be. For example, to determine when you will arrive in Dallas, you must also know how long you will be driving at that rate. You must multiply the miles per hour (the rate) by the number of hours (the time) to find the total miles you will travel. It makes no difference whether you go 50 mph for 2 hours or 25 mph for 4 hours—the end result will be the same distance covered.

Likewise, whether the x-ray tube emits 1 million x-rays per second for 1 second or 0.5 million x-rays per second for 2 seconds, the resultant total exposure to the film will be the same. As a radiologic technologist, your first concern is to produce adequate density on the film for a visible image. This depends on how "fast" the x-rays are being emitted *and* how long the tube is left on. It depends on the mA multiplied by the time—the total mAs.

Because many combinations of mA and time can be used to achieve the same total mAs, radiologic technologists must become skilled at computing these numbers so they can adapt to different equipment and different situations. Some would argue that mAs conversion charts are often available on the wall in the control booth and that all you have to do is look this information up. However, such charts are almost never found on mobile (portable) machines or in surgery, and often they do not match the equipment in the department.

Suppose you normally use 400 mA and 1/80 second for an ankle radiograph in the department and you are called to do a portable ankle radiograph using a mobile unit with a maximum of 300 mA available. It is a time-saving and repeat-avoiding skill to be able to quickly and mentally determine the total mAs value to be 5 mAs and by doing so to realize that for this value to be obtained at 300 mA, a time of 1/60 second is needed.

Such mental math should be second nature to every radiologic technologist. It is not as hard as you might think; it just requires practice. The drills that follow are designed to provide the practice needed to develop that skill.

This section first focuses on total mAs conversions using decimals (because most modern equipment uses decimal timers); then several drills on conversions using fractional times are provided. After that, conversion of fractions to decimals—and vice versa—is reviewed. This is helpful because radiologic technologists often must adjust from equipment that uses decimal timers to equipment that uses fractional timers and then back again.

On x-ray machines, the most used mA stations are provided in multiples of 100. On the exposure timers, the most used decimal times consist of two digits after the decimal, that is, they are "hundredths" (e.g., 0.25, 0.05). This provides an easy starting point for practicing decimal conversions: All you must do is to get into the habit of moving the decimal point on the exposure time two places to the right in your mind's eye; then ignore the two zeros on the mA station while multiplying. You are simply cancelling the hundreds with hundredths.

For example, find the total mAs for the following:
200 mA at 0.05 s

Moving the time decimal two places to the right, you have 5. Ignoring the two zeros on the mA, you have 2. This is simply 2 × 5, or 10 mAs.

Think of 300 mA at 0.080 second (ignore the last zero) as simply 3 × 8, which is 24 mAs; 100 mA at 0.025 second is 1 × 2.5, or 2.5 mAs. Examine these three examples carefully before going on.

If three digits follow the decimal, as in 0.008 second, you will use the same method, but you will still be dealing with a decimal when multiplying. For example, 200 mA at 0.008 second should be 2 × 0.8, which gives a total of 1.6 mAs. However, relatively few time settings on x-ray machines are given in the thousandths like this.

243

If there is only one digit behind the decimal point, such as 0.4 second, again move the decimal two places over. This time it will add a zero to your time number, so you will consider 0.4 as 40. Hence, 200 mA at 0.4 second will be 2 × 40, for a total of 80 mAs. Think of 100 mA at 0.2 second as 1 × 20, or 20 mAs; 500 at 0.8 is 5 × 80, or 400 mAs.

If two nonzero numbers are present after the decimal, you will simply ignore the decimal. That is, 0.16 will be thought of as 16. Three positive numbers after the decimal keep the decimal in the problem: 300 mA at 0.125 is 3 × 12.5. Multiply 3 × 12 first for 36, and then add 3 halves for a total of 37.5 mAs.

On most x-ray machines, a repeating pattern is available in the time settings. Note for example the following times in order from one common brand of equipment: .002 s, .003, .004, .005, .007, .01, .015, .02, .025, .03, .035, .05, .07, .1, .15, .2, .25, .3, .35, .5, .7, 1, 2, and 4. One pattern you will see is that between a 5 and a 1, there is always a 7. Table MT-1 simply reorganizes these numbers so you can see the repetition.

Consider the recurring sevens on this machine: .007, .07, and .7. Once you become familiar with mAs values at, for example, the .07 time, you can easily do figuring with the other two "seven" times by simply moving the decimal point in your answer.

As was previously discussed, you should be thinking of 200 mA at 0.07 second as 2 × 7, for 14 mAs total.

Think of 200 mA at 0.007 also as 2 × 7, only with a decimal added in the answer: 1.4 mAs.

Think of 200 mA at 0.7 second as 2 × 7 with a zero added, or 2 × 70, for 140 mAs.

The act of writing down something helps you to remember it, even if you never again refer to your note. An excellent exercise for memorizing mAs values on a particular machine is to jot down the available times in just the format shown in Table MT-1. Write at the top the mA station you use most often, perhaps 200 or 300 mA,

TABLE MT-1 Decimal exposure times available on a typical x-ray machine

		.01	.1	1
.015	.15			
.002	.02	.2		2
	.025	.25		
.003	.03	.3		
	.035	.35		
.004			4	
.005	.05	.5		
.007	.07	.7		

and then write to the side of each time setting the total mAs produced at that mA station. When you are through, look at the pattern of mAs values. Note the repeating patterns.

Do the following part of this exercise on your own, calculating total mAs values mentally. If you get stuck on one, review the instructions above for help. Do not check your answers after each question; do the whole exercise first, figuring the problems in your head and then writing the answer down. When you have completed the exercise, check your answers and correct the ones you missed.

To benefit from this drill, *do not figure your calculations on paper—do them mentally,* and then write down your answer. Do not look at the answers after trying each question; try the entire exercise, write your answers down, and then check all your answers with the Math Tutor Answer Key.

Name _____

Date _____

Working With Fractional Timers

EXERCISE 1: CALCULATING TOTAL mAs VALUES

	mA	×	Time(s)	=	mAs
1.	100	@	0.05	=	_____
2.	100	@	0.064	=	_____
3.	100	@	0.019	=	_____
4.	100	@	0.125	=	_____
5.	100	@	0.8	=	_____
6.	200	@	0.02	=	_____
7.	200	@	0.05	=	_____
8.	200	@	0.064	=	_____
9.	200	@	0.15	=	_____
10.	200	@	0.015	=	_____
11.	200	@	0.125	=	_____
12.	200	@	0.3	=	_____
13.	200	@	0.4	=	_____
14.	200	@	0.008	=	_____
15.	200	@	0.003	=	_____
16.	200	@	0.035	=	_____
17.	300	@	0.03	=	_____
18.	300	@	0.07	=	_____
19.	300	@	0.7	=	_____
20.	600	@	0.05	=	_____
21.	600	@	0.25	=	_____
22.	600	@	0.8	=	_____
23.	600	@	0.006	=	_____
24.	600	@	0.008	=	_____
25.	300	@	0.1	=	_____

	mA	×	Time(s)	=	mAs
26.	300	@	0.3	=	_____
27.	300	@	0.04	=	_____
28.	300	@	0.015	=	_____
29.	300	@	0.25	=	_____
30.	300	@	0.025	=	_____
31.	300	@	0.15	=	_____
32.	300	@	0.006	=	_____
33.	300	@	0.004	=	_____
34.	400	@	0.01	=	_____
35.	400	@	0.04	=	_____
36.	400	@	0.07	=	_____
37.	400	@	0.16	=	_____
38.	400	@	0.016	=	_____
39.	400	@	0.33	=	_____
40.	400	@	0.8	=	_____
41.	400	@	0.7	=	_____
42.	400	@	0.007	=	_____
43.	500	@	0.08	=	_____
44.	500	@	0.03	=	_____
45.	500	@	0.2	=	_____
46.	500	@	0.7	=	_____
47.	500	@	0.007	=	_____
48.	500	@	0.125	=	_____

Be sure to review those problems you answered incorrectly and to go back to the instructions just given, if necessary.

Working With Fractional Timers

EXERCISE 2: THE 100 mA STATION

Exposure timers that read in fractions are becoming rare. They are somewhat more difficult to convert mentally than those that read in decimals, but they also tend to follow patterned sequences. If you memorize just a few pairs of numbers, you can do most of them.

For this unit, we will do practice drills for each mA station separately. At each mA station, certain pairs of numbers always go together. For example, at the 100 mA station, fives and twos always go together:

100 mA at ½ s 50 mAs
100 mA at ⅕ s 20 mAs
100 mA at 1/50 s 2 mAs
100 mA at 1/20 s 5 mAs

Note that these numbers are rounded up or down to make it easier to memorize them. For example, 100 mA at ⅙ second is actually 16.67 mAs and would normally round up to 17. However, it is easier to remember 16 because the mind associates the sixes in ⅙ with those in 16. The results are close enough for any radiographic technique. Likewise, ⅛ of 100 is actually 12.5, and 1/12 of 100 is actually 8.33. In these units on fractions, all answers will be rounded out. The goal is for you to *mentally* derive a good estimated technique, not an exact answer.

Memorizing the pairs of numbers will not tell you where to put any decimal points—you will have to learn that by practice.

It is important to solve these problems mentally, not on paper. After you have completed this entire exercise, check your answers and review the questions you missed.

Zero may be added or a decimal point moved, but a time fraction that uses a 5 will always result in a total mAs involving a 2, and vice versa.

At the 100 mA station, the following pairs of numbers always go together; commit them to memory before you go on. The best way to memorize them is to get a study partner to drill you as if it were an oral test: 3 and 33 × 4 and 25 × 5 and 2 × 6 and 16 × 7 and 15 × 8 and 12.

	mA	×	Time(s)	=	mAs
1.	100	@	½	=	_____
2.	100	@	1/20	=	_____
3.	100	@	1/50	=	_____
4.	100	@	⅕	=	_____
5.	100	@	⅛	=	_____
6.	100	@	1/80	=	_____
7.	100	@	1/12	=	_____
8.	100	@	1/120	=	_____
9.	100	@	1/7	=	_____
10.	100	@	1/15	=	_____
11.	100	@	1/40	=	_____
12.	100	@	⅓	=	_____
13.	100	@	1/30	=	_____
14.	100	@	⅙	=	_____
15.	100	@	1/60	=	_____
16.	100	@	⅔	=	_____

Working With Fractional Timers

EXERCISE 3: THE 200 mA AND 50 mA STATIONS

Having memorized the number pairs for the 100 mA station, you can figure the total mAs for most time settings at the 200 mA station simply by doubling the answer you would get at 100 mA. For example, once it becomes second nature to you that 100 mA at $\frac{1}{60}$ second is 1.7 mAs, whenever you see 200 mA at $\frac{1}{60}$ second, you can simply double 1.7 in your mind for a total of 3.4 mAs.

You can cope with the 50 mA station in a similar fashion: Simply cut in half the answer you would get at the 100 mA station. If 100 mA at $\frac{1}{30}$ second is 3.3 mAs, 50 mA at $\frac{1}{30}$ second will be approximately 1.6 or 1.7 mAs.

Practice these conversions for typical fractions in this exercise. Carefully correct and review your answers with the Math Tutor Answer Key after you have completed the entire exercise.

	mA	×	Time(s)	=	mAs
1.	200	@	$\frac{1}{8}$	=	_____
2.	50	@	$\frac{1}{20}$	=	_____
3.	200	@	$\frac{1}{5}$	=	_____
4.	200	@	$\frac{1}{50}$	=	_____
5.	50	@	$\frac{1}{8}$	=	_____
6.	200	@	$\frac{1}{80}$	=	_____
7.	200	@	$\frac{1}{12}$	=	_____
8.	200	@	$\frac{1}{120}$	=	_____
9.	50	@	$\frac{1}{12}$	=	_____
10.	50	@	$\frac{1}{120}$	=	_____

	mA	×	Time(s)	=	mAs
11.	50	@	$\frac{1}{7}$	=	_____
12.	200	@	$\frac{1}{15}$	=	_____
13.	200	@	$\frac{1}{40}$	=	_____
14.	50	@	$\frac{1}{3}$	=	_____
15.	50	@	$\frac{1}{30}$	=	_____
16.	200	@	$\frac{1}{3}$	=	_____
17.	200	@	$\frac{1}{30}$	=	_____
18.	200	@	$\frac{1}{6}$	=	_____
19.	200	@	$\frac{1}{60}$	=	_____
20.	200	@	$\frac{2}{3}$	=	_____
21.	50	@	$\frac{1}{6}$	=	_____
22.	50	@	$\frac{1}{60}$	=	_____
23.	50	@	$\frac{1}{80}$	=	_____
24.	200	@	$\frac{1}{7}$	=	_____

Working With Fractional Timers

EXERCISE 4: THE 300 mA STATION

The 300 mA station is a different number and produces its own unique number pairs when using a fractional timer. For example, at the 300 mA station, fives and sixes always go together: $\frac{1}{5}$ second yields 60 mAs total, whereas $\frac{1}{6}$ second produces 50 mAs. The following pairs of numbers always go together when using 300 mA. Commit these to memory, and drill with a study partner if you can:

5 and 6
15 and 20
12 and 25

Remember that at the 100 mA station, sevens always pair with fifteens. One seventh of 100 is about 15. So think of this as the following:

3 sets of 15
= Approximately 45 mAs
= 300 mA at $\frac{1}{8}$ s

Remember that at the 100 mA station, eights always pair with twelves. So think of this as the following:

3 sets of 12
= Approximately 36 mAs

Other combinations can be made, but these three pairs are very common. For other times, such as $\frac{1}{8}$ second or $\frac{1}{7}$ second, it is easier to simply use the paired number you memorized for the 100 mA station and then triple that number. Here are some examples:

300 mA at $\frac{1}{7}$ s

With these tips and with the previous exercises completed, you should be able to figure most mAs values for the 300 mA station in your head.

Proceed to solve the following problems mentally and write only your answers down. Check and review your answers using the Math Tutor Answer Key.

	mA	×	Time(s)	=	mAs
1.	300	@	$\frac{1}{5}$	=	_____
2.	300	@	$\frac{1}{6}$	=	_____
3.	300	@	$\frac{1}{50}$	=	_____
4.	300	@	$\frac{1}{60}$	=	_____
5.	300	@	$\frac{1}{20}$	=	_____
6.	300	@	$\frac{1}{2}$	=	_____
7.	300	@	$\frac{1}{15}$	=	_____
8.	300	@	$\frac{1}{12}$	=	_____
9.	300	@	$\frac{1}{120}$	=	_____
10.	300	@	$\frac{1}{25}$	=	_____
11.	300	@	$\frac{1}{4}$	=	_____
12.	300	@	$\frac{1}{40}$	=	_____
13.	300	@	$\frac{1}{8}$	=	_____
14.	300	@	$\frac{1}{80}$	=	_____
15.	300	@	$\frac{1}{7}$	=	_____
16.	300	@	$\frac{2}{30}$	=	_____

Working With Fractional Timers

EXERCISE 5: THE 400, 500, AND 600 mA STATIONS

Number pairs also can be made for the higher (400, 500, and 600) mA stations, but once you become comfortable with fractions at those stations up to 300 mA, this would be unnecessary. For the 600 mA station, the total mAs values learned at the 300 mA station can simply be doubled. The same thing can be done with the 400 mA station by doubling the results from the 200 mA station.

Any of these can be solved by going back to the number pairs you memorized for the 100 mA station. Whenever you get stuck, use the approach of solving for the 100 mA station and then multiplying the result by the first digit of the mA. Take the following example:

500 mA at $\frac{1}{20}$ s

You may recognize right away that the answer is 25 mAs. Or, you may mentally remove a zero from both the mA and the time, yielding the following:

= 50 at $\frac{1}{2}$ s
= 25 mAs

But *if you are not comfortable* with these other approaches, *go back to the 100 mA number pairs* you memorized. Remembering that 2 and 5 always go together and that $\frac{1}{20}$ of 100 is 5, think of this problem as follows:

500 mA at $\frac{1}{20}$ s
= 5 *sets* of 5
= 25 mAs

Proceed to the following questions, and then check and review your answers using the Math Tutor Answer Key.

	mA	×	Time(s)	=	mAs
1.	400	@	$\frac{1}{20}$	=	_____
2.	500	@	$\frac{1}{20}$	=	_____
3.	600	@	$\frac{1}{20}$	=	_____
4.	400	@	$\frac{1}{5}$	=	_____
5.	600	@	$\frac{1}{5}$	=	_____
6.	400	@	$\frac{1}{50}$	=	_____
7.	600	@	$\frac{1}{50}$	=	_____
8.	500	@	$\frac{1}{4}$	=	_____
9.	600	@	$\frac{1}{4}$	=	_____
10.	500	@	$\frac{1}{40}$	=	_____
11.	600	@	$\frac{1}{40}$	=	_____
12.	600	@	$\frac{1}{30}$	=	_____
13.	400	@	$\frac{1}{30}$	=	_____
14.	400	@	$\frac{1}{60}$	=	_____
15.	400	@	$\frac{1}{7}$	=	_____
16.	400	@	$\frac{2}{8}$	=	_____
17.	400	@	$\frac{1}{80}$	=	_____
18.	500	@	$\frac{1}{8}$	=	_____
19.	600	@	$\frac{1}{12}$	=	_____
20.	600	@	$\frac{1}{120}$	=	_____
21.	500	@	$\frac{1}{12}$	=	_____
22.	400	@	$\frac{1}{120}$	=	_____
23.	400	@	$\frac{1}{15}$	=	_____
24.	500	@	$\frac{1}{15}$	=	_____
25.	400	@	$\frac{1}{25}$	=	_____
26.	500	@	$\frac{1}{25}$	=	_____
27.	600	@	$\frac{1}{25}$	=	_____
28.	400	@	$\frac{1}{3}$	=	_____

Working With Fractional Timers

EXERCISE 6: COMPLEX FRACTIONS

If you have completed all of the previous sections, you are ready to move on to fractional times that involve numerators other than "1" on the top, such as ⅖ or 7/20. These are not as hard as they might seem at a glance. You must do them in two steps: First, divide the bottom (denominator) into the mA station, and then think of the top number as the number of "sets."

Solve the following example:

200 mA at ⅖ s

First, consider the top (numerator) of the fraction as a "1"; in other words, find ⅕ of 200. When you have this number, multiply it by the top of the fraction, thinking in "sets," as follows:

⅕ of 200 = 40
2 sets of 40 = 80 mAs

Think of 200 mA at 7/20 second as 7 sets of 10, and think of 300 mA at 3/15 second as 3 sets of 20. Using this approach, solve all of the following problems mentally, and then check and review your answers.

	mA	×	Time(s)	=	mAs
1.	100	@	⅖	=	_____
2.	100	@	2/15	=	_____
3.	100	@	3/15	=	_____
4.	100	@	3/20	=	_____
5.	100	@	7/20	=	_____
6.	200	@	¾	=	_____
7.	200	@	⅖	=	_____
8.	200	@	⅗	=	_____
9.	200	@	⅘	=	_____
10.	200	@	3/10	=	_____

	mA	×	Time(s)	=	mAs
11.	200	@	7/10	=	_____
12.	200	@	2/15	=	_____
13.	200	@	3/15	=	_____
14.	200	@	3/20	=	_____
15.	200	@	7/20	=	_____
16.	400	@	⅖	=	_____
17.	400	@	⅗	=	_____
18.	400	@	⅘	=	_____
19.	400	@	3/10	=	_____
20.	400	@	7/10	=	_____
21.	300	@	⅔	=	_____
22.	300	@	⅖	=	_____
23.	300	@	⅗	=	_____
24.	300	@	⅘	=	_____
25.	300	@	3/10	=	_____
26.	300	@	7/10	=	_____
27.	300	@	2/15	=	_____
28.	300	@	3/15	=	_____
29.	300	@	3/20	=	_____
30.	400	@	3/20	=	_____
31.	400	@	7/20	=	_____
32.	500	@	⅖	=	_____
33.	500	@	3/10	=	_____
34.	500	@	⅕	=	_____
35.	500	@	3/20	=	_____
36.	600	@	⅖	=	_____
37.	600	@	⅗	=	_____
38.	600	@	3/10	=	_____
39.	600	@	3/20	=	_____
40.	600	@	3/15	=	_____

Timers: Converting Fractions Into Decimals and Vice Versa

EXERCISE 7: CONVERTING FRACTIONS INTO DECIMALS

A radiologic technologist who is used to working with decimal timers should be able to quickly adapt to an x-ray machine that employs a fractional timer. The reverse is also true, and both types of machines are commonly found. It turns out that the mathematics used for doing this is very similar to the mathematics used for mAs conversions.

For example, in converting the fraction ⅙ into a decimal number, 6 is simply divided into 1.00 for an answer of 0.16. Note how similar this operation is to taking ⅙ second at 100 mA to obtain 16 mAs. The only difference is the placement of the decimal point.

You should recall from "Working With Fractional Timers" that certain number pairs always go together; one of these pairs was 6 and 16. When fractions are converted to decimals and back, these number pairs always apply: ⅙ = 0.16, ¹⁄₁₆ = 0.6. (Although the sixteens are actually 16.6666, we are rounding down rather than up because this results in an easy memory device: associating the sixes.) Once again, the list of number pairs that always go together is as follows:

3 and 33
4 and 25
5 and 2
6 and 16
7 and 15
8 and 12

Committing these number pairs to memory will be of great help in solving technique problems in your head.

To change a fraction into a decimal, simply divide the numerator (top) by the denominator (bottom). However, you first need to place a decimal point to the right of the numerator and then add as many zeros as needed to complete the division. For example, to find the decimal equivalent for ³⁄₂₀, you need to complete the following steps.

Temporarily remove the decimal, and remove the extra zeros:

= 1.5

Now, "replacing" the decimal moves it one place to the left in the answer:

= 0.15

If you are comfortable with the mA station exercises in "Working With Decimal Timers" and "Working With Fractional Timers," you will find it even easier to pretend that the numerator is an mA station, in multiples of 100. The following example illustrates.

Think of the numerator (3.0) as the 300 mA station (recall from "Working With Fractional Timers" that at 300 mA, 15 and 20 always go together):

= 15

Now, since you added two zeros to the numerator above, you must move the decimal two places to the left in your answer:

= 0.15

In this exercise, convert each fraction listed into its decimal equivalent. Rely as much as you can on the skills developed in "Working With Decimal Timers" and "Working With Fractional Timers." For unusual fractions or where these skills do not apply, simply divide the numerator by the denominator. Do the entire exercise, and then review your answers using the Math Tutor Answer Key.

	Fraction		Decimal			Fraction		Decimal
1.	¾	=	_____		16.	¹⁄₈₀	=	_____
2.	⅔	=	_____		17.	¹⁄₁₀₀	=	_____
3.	¼	=	_____		18.	¹⁄₂₀₀	=	_____
4.	⅕	=	_____		19.	⁷⁄₁₀	=	_____
5.	⅙	=	_____		20.	²⁄₁₅	=	_____
6.	⅐	=	_____		21.	³⁄₂₀	=	_____
7.	⅛	=	_____		22.	⅖	=	_____
8.	¹⁄₁₂	=	_____		23.	⅗	=	_____
9.	¹⁄₁₅	=	_____		24.	⅘	=	_____
10.	¹⁄₂₀	=	_____		25.	⅓	=	_____
11.	¹⁄₂₅	=	_____		26.	³⁄₁₅	=	_____
12.	¹⁄₃₀	=	_____		27.	⁷⁄₂₀	=	_____
13.	¹⁄₄₀	=	_____		28.	¹⁄₁₅₀	=	_____
14.	¹⁄₅₀	=	_____		29.	⅜	=	_____
15.	¹⁄₆₀	=	_____		30.	⁵⁄₁₆	=	_____

Part One **Basic mAs and Time Conversions**

Timers: Converting Fractions Into Decimals and Vice Versa

EXERCISE 8: CONVERTING DECIMALS INTO FRACTIONS

Converting a decimal number into a fraction requires three steps. First, find the numerator (top of the fraction) by simply writing out all of the nonzero figures to the right of the decimal point. Then, to find the denominator (bottom of the fraction), write 1 for the decimal point and a zero for each decimal place after it. For example, to find the fractional equivalent for 0.0125, the following steps are needed:

For the numerator, write out nonzero figures to the right of the decimal point: 125 is the numerator.

For the denominator, write a 1 in place of the decimal point. There are four figures or decimal places to the right of the decimal point (0.0125), so you will write four zeros after the 1; 10,000 is the denominator. The fraction is as follows:

125
10,000

Finally, reduce the fraction (if possible) to its lowest common denominator. In the preceding example, 125 and 10,000 do not have a lower common denominator, and the fraction cannot be reduced. The following is an example of a decimal number that can be reduced after it is converted into a fraction:

0.6

For the numerator, write the nonzero figures to the right of the decimal point: 6 is the numerator. For the denominator, write a 1 for the decimal point and a zero for each place after it; 10 is the denominator. The fraction is as follows:

⁶⁄₁₀

Six and 10 share a common denominator: They are both divisible by 2. Reduce the fraction by dividing both numbers by 2:

⅗

This fraction cannot be further reduced, and it is the final answer.

In this exercise, convert the decimal numbers listed into equivalent fractions. Some of these problems are easily solved by computing them, whereas *others are better solved by simply recognizing the number pairs listed in Exercise 2*. Do the entire exercise, and then check and review your answers using the Math Tutor Answer Key.

	Decimal		Fraction
1.	0.05	=	_____
2.	0.0333	=	_____
3.	0.2	=	_____
4.	0.75	=	_____
5.	0.025	=	_____
6.	0.6667	=	_____
7.	0.143	=	_____
8.	0.002	=	_____
9.	0.08	=	_____
10.	0.167	=	_____
11.	0.125	=	_____
12.	0.6	=	_____
13.	0.0625	=	_____
14.	0.00833	=	_____

Name _____

Date _____

Finding mA and Time Combinations for Desired mAs

EXERCISE 9: WARM-UP CALCULATIONS

Common mathematics problems that a radiologic technologist faces in daily practice include the following:

1. Having a desired total mAs in mind and trying to mentally determine an mA-time combination that will yield that total
2. Mentally applying the 15% rule for peak kilovoltage (kVp) to adjust techniques
3. Mentally applying the inverse square law for distance changes

The following exercises will help you to develop the ability to do all three of these types of problems in your head. If you have trouble following the instructions on any of these, you may wish to review "Part One: Basic mAs and Time Conversions."

Probably the most common mathematics problem a radiologic technologist faces every day is that of having a desired total mAs in mind and trying to mentally determine an mA-time combination that will yield that total.

This is exactly the reverse of the exercises in Part One, and if you have completed the previous exercises, you will see how they help you in this one. The same number pairs are used. The only difference is that now you must decide whatever mA station your desired total mAs will divide into easily. With a little practice, the correct time fraction will then come to mind.

One unique thing about fractions (and something that you will not find when working with decimals) is that some of the answers can be found only in "complex fractions" as we have defined them. To solve these, you must again learn to think in "sets," such as using two sets of 20 mAs to obtain 40 mAs.

For example, how would you obtain 80 mAs using the 200 mA station? Because 80 does not divide *evenly* into 200, no usable fraction with a "1" on top as the numerator can be found. If you simply divide it out, you will get 2.5 as the denominator, resulting in a fraction of ½.₅; this is a complex fraction that will not be found on the timer knob. However, if you learn to recognize that 80 is 2 sets of 40, you can find a usable time.

First, divide 40 mAs into 200 mA. This will equal 5, and 5 is the denominator of your fraction.

In other words, the fraction used to obtain 40 mAs is ⅕.

Now, simply go back and take *2 sets* of ⅕ by changing the numerator to 2.

The answer is ⅖ second.
80 mAs = 200 mA at ⅖ second
(80 mAs = 2 sets of 40 mAs)

This exercise will "warm you up" for finding these sets of numbers. For each total mAs listed, express it as so many sets of a smaller number that will easily divide into one of the typical mA stations. There are *one* or *two* answers to each problem but no more because for that smaller number, you must choose a number that does not require further reduction. For example:

120 mAs can be expressed as _____ sets of _____.

If you use 6 sets of 20, this ratio can then be reduced to 3 sets (of 40), so 6 sets of 20 is not a good answer. One good answer is *3 sets of 40,* because this number of sets cannot be further reduced. Another good answer is *2 sets of 60,* because again, this number of sets cannot be further reduced. (One set of 120 is absurd, because there is no 120 mA station available.)

Note that sets of 40 will be evenly divisible into the 200 mA station, whereas sets of 60 will be divisible into the 300 mA station.

It sounds complicated at first, but try the following part of this exercise and you will find it is not as hard as you might have expected.

1. 80 mAs can be expressed as _____ sets of _____.
2. 45 mAs can be expressed as _____ sets of _____.
3. 66 mAs can be expressed as _____ sets of _____.
4. 75 mAs can be expressed as _____ sets of _____.
5. 180 mAs can be expressed as _____ sets of _____.
6. 120 mAs can be expressed as _____ sets of _____ or as _____ sets of _____.
7. 160 mAs can be expressed as _____ sets of _____ or as _____ sets of _____.
8. 240 mAs can be expressed as _____ sets of _____ or as _____ sets of _____.
9. 90 mAs can be expressed as _____ sets of _____.
10. 320 mAs can be expressed as _____ sets of _____.

Check your answers in the Math Tutor Answer Key.

In Exercises 10 and 11, the total mAs desired is given, along with the mA station to be used. You must mentally decide which time to use. Use only those times that are available on most x-ray machines. In Exercise 10, your times must be expressed as fractions. In Exercise 11, use decimals. Do the exercises mentally, and then check your answers.

Finding mA and Time Combinations for Desired mAs

EXERCISE 10: CALCULATIONS USING FRACTIONS

Total mA	=	mA	×	Seconds
1. 4 mAs	=	100 mA	×	_____
2. 2.5 mAs	=	100 mA	×	_____
3. 66 mAs	=	100 mA	×	_____
4. 7 mAs	=	100 mA	×	_____
5. 17 mAs	=	100 mA	×	_____
6. 8 mAs	=	100 mA	×	_____
7. 3.3 mAs	=	100 mA	×	_____
8. 1.7 mAs	=	100 mA	×	_____
9. 1.25 mAs	=	100 mA	×	_____
10. 0.8 mAs	=	100 mA	×	_____
11. 40 mAs	=	100 mA	×	_____
12. 5 mAs	=	150 mA	×	_____
13. 2.5 mAs	=	50 mA	×	_____
14. 25 mAs	=	50 mA	×	_____
15. 25 mAs	=	200 mA	×	_____
16. 40 mAs	=	200 mA	×	_____
17. 120 mAs	=	200 mA	×	_____
18. 5 mAs	=	200 mA	×	_____
19. 2.5 mAs	=	200 mA	×	_____
20. 14 mAs	=	200 mA	×	_____
21. 50 mAs	=	300 mA	×	_____
22. 6 mAs	=	300 mA	×	_____
23. 20 mAs	=	300 mA	×	_____
24. 2.5 mAs	=	300 mA	×	_____
25. 45 mAs	=	300 mA	×	_____
26. 180 mAs	=	300 mA	×	_____
27. 240 mAs	=	300 mA	×	_____
28. 75 mAs	=	300 mA	×	_____
29. 80 mAs	=	400 mA	×	_____
30. 240 mAs	=	400 mA	×	_____

263

Finding mA and Time Combinations for Desired mAs

EXERCISE 11: CALCULATIONS USING DECIMALS

Total mA	=	mA	×	Seconds
1. 4 mAs	=	100 mA	×	_____
2. 2.5 mAs	=	100 mA	×	_____
3. 66 mAs	=	100 mA	×	_____
4. 7 mAs	=	100 mA	×	_____
5. 16 mAs	=	100 mA	×	_____
6. 8 mAs	=	100 mA	×	_____
7. 3.3 mAs	=	100 mA	×	_____
8. 1.7 mAs	=	100 mA	×	_____
9. 40 mAs	=	100 mA	×	_____
10. 2.5 mAs	=	50 mA	×	_____
11. 1.25 mAs	=	50 mA	×	_____
12. 25 mAs	=	200 mA	×	_____
13. 40 mAs	=	200 mA	×	_____
14. 120 mAs	=	200 mA	×	_____
15. 5 mAs	=	200 mA	×	_____
16. 2.5 mAs	=	200 mA	×	_____
17. 14 mAs	=	200 mA	×	_____
18. 50 mAs	=	300 mA	×	_____
19. 6 mAs	=	300 mA	×	_____
20. 21 mAs	=	300 mA	×	_____
21. 180 mAs	=	300 mA	×	_____
22. 75 mAs	=	300 mA	×	_____
23. 80 mAs	=	400 mA	×	_____
24. 240 mAs	=	400 mA	×	_____

Part Two **Mathematics of Radiographic Techniques**

Technique Adjustments

Name _____

Date _____

EXERCISE 12: APPLYING THE 15% RULE FOR KVp, APPLYING THE RULE IN STEPS, AND APPLYING THE RULE IN PORTIONS

Radiologic technologists often must adjust techniques using the 15% rule for kVp to increase penetration or change the contrast on the radiograph while maintaining overall density. The ability to make these adjustments mentally should be second nature to the radiologic technologist. It is not very difficult to develop this ability, but it does require practice and repetition. The following drills will help you develop this ability.

The rule states that a 15% adjustment in kVp will change the resultant image density by a *factor of 2*. A 15% increase will double the film density, and a 15% reduction will cut the image density to one-half the original. This is an approximation, but it works very well and is the only practical rule of thumb for predicting the effects of kVp on the ultimate darkness of the radiograph.

To find 15% of the original kVp mentally, think of the operation as taking 10% first and then adding half as much again. For example, to find 15% of 80 kVp:

$80 \times 10\% = 8$	Take 10% of the kVp.
$\frac{8}{2} = 4$	Figure one half of 8.
$8 + 4 = 12$	Add these two numbers.
$80 \times 15\% = 12$	

Fifteen percent of 60 kVp would be $6 + 3 = 9$. Fifteen percent of 120 would be $12 + 6 = 18$. This number is added to the original kVp to double film density, and it is subtracted to obtain one half of the original density.

In the above example that uses 80 kVp, what new total kVp would compensate for cutting the mAs to one half? The answer is 92 kVp (80 + 12). What would the new kVp be if, because of overpenetration, a radiograph turned out twice to be too dark and you wished to cut the density in half? The answer is 68 kVp.

You should also become comfortable with applying the 15% rule in steps and in portions.

A common misconception is that an adjustment of 10 kVp changes density by a factor of 2. This stems from the fact that 15% of 70 is 10.5, and 70 may be considered an "average" kVp for radiographic procedures. However, a 10 kVp change in the range of 40 kVp will almost double the density twice, whereas a 10 kVp change in the range of 100 kVp is only two thirds of the change needed to double or halve the density. For accuracy, it is important to use the 15% rule as prescribed rather than the "10 kVp rule."

Sometimes the desired adjustment in image density is much greater than a doubling or halving. Suppose you need to repeat an extremely light radiograph caused by underpenetration and the density has to be increased fourfold. Always translate the desired changes into terms of doubling (factors of two), and you can apply the rule.

To produce a radiograph that is four times darker, think of this change as two doublings. To obtain two doublings, you will need to increase 15% kVp *in two steps*. (It is not as accurate to simply make a 30% change, and the greater the change, the less accurate this approach is.) For example, if the original radiograph was exposed using 80 kVp:

$80 \times 15\% = 12$
Step 1: Increase by 15% of the original kVp.
$80 + 12 = 92$
This increase achieves the first doubling.
$92 \times 15\% = 14$
Step 2: Increase by 15% of the *adjusted kVp, not the original kVp*.
$92 + 14 = 106$
This increase achieves the second doubling.

A fourfold increase in image density will result from 106 kVp. This would also compensate for a reduction of mAs to one fourth of the original.

Only rarely is kVp adjusted by more than 1 set of 15%, especially for reductions that might result in an underpenetrated radiograph, regardless of increases in mAs. It is to be emphasized that mAs, not kVp, is the primary density control for radiographs, and that kVp is changed only to adjust for penetration, scatter radiation levels, image contrast, or grayscale. Nonetheless, when such adjustments are made, the mAs often must be compensated to maintain density, and the 15% rule comes into play.

One practical example of a kVp adjustment made using two steps of 15% is found in deriving a barium technique (upper gastrointestinal [GI] or solid column barium enema) from a routine abdomen technique. If the technique for an anteroposterior (AP) projection of the abdomen were 30 mAs and 80 kVp, the following

267

calculations would allow adequate penetration of the same abdomen when the gastrointestinal tract is filled with barium:

30 mAs @ 80 kVp
Routine AP abdomen.
15 mAs @ 92 kVp
First step: Increase of 15% (12 kVp), accompanied by one-half the mAs to maintain a density of 15 mAs @ 92 kVp
Second step: Increase (14 kVp) is 15% of 92, with another halving of the mAs to 7.5 mAs.

For a solid column barium procedure (not air contrast), approximately 7 mAs at about 110 kVp would provide good penetration through the barium while keeping overall image density at an optimum level. (For an air contrast technique, simply reduce by 10 to 15 kVp, with the mAs still at about 7.)

The image density on a radiograph must be changed by at least one third (about 30%) for the human eye to detect any difference. In practice, efforts to increase overall radiographic technique by less than 50% or to decrease it by less than 30% are wasted. Changes such as these can be made with the use of the 15% rule in portions.

Suppose you wish to reduce the density but decide that cutting it in half would be too much. You must reduce overall technique by at least one third to make any visible difference. Taking one third of 15%, we can derive a kVp change of about 5%. The kVp must be reduced by a minimum of 5% to lighten up the image. To find 5% of the original kVp, think of it as one half of 10%. For this problem, if the original kVp was 120 kVp, the solution would be as follows:

120 × 10% = 12
Figure 10% of the kVp.
12 × ½ = 6
Take one half of that amount.
120 − 6 = 114

Subtract this number from the original kVp.
The kVp must be reduced at least to 114 for the density to be visibly lightened up in this case.

Although a 2 kVp adjustment may visibly change image density in the 40 kVp range, the same adjustment will not make a visible difference in higher ranges. The change must be at least 5%.

Consider an increase in density of 50% (1.5 times denser than the original). You will recall the recommendation to think of technique changes in terms of doublings or halvings. In this context, such a 50% increase

should be thought of as *halfway to doubling*. (Similarly, a 25% reduction in overall technique would be *halfway to cutting it in half*.) Because a 15% increase in kVp will double the density, one half of 15% should bring the density halfway to a doubling. In other words, to increase the density by 50%, increase the kVp by one half of 15%.

For example, suppose a radiograph taken at 80 kVp comes out a bit light. Doubling the density would be too much. You decide to increase the density by about one half (50%):

80 × 15% = 12
Find 15% of the kVp.
12 × ½ = 6
Find one half of that amount.
80 + 6 = 86
Add this number to the original kVp.
For a radiograph that is 50% darker, increase kVp to 86.

Complete the following exercise using the 15% rule. Some problems will require you to apply the rule in sequential steps, and in some, the rule will have to be applied in portions of one third or one half of 15%. Finish the entire exercise, and then check and review your answers using the Math Tutor Answer Key.

1. What is 5% of 120?
2. What is 5% of 90?
3. What is 5% of 80?
4. What is 5% of 50?
5. What is 5% of 60?
6. What is 15% of 70?
7. What is 15% of 40?
8. What is 15% of 60?
9. What is 15% of 110?
10. What is one half of 15% of 40?
11. What is one half of 15% of 70?
12. What is one half of 15% of 80?
13. What is one half of 15% of 50?
14. What is one half of 15% of 90?
15. What is one half of 15% of 120?
16. Starting at 120 kVp, what new kVp would result in a density that is one half as dark as the original?
17. Starting at 40 kVp, what new kVp would result in a density that is twice as dark as the original?
18. Starting at 60 kVp, what new kVp would result in a density that is 50% darker than the original (halfway to double the original)?
19. Starting at 80 kVp, what new kVp would result in a density that is about 75% (halfway to one half) of the original?

Technique Adjustments

EXERCISE 13: ADJUSTING FOR DISTANCE CHANGES, THE INVERSE SQUARE LAW, AND THE SQUARE LAW: RULES OF THUMB FOR DISTANCE CHANGES

As described in the textbook, radiologic technologists should be completely familiar with the inverse square law. It describes the relationship between radiation quantity or intensity in the x-ray beam and distance from the x-ray tube. Because the x-ray beam "fans out" over larger areas with increasing distance, the concentration of x-rays decreases at a rate inversely proportional to the square of the distance. The formula is as follows:

$$I_2 = I_1 \left(\frac{D_1}{D_2} \right)^2$$

where I_1 is the original quantity or concentration of x-rays, I_2 is the new radiation quantity after the distance change, and D_1 and D_2 are the old and new distances (source-to-image receptor distances [SIDs]), respectively.

The inverse square law can be used to predict radiation exposure to the patient, operator, or film. Because the density produced on the film is generally directly proportional (or "reciprocal") to the exposure, the inverse square law can be used to predict image density changes when distance is altered. Some of the questions in the following exercise apply this formula.

However, this section also focuses on two derivations from the inverse square law that are extremely helpful in daily practice: the "square law" and rules of thumb for distance changes.

Whereas the inverse square law is used to predict image density, the square law is used to compensate technique so that density is maintained when distance changes. The formula for the square law is as follows:

$$mAs_2 = mAs_1 \left(\frac{D_2}{D_1} \right)^2$$

where mAs_1 is the original mAs used at D_1 (the original SID), and mAs_2 is the new mAs needed to maintain equal density if the SID is changed to D_2.

When the original mAs is not given or known, place a 1 in the formula for "mAs_1" and solve for mAs_2. The resulting number will be the *factor* by which mAs should be changed. A result of 2.0 would indicate that the original mAs, whatever it was, should be doubled. A result of 0.5 would indicate that it should be cut in half, and so forth.

As an example, suppose the SID is increased from the usual 40 inches to 60 inches. The technique chart is written for 40 inches. What change would have to be made in the overall technique taken from the chart to maintain adequate image density at 60 inches?

Because the actual mAs is not given, use a 1 for "mAs_1." D_1 is 40 inches, and D_2 is 60 inches.

First, square the distances.
1600 (mAs_2) = 3600 (mAs_1)
Then cross-multiply.
Isolate mAs_2 by dividing both sides of the equation by 1600.
mAs_2 = 2.25 (mAs_1)

This makes 2.25 the *factor* by which mAs should be changed.

The 40-inch technique should be increased 2.25 times to maintain density at 60 inches SID.

The solutions to square law problems are always the inverse of those for solving inverse square law problems. For example, if a distance change would result in twice as dark a film by the inverse square law, then the technique that would be required to maintain the original density at the new distance would be one half the mAs. If the density change can be predicted, simply invert this change to find the technique adjustment.

Although the inverse square law is important to understand, in practice, radiologic technologists rarely use a calculator or a pencil to apply it accurately. Rather, when doing a mobile procedure at 60 inches SID, for example, they will likely make a mental estimate of the increase in technique required as compared with the usual 40-inch SID. This section provides some simple rules of thumb that, if committed to memory, will greatly improve your accuracy in making this kind of technique adjustment.

A handful of distances (30, 40, 60, 72, and 96 inches) can be applied to more than 95% of radiographic procedures. By taking the most commonly used 40 inches as a standard and comparing the others with it, rules of thumb are easily derived and learned.

It helps to think of distance changes in factors of two; that is, doublings and halvings. For example, the square law formula shows that if SID is increased from

269

40 inches to 80 inches (a doubling), the technique must be increased by four times to maintain density. However, by thinking of this quadrupling of the technique as two doublings, rules of thumb can be formulated for other distance changes.

For example, think of increasing the SID from 40 inches to 60 inches as going halfway to doubling the SID; that is, 60 inches is halfway from 40 to 80. Because 80 inches would require two doublings of technique, 60 inches will require one half of that increase, or one doubling. For a 60-inch projection, double the mAs used at 40 inches.

In a similar manner, 30 inches can be considered as halfway to cutting 40 inches in half. A 20-inch distance would require one fourth of the overall technique, or two halvings. Thus, 30 inches requires only one halving of the 40-inch technique.

Table MT-2 summarizes these rules of thumb for the most often used distances. A column listing the actual solution based on the square law formula is provided as well, so you can see how close these rules of thumb are for accuracy. If you keep in mind that density must be changed by at least 30% for a visible difference to be seen, the rules of thumb are clearly accurate enough for practical use.

By far the most useful of these rules of thumb will be those for 60 inches and 72 inches because these distances are frequently used in mobile procedures and in the radiology department. For mobile procedures, the rules of thumb can be taken one step further to derive a technique for 50 inches SID.

If you consider 50 as halfway to 60, the technique would be increased halfway to a doubling, or increased by 50%. By the square law formula, the needed increase is 1.57 times the original. The rule of thumb rounds it to 1.5 times. *Radiologic technologists assigned to mobile units should remember that, compared with the usual 40-inch technique, a 50-inch SID requires a 50% increase in overall technique (preferably using mAs), a 60-inch distance requires a doubling, and a 72-inch distance requires a tripling.*

Because chest radiography is commonly performed with the 72-inch SID, it is important to emphasize that the 72-inch distance requires three times the 40-inch technique, and that a 40-inch distance requires one third of the 72-inch technique. This relationship is frequently encountered when upright or decubitus abdomen radiographs are taken along with chest radiographs. *Remember that the relationship between a 40-inch SID and a 72-inch SID is a factor of 3.*

These rules of thumb also can be used to solve for density problems if you remember to invert them (make fractions out of them). For example, if the distance is increased from 40 inches to 72 inches and the technique is not compensated for this change, how dark will the radiograph be? Simply invert the factor for 72 inches that is found in Table MT-2. The answer is that the new radiograph will have one third the density of the original. A radiograph taken at 60 inches without compensating technique would be one half as dense, and so forth.

Complete the following exercise as directed. The first 13 questions should be done mentally, using rules of thumb. Note that those starting at 60 inches or 30 inches also can be solved in your head if you analyze the distance changes as doubling, halving, halfway to doubling, or halfway to halving. Questions 14 to 25 employ the square law to find a new mAs that will compensate for the change in distance.

After completing the entire exercise, carefully check and review your answers using the Math Tutor Answer Key.

TABLE MT-2 Rules of thumb for distance changes starting at 40 inches

New distance (in)	Technique change computed by square law	Rule of thumb technique change
30	0.56	1/2
40	1.0 (standard)	1
60	2.25	2×
72	3.24	3×
80	4.0	4×
96	5.76	6×

Name _____

Date _____

Technique Adjustments

EXERCISE 13: ADJUSTING FOR DISTANCE CHANGES, THE INVERSE SQUARE LAW, THE SQUARE LAW: RULES OF THUMB FOR DISTANCE CHANGES

Use the technique rules of thumb to solve these problems:

	From:	To maintain density:
1.	25 mAs 40-in SID	_____ mAs 72-in SID
2.	15 mAs 40-in SID	_____ mAs 60-in SID
3.	7.5 mAs 40-in SID	_____ mAs 80-in SID
4.	6 mAs 40-in SID	_____ mAs 96-in SID
5.	60 mAs 40-in TFD	_____ mAs 20-in TFD
6.	2.5 mAs 30-in TFD	_____ mAs 60-in TFD
7.	30 mAs 40-in TFD	_____ mAs 30-in TFD
8.	12.5 mAs 30-in TFD	_____ mAs 45-in TFD
9.	30 mAs 80 kVp 40-in TFD	120 mAs _____ mAs 60-in TFD

Use the density rules of thumb to solve these problems:

	From:	To:
10.	40-in TFD Density = 1	20-in TFD Density = _____
11.	60-in TFD Density = 1	45-in TFD Density = _____
12.	40-in TFD Density = 1	80-in TFD Density = _____
13.	30-in TFD Density = 1	45-in TFD Density = _____

Use the square law to solve these problems:

	From:	To maintain density:
14.	10 mAs 40-in TFD	_____ mAs 100-in TFD
15.	5 mAs 60-in TFD	_____ mAs 50-in TFD
16.	2.5 mAs 72-in TFD	_____ mAs 40-in TFD
17.	2.5 mAs 60-in TFD	_____ mAs 20-in TFD
18.	2.5 mAs 80 kVp 60-in TFD	2.5 mAs _____ kVp 42.5-in TFD
19.	180 mAs 36-in TFD	20 mAs _____ TFD
20.	45 mAs 90-in TFD	5 mAs _____ TFD
21.	30 mAs 20-in TFD	120 mAs _____ TFD
22.	5 mAs 20-in TFD	45 mAs _____ TFD
23.	12 mAs 96-in TFD	_____ mAs 30-in TFD
24.	25 mAs 96-in TFD	_____ mAs 40-in TFD
25.	40 mAs 80-in TFD	_____ mAs 36-in TFD

Use the inverse square law to solve these problems:

	From:	To:
26.	40-in TFD Density = 1	72-in TFD Density = _____
27.	60-in TFD Density = 1	72-in TFD Density = _____
28.	50-in TFD Density = 1	36-in TFD Density = _____
29.	72-in TFD Density = 1	96-in TFD Density = _____

271